ABBAS CHOTHIA, M.D.
2007.

ABBAS CHOTHIA, M.D.
2007.

Cardiac CT Imaging

Matthew J. Budoff and Jerold S. Shinbane *Editors*
Associate Editors Stephan Achenbach,
Paolo Raggi, and John A. Rumberger

Cardiac CT Imaging

Diagnosis of Cardiovascular Disease

With 299 Figures
including 168 Color Plates

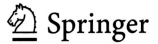 Springer

Editors:

Matthew J. Budoff, MD, FACC, FAHA
Los Angeles Biomedical Research
Institute at Harbor-UCLA
Medical Center
Torrance, CA
USA

Jerold S. Shinbane, MD, FACC
Division of Cardiovascular
Medicine
University of Southern California
Keck School of Medicine
Los Angeles, CA
USA

Associate Editors:

Stephan Achenbach, MD, FESC
Department of Internal Medicine II
University of Erlangen
Erlangen, Germany

Paolo Raggi, MD
Department of Cardiology
Tulane University School of Medicine
New Orleans, LA, USA

John A. Rumberger, PhD, MD
Cardiovascular Disease
The Ohio State University
Dublin, OH, USA

British Library Cataloguing in Publication Data
Cardiac CT imaging : diagnosis of cardiovascular disease
   1. Heart – Tomography   2. Cardiovascular system – Diseases – Diagnosis
   I. Budoff, Matthew J.   II. Shinbane, Jerold   III. Rumberger, John A.   IV. Raggi, Paolo   V. Achenbach, S.
(Stephan)
   616.1′2′075722
ISBN-10: 1846280281

Library of Congress Control Number: 2005928171

ISBN-10: 1-84628-028-1   e-ISBN 1-84628-146-6
ISBN-13: 978-1-84628-028-3

Printed on acid-free paper

Printed in Singapore.   (BS/KYO)

9 8 7 6 5 4 3 2

Springer Science+Business Media
springeronline.com

Dedication

If I have been able to see further, it was only because I stood on the shoulders of giants.
Sir Isaac Newton

To fully appreciate the current stature of cardiac computed tomography (CT) as both a radiological procedure and cardiology tool, one must acknowledge the pioneering efforts of the original luminaries in the field. British-born visionary David G. King was the lead engineer in the development of the original CT scanner that resulted in a Nobel Prize for his colleague, Sir Godfrey Hounsfield. Their combined "broad shoulders" became a springboard for the worldwide development and commercial success of CT. King introduced CT imaging to the United States, installing and commissioning a "head scanner" at the Mayo Clinic in 1973. David King's scientific career began at the EMI Research Labs in Middlesex (UK). It ended at General Electric, after he shepherded electron beam tomography at Imatron. He became the intellectual centerpiece of a fertile "brain trust," which stimulated the research and coordinated the clinical activities of a new generation of cardiologists and radiologists. The authors dedicate this edition to David King, an inspirational friend and the "father of coronary calcium imaging."

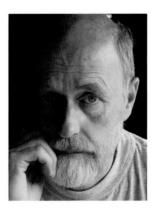

David G. King (1946–2004)
Scientist, Mentor, Friend

Foreword

Cardiac CT has finally come of age. After nearly 30 years of development and growth, tomographic X-ray is being embraced by cardiologists as a useful imaging technology. Thirty years ago, Doug Boyd envisioned a unique CT scanner that would have sufficient temporal resolution to permit motion-artifact-free images of the heart. In the late 1970s I had the good fortune to work closely with Dr. Boyd, Marty Lipton, and Bob Herkens who had the vision to recognize the potential of CT imaging for the diagnosis of heart disease. In the early 1980s, when electron beam CT became available, others, including Mel Marcus, †John Rumberger, Arthur Agatston, and †Dave King, were instrumental in making clinical cardiologists aware of the potential of cardiac CT.

In 1985 several investigators recognized the potential of cardiac CT for identifying and quantifying coronary artery calcium. Now, 20 years later, there is wide recognition of the value of coronary calcium quantification for the prediction of future coronary events in asymptomatic people. It has been a long and arduous road, but finally widespread screening may significantly reduce the 150,000 sudden deaths and 300,000 myocardial infarctions that occur each year in the United States as the first symptom of heart disease.

In the late 1970s, it was thought that a 2.4-sec scan time was very fast CT scanning. With the development of electron beam technology, scan times of 50 msec became possible giving rise to terms such as fast CT, ultrafast CT and RACAT (rapid acquisition computed axial tomography). Now, with the development of multidetector scanners capable of 64, 128, 256, and beyond simultaneous slices, spatial resolution is approaching that of conventional cineangiography and the holy grail, non-invasive coronary arteriography, appears attainable.

In this book, Drs. Matt Budoff and Jerold Shinbane, preeminent leaders in the field of cardiac CT, have described the many and varied uses of the technology in the diagnosis of cardiovascular disease. The book clearly documents that cardiac CT has not only arrived but has become a very valuable and potent diagnostic tool.

Bruce H. Brundage, MD MACC
Medical Director
Heart Institute of the Cascades
Professor of Medicine Emeritus
UCLA School of Medicine

†Deceased

Preface

Since its introduction in the early 1970s, computed tomography (CT) has become a robust modality to evaluate extracranial, thoracic, and abdominal vascular distributions. It has become a gold standard to non-invasively image the aorta, pulmonary arteries, great vessels, renal and peripheral arteries. However, cardiac anatomy evaluation with this modality was not possible, due to rapid cardiac motion and slow image acquisition times. Since the introduction of the first dedicated cardiac CT scanner, the electron beam CT (EBCT), the diagnosis and workup of cardiac structures has become possible. The lack of movement of the X-ray source allowed for images at a rate of 20 per second – 100 times faster than conventional CT at that time. Dr. Douglas Boyd, the inventor of EBCT, created this technology specifically with cardiac imaging in mind, and first published clinical data in 1982 [1]. However, limited reimbursement, high cost of acquisition, and very limited industry support kept this technology from expanding. The number of EBCT scanners in operation at any time never exceeded 100 worldwide, and physician exposure to the technology was very limited. Despite these hurdles, functional cardiac analysis (wall motion, cardiac output, wall thickening, and ejection fraction), perfusion imaging, non-invasive angiography, and coronary calcium assessment were validated, each with at least ten years of experience. To date, over 1000 scientific papers have been published in English, and three scientific statements from the American Heart Association have been written specifically on this modality. With the advent of helical CT in the mid-1990s and multidetector CT (MDCT) in 1999, the widespread availability of scanners to thousands of centers created a marked increase in utilization of and interest in cardiac CT. By 2004, three professional societies were vying for membership of potential cardiac CT physicians, and guidelines and credentialing standards were developed at a record pace.

Despite coronary calcium reports since 1989, and non-invasive coronary angiographic imaging reports with EBCT since 1995 [2], these applications did not gain widespread appeal until studies with MDCT became available. The preliminary studies (with subsecond single slice "helical" CT), had very limited cardiac applications and significant motion artifacts. The comparisons to EBCT were modest at best, and most investigators were quite concerned about applying the results of helical CT to clinical patients [3]. The early exposure MDCT, specifically the 4-slice scanner, was also disappointing with limited temporal resolution, volume coverage, collimation, and z-axis imaging. Due to the rapid coronary motion and limited scan speeds available with these early scanners, accurate and reliable imaging of the heart and coronary arteries has been significantly limited [4]. Diagnostic accuracy for cardiac 4-slice MDCT angiography, the most promising new application of these machines, was severely limited. Several studies reported diagnostic rates of only 30%, mostly due to cardiac motion [5]. However, evolution of MDCT with increased detectors, allowing for thinner slices and improved spatial resolution, has made this a most robust technology. Cardiac CT (with either MDCT or EBCT) offers several advantages over other diagnostic methodologies and is quite complementary to more common or traditional tests performed today. Clearly, the ability to see the lumen and vessel wall adds quite a lot to the assessment of the cardiac patient. Yet cardiac CT does not readily afford functional assessment of the patient under stress (exercise), and that information, garnered most commonly with treadmill testing, stress thallium, or echocardiography, adds vital information to the cardiac assessment. Thus, cardiac CT has been seen as a mostly complementary modality, adding anatomic information to the functional data acquired with stress testing.

Magnetic resonance imaging garnered quite a bit of interest in the early 1990s with the promise of a non-invasive angiogram with high accuracy. However, the next decade brought little improvement in the diagnostic accuracy of this technique, most likely due to limitations in slice thickness, temporal and spatial resolution. As compared to MRI, EBCT and MDCT allow for higher spatial and temporal resolution. The ease of use and robustness allow for fairly easy application to a variety of cardiac diagnoses. This book will highlight the vast array of cardiac (and vascular) applications of CT, updating the reader on the methodology employed by a variety of experts with a cumulative 100 or more years of cardiac CT experience.

We are forever indebted to the experts (both cardiologists and radiologists) who have spent the last 10 to 20 years of their lives dedicated to studying and publishing in this particular field of interest. Some of the experts who originated this work in the mid-1980s and allowed us to progress to where we are today include Bruce Brundage, William Stanford, Ralph Haberl, Geoff Rubin, Robert Detrano, Warren Janowitz, Arthur Agatston, John Rumberger, Marty Lipton, and Ruping Dai. This is clearly a very incomplete list, yet these are some of the early investigators who had to literally fight against a medical community that thought cardiac CT posed a threat to their more traditional tests. There has been significant controversy regarding cardiac CT over the years, with raging debates at national meetings and policies by the professional organizations sometimes swayed against the technology more by emotion than science.

The pathway that cardiac CT had to endure over the last 20 years is reminiscent of a quote by Arthur Schopenhauer. He stated:

> *All truth passes through three stages.*
> *First, it is ridiculed.*
> *Second, it is violently opposed.*
> *Third, it is accepted as being self-evident.*

A prominent cardiologist and past president of the American College of Cardiology recently told me that he thought some of the early investigators in the 1980s were clearly out of their mind when suggesting widespread use of cardiac CT, whether for coronary calcium assessment as a "mammogram of the heart," or CT angiography as a possible replacement for some conventional angiograms (ridicule stage). Violent opposition to this modality came in the late 1990s, when debates at the American College of Cardiology and AHA centered on the inappropriate advertising of these tests, rather than the science. Today, we are approaching the third stage, with the acceptance that cardiac CT has an important role in risk stratification (coronary artery calcification) and diagnosis of obstructive coronary artery disease (CT angiography).

As you will see, cardiac CT has matured significantly. It has become a powerful risk stratifying tool for the early detection of atherosclerosis, a possible substitute for coronary angiography or non-invasive exercise testing in certain clinical situations, and a powerful tool to image the heart for congenital heart disease, pre- and post-electrophysiologic testing and peripheral angiography. Future directions include possibly replacing some conventional catheterizations, and non-invasive tracking of atherosclerosis (progression/regression of either calcified plaque or non-calcified or "soft plaque"). The promise of CT includes non-invasive coronary plaque characterization, as well as accurate stenosis identification. It is highly likely that if these goals are obtained, CT coronary angiography may become the most valuable tool to evaluate the coronary arteries non-invasively. It is possible that direct non-invasive CT visualization of the arteries will partially replace both nuclear cardiology and diagnostic angiography in certain clinical situations, with a subsequent increase in coronary revascularizations.

Matthew J. Budoff, MD, FACC, FAHA
Jerold S. Shinbane, MD, FACC

References

1. Boyd DP, Lipton MJ. Cardiac computed tomography. Proc IEEE 1982;71;298–307.
2. Moshage WEL, Achenbach S, Seese B, Bachmann K, Kirchgeorg M. Coronary artery stenoses: Three-dimensional imaging with electrocardiographically triggered, contrast agent-enhanced, electron beam CT. Radiology 1995;196:707–714.
3. Budoff MJ, Mao SS, Zalace CP, Bakhsheshi H, Oudiz RJ. Comparison of spiral and electron beam tomography in the evaluation of coronary calcification in asymptomatic persons. Int J Cardiol 2001;77:181–188.
4. Budoff MJ, Achenbach S, Duerinckx A. Clinical Utility of Computed Tomography and Magnetic Resonance Techniques for Noninvasive Coronary Angiography. J Am Coll Cardiol 2003;42;1867–1878.
5. Achenbach S, Ulzheimer S, Baum U, et al. Non-invasive coronary angiography by retrospectively EcG-gated multislice spiral CT. Circulation 2000;102:2823–2828.

Acknowledgments

I would like to first thank Bruce Brundage MD, without whom as a mentor and friend, I never would have gotten into this field. He was a true visionary, who 20 years ago was already foreseeing the day when cardiac CT would become a mainstream test in Cardiology, as it now finally is. I would also like to thank my colleagues (mostly the other contributors and editors of this book) and researchers (Drs Songshou Mao, Lu Bin, Junichiro Takasu and others) who have taught me more about cardiac CT than I will ever teach them. Without their dedication and commitment, we would never be looking at the wealth of knowledge and understanding we have today. I would also like to thank the vendors (of both CT and workstations), who have provided insight, support and scientific knowledge to get us to where we are today. When we started doing CT angiography in 1995, it took us 3 weeks to reconstruct these images, now it takes 30 seconds. Some specific people who have particularly helped me in this regard: DeAnn Haas (General Electric), Philip Prather (Phillips Medical Systems), Robb Young (Toshiba) as well as Robert Taylor (TeraRecon) and Tina and Jason Young (NeoImagery Technologies).

Most importantly, I would like to thank my family, who have put up with me writing or editing this book for the past 8 months, working at times when I should have been with them. Thank you, Vicky, Daniel, and Garrett. Your support has made this book possible.

Matthew J. Budoff, MD, FACC, FAHA

I would like to thank Matthew Budoff for introducing me to the art and science of cardiovascular CT, and having the vision to see the applications for a multitude of disciplines within Cardiovascular Medicine. Your intelligence and enthusiasm have truly moved the field in novel directions. I would also like to thank Songshou Mao for his great insights and expertise in defining cardiovascular CT techniques. To the Harbor-UCLA EBCT Center staff, thank you for your excellence in providing CT services. Thank you to my family for your encouragement throughout my career. Most of all, to Rosemary, Anna, and Laura, thank you for your love and support.

Jerold S. Shinbane, MD, FACC

Contents

Contributors

Jamil AboulHosn, MD
Ahmanson/UCLA
Adult Congenital Heart
Disease Center,
David Geffen School of
Medicine at UCLA,
Los Angeles, CA, USA

Stephan Achenbach, MD, FESC
Department of Internal Medicine II
University of Erlangen
Erlangen, Germany

Daniel S. Berman
Department of Imaging
Cedars-Sinai Medical Center
Los Angeles, CA, USA

Matthew J. Budoff, MD, FACC, FAHA
Los Angeles Biomedical Research
Institute
Harbor-UCLA Medical Center,
Torrance, CA, USA

Patrick M. Colletti, MD
Department of Radiology
USC Keck School of Medicine
LAC + USC Imaging Science Center
Los Angeles, CA, USA

Raimund Erbel, MD
Department of Cardiology
University Clinic Essen
Essen, Germany

Guido Germano, PhD, MBA
Artificial Intelligence in Medicine (AIM)
Program
Cedars-Sinai Medical Center
Los Angeles, CA, USA

Rory Hachamovitch, MD, MSC
Division of Cardiovascular Medicine,
USC Keck School of Medicine
Los Angeles, CA, USA

Harvey S. Hecht, MD, FACC
Cardiac Computed Tomography
Lenox Hill Heart and Vascular
Institute
New York, USA

Songshou Mao, MD
Department of Cardiology
Los Angeles Biomedical Research
Institute
Harbor-UCLA Medical Center
Torrance, CA, USA

Stefan Möhlenkamp, MD
Department of Cardiology
Westdeutsches Herzzentrum Essen
Essen, Germany

Khurram Nasir, MD, MPH
Department of Cardiology
Johns Hopkins University
Baltimore, MD, USA

Ronald J. Oudiz, MD
Division of Cardiology
Harbor-UCLA Medical Center
Torrance, CA, USA

Gerald M. Pohost, MD, FACC, FAHA
Division of Cardiovascular Medicine
USC Keck School of Medicine
Los Angeles, CA, USA

Paolo Raggi, MD
Department of Cardiology
Tulane University School of
Medicine
New Orleans, LA, USA

M. Leila Rasouli, MD
Department of Cardiology
Harbor-UCLA Medical Center
Newport Coast, CA, USA

Alan Rozanski, MD
Department of Medicine
St. Luke's Roosevelt Hospital Center
New York, NY, USA

John A. Rumberger, PhD, MD
Cardiovascular Disease
The Ohio State University
Dublin, Ohio, USA

Thomas Schlosser, MD
Department of Diagnostic and
Interventional Radiology and
Neuroradiology
University Clinic Essen
Essen, Germany

Axel Schmermund, MD
Internal Medicine and Cardiology
Cardioangiologisches Centrum
Bethanien
Frankfurt am Main, Germany

Jeffrey M. Schussler, MD, FACC, FSCAI
Cardiovascular Disease (Internal
Medicine)
Baylor University Medical Center
Dallas, Texas, USA

David M. Shavelle, MD
Division of Cardiology, Department of
Medicine
Harbor-UCLA Medical Center
Torrance, CA, USA

Leslee J. Shaw, PhD
Department of Medicine
Cedars-Sinai Medical Center
Los Angeles, CA, USA

Jerold S. Shinbane, MD, FACC
Division of Cardiovascular
Medicine
USC Keck School of
Medicine
Los Angeles, CA, USA

Junichiro Takasu, MD, PhD
Department of Medicine
Harbor-UCLA Medical Center
UCLA School of Medicine,
Torrance, CA, USA

Philip H. Tseng, BS
Department of Cardiology
Los Angeles Biomedical Research
Institute
Harbor-UCLA Medical Center
Torrance, CA, USA

Nathan D. Wong, PhD
Heart Disease Prevention Program,
Department Medicine
University of California Irvine
Irvine, CA, USA

1

Computed Tomography

Matthew J. Budoff

Overview of X-ray Computed Tomography

The development of computed tomography (CT), resulting in widespread clinical use of CT scanning by the early 1980s, was a major breakthrough in clinical diagnosis. The primary advantage of CT was the ability to obtain thin cross-sectional axial images, with improved spatial resolution over echocardiography, nuclear medicine, and magnetic resonance imaging. This imaging avoided superposition of three-dimensional (3-D) structures onto a planar 2-D representation, as is the problem with conventional projection X-ray (fluoroscopy). The increased contrast resolution of CT is the reason for its increase in sensitivity for atherosclerosis and coronary artery disease (CAD). Localization of structures (in any plane) is more accurate and easier with tomography than with projection imaging like fluoroscopy. Furthermore, the images, which are inherently digital and thus quite robust, are amenable to 3-D computer reconstruction, allowing for ultimately nearly an infinite number of projections.

The basic principle of CT is that a fan-shaped, thin X-ray beam passes through the body at many angles to allow for cross-sectional images. The corresponding X-ray transmission measurements are collected by a detector array. Information entering the detector array and X-ray beam itself is collimated to produce thin sections while avoiding unnecessary photon scatter (to keep radiation exposure and image noise to a minimum). The data recorded by the detectors are digitized into picture elements (pixels) with known dimensions. The gray-scale information contained in each individual pixel is reconstructed according to the attenuation of the X-ray beam along its path using a standardized technique termed "filtered back projection." Gray-scale values for pixels within the reconstructed tomogram are defined with reference to the value for water and are called "Hounsfield units" (HU; for the 1979 Nobel Prize winner, Sir Godfrey N. Hounsfield), or simply "CT numbers." Dr Hounsfield is credited with the invention of the CT scanner in the late 1960s. Since CT uses X-ray absorption to create images, the differences in the image brightness at any point will depend on physical density and the presence of atoms with a high difference in anatomic number like calcium, and soft tissue and water. The absorption of the X-ray beam by different atoms will cause differences in CT brightness on the resulting image. Blood and soft tissue (in the absence of vascular contrast enhancement) have similar density and consist of similar proportions of the same atoms (hydrogen, oxygen, carbon). Bone has an abundance of calcium. Fat has an abundance of hydrogen. Lung contains air which is of extremely low physical density. The higher the density, the brighter the structure on CT. Calcium is bright white, air is black, and muscle or blood is gray. Computed tomography, therefore, can distinguish blood from air, fat and bone but not readily from muscle or other soft tissue. The densities of blood, myocardium, thrombus, and fibrous tissues are so similar in their CT number, that non-enhanced CT cannot distinguish these structures. Thus, the ventricles and other cardiac chambers can be seen on non-enhanced CT, but delineating the wall from the blood pool is not possible (Figure 1.1). Investigators have validated the measurement of "LV size" with cardiac CT, which is the sum of both left ventricle (LV) mass and volume [1]. Due to the thin wall which does not contribute significantly to the total measured volume, the left and right atrial volumes can be accurately measured on non-contrast CT [2].

The higher spatial resolution of CT allows visualization of coronary arteries both with and without contrast enhancement. The ability to see the coronary arteries on a non-contrast study depends upon the fat surrounding the artery (of lower density, thus more black on images), providing a natural contrast between the myocardium and the epicardial artery (Figure 1.1). Usually, the entire course of each coronary artery is visible on non-enhanced scans (Figure 1.2). The major exception is bridging, when the coronary artery delves into the myocardium and cannot be distinguished without contrast. The distinction of blood and soft tissue (such as the left ventricle, where there is no air or fat to act as a natural contrast agent) requires injection of contrast with CT. Similarly, distinguishing the

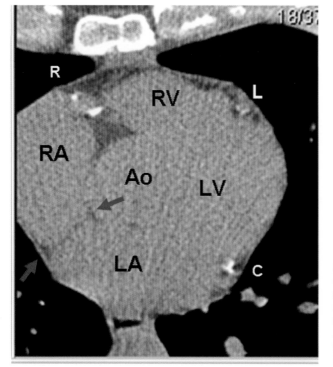

Figure 1.1. A non-contrast CT scan of the heart. Quite a bit of information can be garnered without contrast. The pericardium is visible as a thin line just below the R and L. The coronary arteries can be seen, and diameters and calcifications are present. The right coronary artery is seen near the R, the left anterior at the L, and the circumflex at the C. The four chambers of the heart are also seen, and relative sizes can be measured from this non-contrast study. The interatrial septum is clearly seen (red arrows). The ascending aorta is also present on this image and can be evaluated. Ao = aorta, L = left anterior descending artery, LA = left atrium, LV = left ventricle, RA = right atrium, RV = right ventricle.

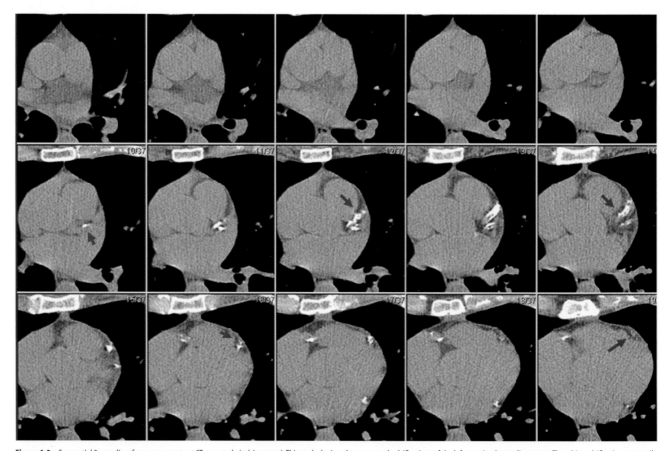

Figure 1.2. Sequential 3 mm slices from a non-contrast CT scan study (calcium scan). This study depicts the course and calcifications of the left anterior descending artery. The white calcifications are easily seen (red arrows) and quantitated by the computer to derive a calcium score, volume or mass with high inter-reader reproducibility.

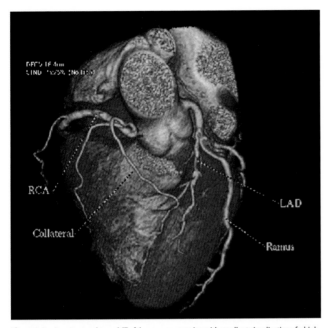

Figure 1.3. A contrast-enhanced CT of the coronary arteries, with excellent visualization of a high-grade stenosis in the mid-portion of the left anterior descending (LAD). A large collateral vessel is seen from the right coronary artery (RCA), but this is quite rare, as usually the collaterals are too small to be well seen on cardiac CT. A large ramus intermedius is well visualized, and the dominant RCA is present. This is but one view of many that can be visualized with cardiac CT, allowing for near-complete visualizations of the coronary tree.

lumen and wall of the coronary artery also requires contrast enhancement. The accentuated absorption of X-rays by elements of high atomic number like calcium and iodine allows excellent visualization of small amounts of coronary calcium as well as the contrast-enhanced lumina of medium-size coronary arteries (Figure 1.3). Air attenuates the X-ray less than water, and bone attenuates it more than water, so that in a given patient, Hounsfield units may range from −1000 HU (air) through 0 HU (water) to above +1000 HU (bone cortex). Coronary artery calcium in coronary atherosclerosis (consisting of the same calcium phosphate as in bone) has CT number >130 HU, typically going as high as +600 HU. It does not go as high as the bony cortex of the spine due to the smaller quantity and mostly inhomogeneous distribution in the coronary artery plaque. Metal, such as that found in valves, wires, stents and surgical clips, has densities of +1000 HU or higher.

Cardiac CT

Cardiac computed tomography (CT) provides image slices or tomograms of the heart. CT technology has significantly improved since its introduction into clinical practice in 1972. Current conventional scanners used for cardiac and cardiovascular imaging now employ either a rotating X-ray source with a circular, stationary detector array (spiral or helical CT) or a rotating electron beam (EBCT). The biggest issue with cardiac imaging is the need for both spatial and temporal resolution. Cardiac magnetic resonance (MR) has been an emerging technique for almost two decades, making little progress toward widespread utilization over this time. Temporal resolution (how long it takes to obtain an image) is inversely related to spatial resolution with cardiac MR. Improving the MR spatial resolution requires prolonging the imaging time. This greatly limits the ability to focus with precision on moving objects, as the viewer needs to settle for either a high resolution image plagued by cardiac motion, or a low resolution image with no motion artifacts. Cardiac CT does not suffer from this inverse relationship, and allows for both high spatial and temporal resolution. Electron beam CT (EBCT – described in detail below) allows for high resolution imaging at 50–100 milliseconds (ms). Multidetector CT (MDCT), with improved spatial resolution, allows for rotation speeds now on the order of 330–400 ms. Thus, EBCT has the best temporal resolution, MDCT the best spatial resolution, and cardiac MR is generally the worst in each category (although in non-moving structures such as the spine, MR, which is inherently a 3-D method, is capable of spatial resolution on the order of microns). The most distinct advantage of cardiac CT over cardiac MR is the improved spatial resolution. The best resolution reported by a cardiac MR study (using the strongest magnet −3 teslas) demonstrated resolution in the x-, y- and z-axes of $0.6 \times 0.6 \times 3$ mm [3]. The best resolution offered by cardiac CT is $0.35 \times 0.35 \times 0.5$ mm, which is almost a factor of 10 better spatial resolution and approaching the ultimate for 3-D tomography of nearly cubic (isentropic) "voxels" – or volume elements. As we consider non-invasive angiography with either CT or MR, we need to remember that both spatial and temporal resolution is much higher with traditional invasive angiography (discussed in more detail below).

Reconstruction algorithms and multi-"head" detectors common to both current electron beam and spiral/helical CT have been implemented enabling volumetric imaging, and multiple high-quality reconstructions of various volumes of interest can be done either prospectively or retrospectively, depending on the method. The details of each type of scanner and principles of use will be described in detail.

MDCT Methods

Sub-second MDCT scanners use a rapidly rotating X-ray tube and several rows of detectors, also rotating. The tube and detectors are fitted with slip rings that allow them to continuously move through multiple 360° rotations. The "helical" or "spiral" mode is possible secondary to the development of this slip-ring interconnect. This allows the X-ray tube and detectors to rotate continuously during image acquisition since no wires directly connect the rotating and stationary components of the system (i.e. no need to unwind the wires). This slip-ring technology was a fundamental breakthrough in conventional CT performing single slice scanning in the 1980s to rapid multislice scanning in the 21st century. With gantry continuously rotating, the table moves the patient through the imaging plane at a predetermined speed. The relative speed of the gantry rotation table motion is the scan pitch. Pitch is calculated as table speed divided by collimator width. Thus, moving the table faster will lead to wider slices and vice versa. A low pitch (low table speed or wide slices) allows for overlapping data from adjacent detectors. Most commonly, physicians use a low table speed and thin imaging, leading to a lot of images, each very thin axial slices which are of great value for imaging the heart with high resolution. The downside is that the slower the table movement (while still rotating the X-ray tube), the higher the radiation exposure.

The smooth rapid table motion or pitch in helical scanning allows complete coverage of the cardiac anatomy in 5 to 25 seconds, depending on the actual number of multi-row detectors. The current generation of MDCT systems complete a 360° rotation in about 3–4 tenths of a second and are capable of acquiring 4–64 sections of the heart simultaneously with electrocardiographic (ECG) gating in either a prospective or retrospective mode. MDCT differs from single detector-row helical or spiral CT systems principally by the design of the detector arrays and data acquisition systems, which allow the detector arrays to be configured electronically to acquire multiple adjacent sections simultaneously. For example, in 16-row MDCT systems, 16 sections can be acquired at either 0.5–0.75 or 1–1.5 mm section widths or 8 sections 2.5 mm thick.

In MDCT systems, like the preceding generation of single-detector-row helical scanners, the X-ray photons are generated within a specialized X-ray tube mounted on a rotating gantry. The patient is centered within the bore of the gantry such that the array of detectors is positioned to record incident photons after traversing the patient. Within the X-ray tube, a tungsten filament allows the tube current to be increased (mA), which proportionately increases the number of X-ray photons for producing an image. Thus, heavier patients can have increased mA, allowing for better tissue penetration and decreased image noise. One of the advantages of MDCT over EBCT is the variability of the mA settings, thus increasing the versatility for general diagnostic CT in nearly all patients and nearly all body segments.

For example, the calcium scanning protocol employed in the National Institutes of Health (NIH) Multi-Ethnic Study of Atherosclerosis is complex [4]. Scans were performed using prospective ECG gating at 50% of the cardiac cycle, 120 kV, 106 mAs, 2.5 mm slice collimation, 0.5 s gantry rotation, and a partial scan reconstruction resulting in a temporal resolution of 300 ms. Images were reconstructed using the standard algorithm into a 35 cm display field of view. For participants weighing 100 kg (220 lb) or greater, the milliampere (mA) setting was increased by 25%.

This is a design difference with current generation EBCT systems, which use a fixed mA. The attenuation map

recorded by the detectors is then transformed through a filtered back-projection into the CT image used for diagnosis (these algorithms are common to both EBCT and MDCT).

MDCT systems can operate in either the sequential (prospective triggered) or helical mode (retrospective gating). These modes of scanning are dependent upon whether the patient on the CT couch is stationary (axial, or sequential mode) or moved at a fixed speed relative to the gantry rotation (helical mode). The sequential mode utilizes prospective ECG triggering at predetermined offset from the ECG-detected R wave analogous to EBCT and is the current mode for measuring coronary calcium at most centers using MDCT. This mode utilizes a "step and shoot modality," which reduces radiation exposure by "prospectively" acquiring images, as compared to the helical mode, where continuous radiation is applied (and hundreds or thousands of images created) and images are "retrospectively" aligned to the ECG tracing. In the sequential mode, a 16- or 64-slice scanner can acquire 16 or 64 simultaneous data channels of image information gated prospectively to the ECG. Thus a 16-channel system can acquire, within the same cardiac cycle, 20 mm in coverage per heartbeat. The promise of improved cardiac imaging from the 64-slice scanner is mostly due to larger volumes of coverage simultaneously (up to 40 mm of coverage per rotation), allowing for less z-axis alignment issues (cranial–caudal), and improved 3-D modeling with only 5–12 seconds of imaging, although each vendor has a different array of detectors, with different slice widths and capabilities (Table 1.1).

Modern MDCT systems have currently an X-ray gantry rotation time of 500 ms or less. The fastest available rotation time is 333 ms. This is clearly suboptimal in faster heart rates, as imaging during systole (or atrial contraction during late diastole) will be plagued by motion artifacts. Reconstruction algorithms have been developed that permit the use of data acquired during a limited part of the X-ray tube rotation (e.g. little more than one half of one rotation or smaller sections of several subsequent rotations) to reconstruct one cross-sectional image (described below). Simultaneous recording of the patient ECG permits the assignment of reconstructed images to certain time

---

Table 1.1. Sample protocols for MDCT angiography: contrast-enhanced retrospectively ECG-gated scan

4-Slice scanner: 4 × 1.0 mm collimation, table feed 1.5 mm/rotation, effective tube current 400 mAs at 120 kV. Pitch = 1.5/4.0 collimation = 0.375. Average scan time = 35 seconds

16-Slice scanner (1.5 mm slices): 16 × 1.5 mm collimation, table feed 3.8 mm/rotation, effective tube current 133 mAs at 120 kV. Pitch = 3.8/24 mm collimation = 0.16. Average scan time = 15–20 seconds

16-Slice scanner (0.75 mm slices): 16 × 0.75 mm collimation, table feed 3.4 mm/rotation, effective tube current 550–650 mAs at 120 kV. Pitch = 3.4/12 mm collimation = 0.28. Average scan time = 15–20 seconds

64-Slice scanner (0.625 mm slices): 64 × 0.6.25 mm collimation, table feed 3.8 mm/rotation, effective tube current 685 mAs at 120 kV. Pitch = 3.8/40 mm collimation = 0.1. Average scan time = 6–10 seconds

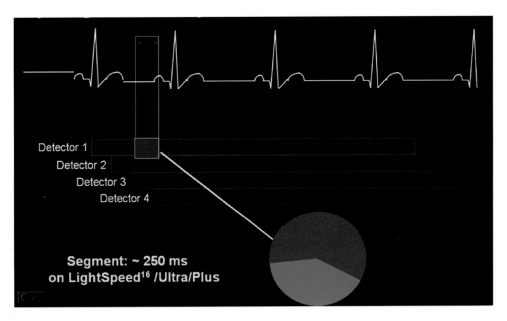

Figure 1.4. A typical acquisition using the "halfscan" method on multidetector CT (Light-Speed16, GE Medical Systems, Milwaukee Wisconsin). This demonstrates an acquisition starting at approximately 50% of the R-R interval. A scanner with a rotation speed of 200 ms takes approximately 250 ms to complete an image, as depicted.

instants in the cardiac cycle. Image acquisition windows of approximately 250 ms can be achieved without the necessity to average data acquired over more than one heartbeat (Figure 1.4). This may be sufficient to obtain images free of motion artifacts in many patients if the data reconstruction window is positioned in suitable phases of the cardiac cycle, and the patient has a sufficiently low heart rate. Motion-free segments on four-slice MDCT decrease from approximately 80% to 54% with increasing heart rates [5].

MDCT Terminology

Isotropic Data Acquisition. The biggest advance that the newest systems provide is thinner slices, important for improving image quality as well as diminishing partial volume effects. The current systems allow for slice thicknesses between 0.5 and 0.75 mm (depending on manufacturer and scan model). Thus, the imaging voxel is virtually equal in size in all dimensions (isotropic). The spatial resolution of current CT systems is 0.35 mm × 0.35 mm, and has always been limited by the z-axis (slice thickness). Current systems allow for isotropic resolution (as reconstructed images can be seen at 0.4 mm), allowing for no loss of data by reconstructing the data in a different plane. This is very important for imaging the coronary, peripheral, and carotid arteries, as they run perpendicular to the imaging plane (each slice only encompasses a small amount of data) and to follow these arteries, one must add multiple slices together in the z-axis. The old limitations of CT (better interpretation for structures that run within the plane it was imaged, i.e. parallel to the imaging plane) are no longer present. There is now no loss of data with reformatting the data with multiplanar reformation (MPR) or volume ren-

dering (VR). Furthermore, the thinner slice imaging allows for less partial volume artifacts, prevalent from dense calcifications and metal objects (such as bypass clips, pacemaker wires, and stents).

Pitch. In the helical or spiral mode of operation, a 16-MDCT system can acquire 16 simultaneous data channels while there is continuous motion of the CT table. The relative motion of the rotating X-ray tube to the table speed is called the scan pitch and is particularly important for cardiac gating in the helical mode. Increased collimator coverage allows for decreasing the pitch, without losing spatial resolution. The definition of pitch for the multidetector systems is the distance the table travels per 360° rotation of the gantry, divided by the dimension of the exposed detector array (the collimation, which is the slice thickness times the number of imaging channels). For example, a 16-slice system, with 16 equal detectors each of 0.625 mm, gives a collimation of 10 mm. Thus, if the table is moving at 10 mm/rotation, the pitch is 1.0. The pitch remains 1.0 if the table moves at 20 mm/rotation and the slices are thicker (1.25 mm each), or if the number of channels increases. Moving the table faster will lead to thicker slices, which will decrease resolution and lead to partial volume effects. If there is no overlap, the pitch is 1. If 50% overlap is desired, the pitch is 0.5, as the table is moved slower to allow for overlapping images. This is necessary with multisector reconstruction. Typical pitch values for cardiac work are 0.25 to 0.4, allowing for up to a 4-fold overlap of images. If the collimation with 64-row scanners increases to 40 mm, the table can move four times faster than the 16-slice scanner, without affecting slice thickness. Thus, the coverage can go up dramatically over a short period of scanning time, by imaging more detectors and increasing the speed of table movement in concert.

Field of View. Another method to improve image quality of the CT angiograph (CTA) is to keep the field of view small. The matrix for CT is 512 × 512, meaning that is the number of voxels in a given field of view. This is significantly better than current MR scanners, accounting for the improved spatial resolution. If the field of view is 15 cm, than each pixel is 0.3 mm. Increasing the field of view to 30 cm (typical for encompassing the entire chest) increases each pixel dimension to 0.6 mm, effectively reducing the spatial resolution 2-fold.

Contrast. Finally, the high scan speed allows substantial reduction in the amount of contrast material. The high speed of the scan allows one to decrease the amount of contrast administered; by using a 16-channel unit with a detector collimation of 0.625 mm and a tube rotation of 0.4 seconds (typical values for a 16-detector coronary CTA), the acquisition interval is around 11–15 seconds, which allows one to reduce the contrast load to 55–75 mL. For a faster acquisition protocol, the contrast delivery strategy needs to be optimized according to the scan duration time. The general rule is the duration of scanning (scan acquisition time) equals the contrast infusion. So, if an average rate of 4 mL/s is used, a 15-second scan acquisition would require 60 mL of contrast. With volume scanners (40- and 64-detector systems), the scan times are reduced to 5–8 seconds, and contrast doses are subsequently reduced as well.

Prospective Triggering. The prospectively triggered image uses a "step and shoot" system, similar to EBCT. This obtains images at a certain time of the cardiac cycle (see Chapter 2), which can be chosen in advance, and then only one image per detector per cardiac cycle is obtained. This reduces contrast requirements, but does not allow for CT angiographic images, as motion artifacts may plague these images. When performing prospective gating, the temporal resolution of a helical or MDCT system is proportional to the gantry speed, which determines the time to complete one 360° rotation. To reconstruct each slice, data from a minimum of 180° plus the angle of the fan beam are required, typically 220° of the total 360° rotation. For a 16-row system with 0.40-second rotation, the temporal resolution is approximately 0.25 seconds or 250 ms for a 50 cm display field of view. By reducing the display field of view to the 20 cm to encompass the heart, the number of views can be reduced to further improve temporal resolution to approximately 200 ms per slice. The majority of MDCT systems in 2005 have gantry speeds of 330 to 500 ms and temporal resolution of 180–300 ms per image when used for measuring coronary calcium or creating individual images for CT angiography, as compared to 50 or 100 ms for EBCT. The newest 64-slice scanners now have rotation gantry speeds down to 330 ms. Although physically faster rotational times may be possible in the future, this is still rotation of an X-ray source (with or without attached detectors) within a fixed radius of curvature. This is subject to the forces and limitations of momentum. This is not an issue when it comes to moving an electron beam as with EBCT.

Retrospective Gating. The ECG is used to add R peak markers to the raw data set. A simultaneous ECG is recorded during the acquisition of cardiac images. The ECG is retrospectively used to assign source images to the respective phases of the cardiac cycle (ECG gating). The best imaging time to minimize coronary motion is from 40% to 80% of the cardiac cycle (early to mid-diastole).

The interval between markers determines the time of each scanned cardiac cycle. Retrospective, phase-specific, short time segments of several R-R intervals are combined to reconstruct a "frozen axial slice." During helical scanning, the patient is moved through the CT scanner to cover a body volume (i.e. the heart). An advantage of the helical acquisition mode is that there is a continuous model of the volume of interest from base to apex, as opposed to the sequential/cine mode in which there are discrete slabs of slices which have been obtained in a "step and shoot" prospective fashion. The obvious detriment to the helical acquisition is the increase in radiation dose delivered to the patient, as continuous images are created, and then "retrospectively" aligned to the ECG tracing to create images at any point of the R-R interval (cardiac cycle).

Halfscan Reconstruction

A multislice helical CT halfscan (HS) reconstruction algorithm is most commonly employed for cardiac applications. Halfscan reconstruction using scan data from a 180° gantry rotation (180–250 ms) for generating one single axial image (Figure 1.4). The imaging performances (in terms of the temporal resolution, *z*-axis resolution, image noise, and image artifacts) of the heartscan algorithm have demonstrated improvement over utilizing the entire rotation (full scan). It has been shown that the halfscan reconstruction results in improved image temporal resolution and is more immune to the inconsistent data problem induced by cardiac motions. The temporal resolution of multislice helical CT with the halfscan algorithm is approximately 60% of the rotation speed of the scanner. The reason it is not 50% of the rotation speed is that slightly more than 180° is required to create an image, as the fan beam width (usually 30°) must be excluded from the window (Figure 1.4). Thus approximately 210° of a rotation is needed to reconstruct an entire image. Central time resolution (the point in the center of the image) is derived by the 180° rotation. MDCT using the standard halfscan reconstruction method permits reliable assessment of the main coronary branches (those in the center of the image field) in patients with heart rates below 65 beats/min [6,7]. The necessity of a low heart rate is a limitation of MDCT coronary angiography using this methodology.

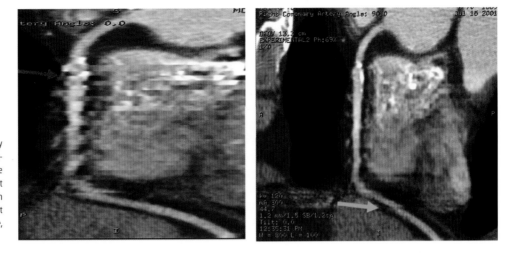

Figure 1.5. LightSpeed16 CT angiography images. On the left is the halfscan reconstruction. On the right, is a reconstructed image using the same dataset, using multisegment reconstruction. There are still some motion artifacts in the distal right (green arrow), but much improved over the halfscan image, which is not interpretable (red arrow).

With halfscan reconstruction, the proportion of the acquisition time per heartbeat is linearly rising from 20% at 60 beats/min to 33% at 100 beats/min. When evaluating the diastolic time, the proportion is much greater. Slower heart rates have longer diastolic imaging. The diastolic time useful for imaging for a heart rate of 60 beats/min is on the order of 500 ms (excluding systole and atrial contraction). Thus, a 250 ms scan will take up 50% of the diastolic imaging time. Increase the heart rate to 100 beats/min (systole remains relatively fixed) and the biggest change is shortening of diastole. Optimal diastolic imaging times are reduced to approximately 100 ms, clearly far too short for a motion-free MDCT scan acquisition of 250 ms (Figure 1.5, left panel). Thus, heart rate reduction remains a central limitation for motion-free imaging of the heart using MDCT. This can be partially overcome by multisegment reconstruction, described below.

Multisegment Reconstruction

The scan window refers to the time when the volume of interest is present in the scan field and is therefore "seen" by the detector. It is the limiting factor for temporal resolution. In multisegment reconstruction, it defines the number of cardiac cycles available and hence the maximum number of segments that can be used to reconstruct one slice. Multisegment reconstruction utilizes a helical scanning technique coupled with ECG synchronization (images are retrospectively aligned to the ECG data acquired to keep track of systolic and diastolic images). Multisegment reconstruction can typically use up 2–4 different segments correlated to the raw data. By using four heartbeats to create an image, the acquisition time can be reduced to a minimum of 65 ms (Figure 1.6).

Figure 1.6. A demonstration of a theoretical image using multisegment reconstruction. The resulting image is constructed of four equal segments from four different detectors. Each is reconstructed from the same point in the cardiac cycle (approximately 50% in this depiction). Four different detectors, each visualizing the same portion of the heart in the same portion of the cardiac cycle, can be used to add together to create one image. In practice, the segments are not always of equal length, and four images are not always available for reconstruction.

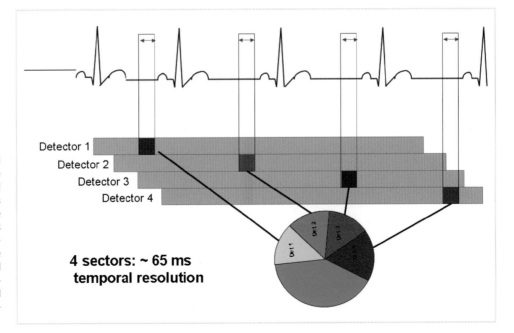

Detector 1
Detector 2
Detector 3
Detector 4

4 sectors: ~ 65 ms temporal resolution

During retrospective segmented reconstruction, views from different rotations are combined to simulate one half-scan rotation (approximately 210° of data is needed to create an image). To calculate the number of segments that can be extracted from a scan window, the number of positions available for reconstruction is determined automatically by a workstation. Each position is extended into a wedge so that the combination of all wedges simulates a halfscan tube rotation. The raw data acquired in this virtual halfscan rotation is sufficient for the reconstruction of one slice. The size of the largest wedge (largest segment) defines the temporal resolution within the image (Figure 1.6). In other words, the subsegment with the longest temporal data acquisition determines the temporal resolution of the overall image. If the four segments used to create an image were of the following size (65 ms, 65 ms, 50 ms, and 100 ms), then the temporal resolution of the reconstructed image is 100 ms.

The use of multisegment reconstruction has allowed for markedly improved effective temporal resolution and image quality. Just to be clear about how this works, let's use an analogy of a pie. Imagine needing just over half of a pie for a picture. To create an image, you can either add together one small slice from several pies (Figure 1.6) or you can take one large piece from one pie (Figure 1.4). The advantage of taking small pieces from each heartbeat is that the temporal resolution goes down proportionally. The difficulty in using this technique is that the pieces of the pie must align properly. Patients with even very slight arrhythmias (especially atrial fibrillation, sinus arrhythmia, or multifocal atrial rhythms), changing heart rates (increased vagal tone during breath-holding, catecholamine response after getting a contrast flush, etc.), or premature beats will cause misregistration to occur. If the heartbeats used are not perfectly regular, the computer will inadvertently add different portions of the cardiac cycle together, making a non-diagnostic image. Thus, there is

still need for regular rhythms with CT angiography, although with higher detector systems (i.e. 64 detectors), the number of heartbeats needed to cover the entire heart goes down to 4–8, reducing the chance of significant changes in heart rates due to premature beats, breath-holding, vagal or sympathetic tone.

By combining information from each of the detector rows, the effective temporal resolution of the images can *theoretically* be reduced to as low as 65 ms. However, to do this requires four perfectly regular beats consecutively and a fast baseline heart rate, and usual reconstructions allow for two to three images to be utilized, yielding an effective temporal resolution of 130–180 ms per slice (Figure 1.7), but with a direct proportional increase in radiation exposure to the patient. This method of segmenting the information of one image into several heartbeats is quite similar to the established prospective triggering techniques used for MRI of the coronary arteries [8,9]. With multisegment reconstruction the length of the acquisition time varies between 10% and 20% of the R-R interval. Since the reconstruction algorithm is only capable of handling a limited number of segments, the pitch (table speed) is often increased for patients with higher heart rates. Thus, fewer images are available with higher heart rates, decreasing the potential success rate with this methodology (see "Speed/Temporal Resolution" below).

Multisegment reconstruction has been shown to improve depiction of the coronary arteries as compared to halfscan reconstruction [10,11] (Figure 1.5). This methodology will improve temporal resolution, but high heart rates will still increase the motion of the coronaries, increasing the likelihood of image blurring and non-diagnostic images (Figure 1.5, right panel still demonstrating some blurring of the mid-distal right coronary artery with heart rates of 70–75 beats/min). It is fairly common for patients with low heart rates at rest to increase the heart rate significantly at the time of CT angiography. This can

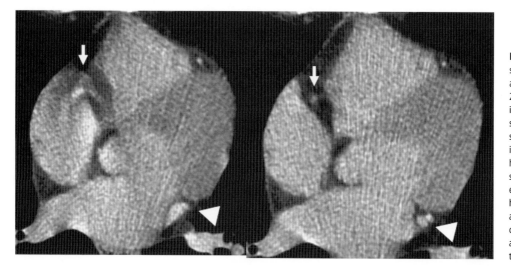

Figure 1.7. The figure on the left demonstrates a standard halfscan reconstruction with a rotation speed of 400 ms (approximate 260 ms image temporal resolution), with image data acquired on a four-channel MDCT system, 1.25 mm slice collimation, 0.6 gantry speed and a heart rate of 72 beats/min. The image to the right demonstrates the same helical scan data but processed with a two-sector reconstruction algorithm resulting in an effective temporal resolution of 180 ms. Note how the proximal right coronary artery (white arrows), as well as the left circumflex and great coronary vein, are now distinguishable (white arrowhead) and motion-free on the multisector reconstructed image.

occur due to three factors: anxiety about the examination, the breath-hold, or the warmth of the contrast infusion to the patient. Thus, there is still a need for somewhat reduced heart rates during MDCT angiography with all current reconstruction systems.

Studies examining the image quality of multisegment and halfscan reconstruction in CT with four [12] and eight [11] detector rows showed similar image quality in both phantoms and patients. However, Dewey et al. [13] demonstrated that the accuracy, sensitivity, specificity, and rate of non-assessable coronary branches were significantly better using multisegment reconstruction in a 16-slice MDCT scanner. The authors attributed the difference to the higher image quality and resulting longer vessel length free of motion artifacts with multisegment reconstruction. The obvious advantage of multisegment reconstruction is achieved by reducing the acquisition window per heartbeat to approximately 160 ms on average, particularly useful for diagnostic images of the right coronary artery and circumflex artery (the two arteries that suffer the most from motion artifacts) [14]. Therefore, MDCT in combination with multisegment reconstruction does not always require administration of beta blockers to reduce heart rate. This improvement simplifies the procedure and expands the group of patients who can be examined with non-invasive coronary angiography using MDCT. The potential is for even greater application with aligning these multiple segments together with 64-slice scanners, further improving the diagnostic rate with MDCT angiography.

Limitations of Multisegment Reconstruction

Heart rates above 65 beats/min demonstrate the biggest benefit of multisegment reconstructions. The benefit of multisegment reconstruction in low heart rates has not been demonstrated, and some experts recommend avoiding this in lower heart rates to minimize radiation exposure. A drawback of multisegment reconstruction is the effective radiation dose, which is estimated to be 30% higher than necessary for halfscan reconstruction, resulting from the lower pitch (slower table speed, increasing the time the X-ray beam is on) needed with multisegment reconstruction. The results of studies indicate that multisegment reconstruction has superior diagnostic accuracy and image quality compared with halfscan reconstruction in patients with normal heart rates (Figure 1.7). Thus, multisegment reconstruction holds promise to make the routine use of beta blockers to reduce the heart rate before CT coronary angiography less necessary as a routine. One further limitation is that certain heart rates cannot undergo multisegment reconstruction if the R-R interval (in milliseconds) is an even multiple of the scanner rotational speed. If the heart rate and the rotation of the scanner are synchronous, the same heart phase always corresponds to the same angle segment, and a partial-scan interval cannot be divided into smaller segments. Finally,

if the heart rate is unexpectedly irregular (i.e. Premature Ventricular Contractions (PVCs) or stress reaction to the dye causing increased heart rate during imaging), multi-segment reconstruction will not be successful and the diagnostic image quality will have to rely on the halfscan reconstruction. Some scanners (Philips Medical Systems is the first to introduce such proprietary software) have intrinsic programs which improve the success rate with multisegment reconstruction at increased heart rates. How well these systems work and how often are clinical questions still being answered.

EBCT Methods

Electron beam computed tomography (GE Healthcare, Waukegan, WI) is a tomographic-imaging device developed over 20 years ago specifically for cardiac imaging. To date, and specifically over the past decade, there has been a huge increase in diagnostic and prognostic data regarding EBCT and coronary artery imaging. In order to achieve rapid acquisition times useful for cardiac imaging, these fourth-generation CT scanners have been developed with a non-mechanical X-ray source. This allows for image acquisition on the order of 50–100 ms, and with prospective ECG triggering, the ability to "freeze" the heart. Electron beam scanners use a fixed X-ray source, which consists of a 210° arc ring of tungsten, activated by bombardment from a magnetically focused beam of electrons fired from an electron source "gun" behind the scanner ring. The patient is positioned inside the X-ray tube, obviating the need to move any part of the scanner during image acquisition (Figure 1.8). EBCT is distinguished by its use of a scanning electron beam rather than the traditional X-ray tube and mechanical rotation device used in current "spiral" single and multiple detector scanners (requiring a

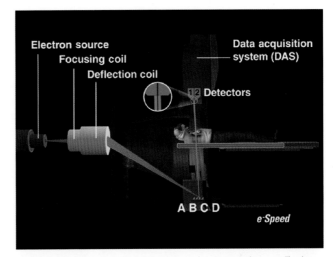

Figure 1.8. Depiction of the e-Speed electron beam computed tomography scanner. The electron source emits a beam, which is steered magnetically through the detection coil, then reflected to tungsten targets (A B C D), where a fan-shaped X-ray beam is created and, after passing through the area of interest, seen by the detectors.

physically moving X-ray source around the patient). EBCT requires only that the electron beam is swept across the tungsten targets to create a fan beam of X-ray, possible in as short as 50 ms per image (20 frames/second). The electron beam is emitted from the cathode, which is several feet superior to the patient's head, and then passes through a magnetic coil, which bends the beam so that it will strike one of four tungsten anode targets. The magnetic coil also steers the beam through an arc of 210°. The X-rays are generated when the electron beam strikes the tungsten anode target, then passes through the patient in a fan-shaped X-ray and strikes the detector array positioned opposite the anodes. This stationary multisource/split-detector combination is coupled to a rotating electron beam and produces serial, contiguous, thin section tomographic scans in synchrony with the heart cycle.

There have been four iterations for EBCT since it was introduced clinically in the early 1980s. Since its initial introduction in 1982, it has been known as "rapid CT," "cine CT," "Ultrafast CT©," Electron Beam CT, and "Electron Beam Tomography©." The overall imaging methods have remained unchanged, but there have been improvements in data storage, data manipulation and management, data display, and spatial resolution. The original C-100 scanner was replaced in 1993 by the C-150, which was replaced by the C-300 in 2000. The current EBCT scanner, the e-Speed (GE/Imatron) was introduced in 2003. The e-Speed is a multislice scanner and currently can perform a heart or vascular study in one-half the total examination time required by the C-150 and C-300 scanners. The e-Speed, in addition to the standard 50 ms and 100 ms scan modes common to all EBCT scanners, is capable of imaging speeds as fast as 33 ms. A major limitation of this modality currently is the slice width, which is limited to 1.5 mm. Current MDCT scanners can obtain images in 0.5–0.75 mm per slice.

Three imaging protocols are used with the EBCT scanner. They provide the format to evaluate anatomy,

cardiovascular function, and blood flow. The imaging protocol used to study cardiovascular anatomy is called the *volume scanning mode* and is similar to scanning protocols employed by conventional CT scanners. Single or dual scans are obtained and then the scanner couch is incremented a predetermined distance. For non-contrast studies, the table increment is usually the width of the scan slice, so that there is no overlap imaging of anatomy. For contrast studies, especially those to be reconstructed three-dimensionally, table incrementation is usually less than the slice width, giving overlap of information to improve spatial resolution (see Chapters 3 and 4). For example, moving the table forward 1 mm, while taking a 1.5 mm slice, gives 33% overlap per image. Using the older scanners, with slice thickness of 3 mm, moving the table only 1.5 mm gives overlap to improve spatial resolution. This scanning mode is utilized with and without contrast enhancement and provides high spatial resolution of cardiovascular anatomy. This technique provides high resolution axial images, and is ideal for evaluation of the aorta, coronary arteries, and congenital heart disease. A 3-D arteriogram reconstructed from tomographic images has the potential for more complete visualization of the coronary arteries (Figures 1.3, 1.9).

The *cine scanning protocol* acquires images in 33 or 50 ms. Each scan is separated by an 8 ms delay, which translates to a scanning rate of 17 scans/s (or 32 f/s). The scanning period is predetermined by the heart rate. Scans are acquired for the duration of the cardiac cycle. Depending on the heart rate, up to 12 cm of the heart can be imaged in a single scanning period. The acquired images are displayed in a cine loop, making assessment of cardiac and valve motion possible. Blood pool contrast enhancement is achieved by injection of contrast medium boluses via a superficial peripheral vein. The bolus amount for each image acquisition period averages 30 mL. The end-systolic images can be compared to the end-diastolic images, allowing for accurate measurement of regional wall thickening

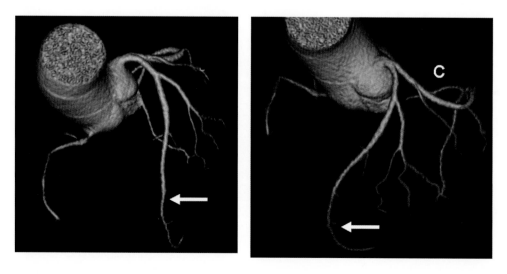

Figure 1.9. A contrast-enhanced electron beam angiogram demonstrating long segments of the left anterior descending (arrow). Images such as seen here can be created which are much more similar to a conventional coronary angiogram, if desired.

and motion, myocardial mass (utilizing the known specific gravity of cardiac tissue), global and regional ejection fraction [15]. Importantly, since blood is being injected into the venous system, simultaneous enhancement of the right and left ventricle allows for excellent visualization of all cardiac chambers simultaneously, and measure of both right and left ventricular function and structure [16]. Cine angiographic studies at lower frame rates of 8/second can be done in conjunction with specialized volume scanning protocols when performing EB coronary angiography.

The *flow mode imaging protocol* acquires a single image gated to the electrocardiogram at a predetermined point in the cardiac cycle (e.g. end-diastole (peak of the R-wave)). Images can be obtained for every cardiac cycle or multiples thereof. Scanning is initiated before the arrival of a contrast bolus at an area of interest (e.g. left ventricular (LV) myocardium) and is continued until the contrast has washed in and out of the area. Time density curves from the region of interest can be created for quantitative analysis of flow (Figure 1.10). The filling of different chambers can be visualized sequentially, allowing for visualization of flow into and out of any area of interest. This was the original methodology employed to assess for graft patency, prior to the ability to create 3-D images. It should be noted that early studies dating back to 1983 have demonstrated saphenous vein graft patency with this technique, achieving an accuracy of approximately 90% as compared to invasive angiography [17]. This technique is still commonly employed to detect shunts (Chapter 16), as well as to determine the length of time it takes for contrast to travel from the arm vein at the site of injection to the central aortic root (allowing for accurate image acquisition of the high resolution contrast-enhanced images, Chapter 4).

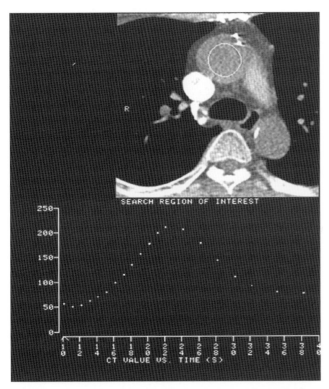

Figure 1.10. A flow or timing study. This study images the same level over time. A region of interest (in this study, the circle is placed in the ascending aorta) defines the anatomy to be measured. The graph below measures the Hounsfield units (HU) of that region of interest on each subsequent image. Initially, there is no contrast enhancement, and the measures are of non-enhanced tissue, around 50–60 HU. Contrast starts to arrive on this study around 16 seconds, and peaks at 22 seconds. The bright white structure next to the ascending aorta is the superior vena cava, filled with unmixed contrast.

Comparisons of EBCT and MDCT Scanners

Spatial Resolution

Spatial resolution compares the ability of the scanners to reproduce fine detail within an image, usually referred to as the high contrast spatial resolution. Spatial resolution is important in all three dimensions when measuring coronary plaque. Even if limited to the proximal coronary arteries, the left system courses obliquely within the x–y imaging plane, while the right coronary artery courses through the x–y imaging plane. Simply put, one axial image may demonstrate 5 or more centimeters of the left anterior descending, while most images will demonstrate only a cross-section of the right coronary artery. For more on cardiac anatomy with examples, see Chapter 3. The in-plane resolution of both EBCT and MDCT systems is nearly equivalent at the same display fields of view. The resolution in z dimension is determined by the collimation in EBCT and the detector width in MDCT (this may be thought of as the measurement of the slice width for individual images from either scanner). This is a "voxel" or volume element and it has the potential to be nearly cubic using MDCT but will always be "rectanguloid" for EBCT (slice width greater than x–y pixel width). Current coronary artery calcification (CAC) scanning protocols use 3 mm thickness for EBCT and vary between manufacturers from 2.5 mm to 3.0 mm for MDCT. For CT angiography, EBCT utilizes 1.5 mm slices, and MDCT most often obtains images with 0.5–0.75 mm per axial slice. Thus, MDCT has a significant advantage in terms of spatial resolution, and results in less partial volume averaging. Also the principles of resolution of say a 1 mm vessel require that the slice width be 1 mm or less. Partial volume averaging occurs when a small plaque has dramatically different CT numbers related to whether it is centered within one slice or divided between two adjacent slices. Thus, thinner slices will have less partial volume averaging. The visualization of smaller lesions is only possible with smaller slice widths. For EBCT, the slice thickness is 1.5 to 3.0 mm, with an in-plane resolution of approximately 7 to 9 line pairs/cm (Figure 1.11). Modern MDCT systems permit simultaneous data acquisition in 16–64 parallel cross-sections with 0.625–0.75 mm collimation each. The in-plane spatial resolution is now as high as 14 line pairs/cm. However, conventional CT angiography still has higher temporal and

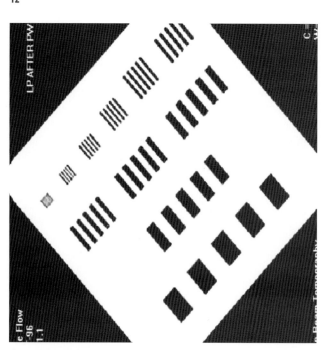

Figure 1.11. Spatial resolution as measured on computed tomography. A phantom is imaged and the smallest line pairs per centimeter are evaluated. Somewhat similar to an eye chart, the thinnest lines clearly seen define the spatial resolution of the scanner.

spatial resolution, allowing for better visualization of the smaller arteries and collateral vessels. Modern angiographic equipment has a resolution of 40 line pairs per centimeter with a six-inch field of view, the usual image magnification for coronary angiography [18]. Thus, invasive coronary angiography still has a 3–4-fold better resolution than current MDCT systems. It is likely to remain this way until the perfection of flat panel detectors for CT – which would be akin to the current state of the art in conventional angiography devices.

Generally, the higher X-ray flux (mAs = tube current × scan time) and greater number and efficiency of X-ray detectors available with MDCT devices leads to images with better signal-to-noise ratio and higher spatial resolution when compared to current EBCT scanners. Early detection of calcified plaque is dependent upon distinguishing the plaque from image noise. MDCT systems have reduced image noise compared to EBCT systems (8–18 noise/HU versus 24 noise/HU). Image noise with EBCT has been shown to have an association with body mass index which may result in falsely identifying noise as calcified plaque or overestimation of true plaque burden. This limitation of EBCT relative to MDCT is the lower power, with EBCT limited to 63 mAs (100 mAs for e-Speed). Typical values for mAs for MDCT angiography is on the order of 300 to 400. While both EBCT and MDCT have difficulties with the morbidly obese patient, MDCT can increase the mAs (and kV) to help with tissue penetration, while EBCT is more limited in this clinical setting.

Speed/Temporal Resolution

Cardiac CT is dependent upon having a high temporal resolution to minimize coronary motion-related imaging artifacts. By coupling rapid image acquisition with ECG gating, images can be acquired in specific phases of the cardiac cycle. Studies have indicated that temporal resolutions of 19 ms are needed to suppress all pulmonary and cardiac motion [19]. Interestingly, temporal resolution needs to be faster to suppress motion of the pulmonary arteries than for cardiac imaging. The study by Ritchie et al. demonstrated the need for 19 ms imaging to suppress pulmonary motion (despite breath-holding), while needing 35 ms imaging to fully suppress motion for cardiac structures. This is most likely due to the accordion motion of the pulmonary arteries, whereby the motion of the heart causes the surrounding pulmonary arteries to be pulled in and out with each beat. This has led to some physicians to use cardiac gating during pulmonary embolism studies to improve resolution down to fourth and fifth generation branches of the pulmonary system.

Cardiac MR motion studies of the coronary arteries demonstrate that the rest period of the coronary artery (optimal diastolic imaging time) varies significantly between individuals with a range of 66–333 ms for the left coronary artery and 66–200 ms for the right coronary artery [20] and that for mapping coronary flow, temporal resolution of 23 ms may be required for segments of the right coronary artery [21,22]. Current generation cardiac CT systems which create images for measuring calcified plaque at 50–100 ms (EBCT) and 180–300 ms (prospectively gated MDCT) cannot totally eliminate coronary artery motion in all individuals. Motion artifacts are especially prominent in the mid-right coronary artery, where the ballistic movement of the vessel may be as much as two to three times its diameter during the twisting and torsion of the heart during the cardiac cycle (Figure 1.12). It should be remembered that the motion of the coronary artery during the cardiac cycle is a 3-D event with translation, rotation, and accordion type movements. Thus portions of the coronary artery pass within and through adjacent tomographic planes during each R-R cycle. Blurring of plaques secondary to coronary motion increases in systems with slower acquisition speeds. The resulting artifacts tend to increase plaque area and decrease plaque density and thus alter the calcium measurements. The artifacts may make those segments of the CT angiogram non-diagnostic, a problem that plagued up to 70% of the early four-slice MDCT system studies [5,12].

The image quality achieved with cardiac CT is determined not only by the 3-D spatial resolution but also by the temporal resolution. The spatial resolution is directly related to the scan slice thickness and the reconstruction matrix. The temporal resolution, which determines the degree of motion suppression, is dependent on the pitch factor (which is determined by the table speed), the gantry rotation time, and the patient's heart rate during the

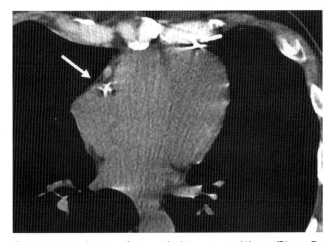

Figure 1.12. A typical motion artifact seen with calcium scans on multidetector CT images. The limited reproducibility of this technique is due to the star artifacts seen on this image (right coronary artery, white arrow). Prospective gating is done, with halfscan reconstruction techniques. In cases of faster heart rates, motion artifacts seen here are commonplace. To limit radiation to a reasonable level for this screening test, no overlap or retrospective images are obtained, so multisegment reconstruction is not possible.

examination. As stated above, utilizing more detectors (i.e. 4- versus 8- versus 16- versus 64-detector/channel systems) can improve the temporal resolution of the images, and reduces scan time (i.e. breath-hold time) and section misregistration.

Radiation Dose

Computed tomography utilizes X-rays, a form of ionizing radiation, to produce the information required for generating CT images. Although ionizing radiation from natural sources is part of our daily existence (background radiation including air travel, ground sources, and television), a role of healthcare professionals involved in medical imaging is to understand potential risks of a test and balance those against the potential benefits. This is particularly true for diagnostic tests that will be applied to healthy individuals as part of a disease screening or risk stratification program. In order for healthcare professionals to effectively advise individuals they must have an understanding of the exposure involved. The use of radiological investigations is an accepted part of medical practice, justified in terms of clear clinical benefits to the patient which should far outweigh the small radiation risks. Diagnostic medical exposures, being the major source of man-made radiation exposure of the population, add up to 50% of the radiation exposure to the population. However, even small radiation doses are not entirely without risk. A small fraction of the genetic mutations and malignant diseases occurring in the population can be attributed to natural background radiation. The concept of "effective dose" was introduced in 1975 to provide a mechanism for assessing the radiation detriment from partial body irradiations in terms of data derived from whole-body irradiations. The effective dose for a radiological investigation is the weighted sum of the doses to a number of body tissues, where the weighting factor for each tissue depends upon its relative sensitivity to radiation-induced cancer or severe hereditary effects. It thus provides a single dose estimate related to the total radiation risk, no matter how the radiation dose is distributed around the body. Adoption of the *effective dose* as a standard measure of dose allows comparability across the spectrum of medical and non-medical exposures. "The effective dose is, by definition, an estimate of the uniform, whole-body equivalent dose that would produce the same level of risk for adverse effects that results from the non-uniform partial body irradiation. The unit for the effective dose is the sievert (Sv)" (www.fda.gov/cdrh/ct/rqu.html). Although it has many limitations, the effective dose is often used to compare the dose from a CT examination, a fluoroscopic examination, and the background radiation one experiences in a year. Units are either millirem (mrem) or millisievert (mSv); 100 mrem equals 1 mSv. The estimated dose from chest X-ray is 0.04 mSv, and the average annual background radiation in the United States is about 300 mrem or 3 mSv [23]. Table 1.2 shows the estimated radiation doses of some commonly used tests.

The Food and Drug Administration (FDA) in describing the radiation risks from CT screening in general used the following language (www.fda.gov/cdrh/ct/risks.html):

In the field of radiation protection, it is commonly assumed that the risk for adverse health effects from cancer is proportional to the amount of radiation dose absorbed and the amount of dose depends on the type of X-ray examination. A CT examination with an effective dose of 10 millisieverts (abbreviated mSv; 1 mSv = 1 mGy in the case of x rays) may be associated with an increase in the possibility of fatal cancer of approximately 1 chance in 2000. This increase in the possibility of a fatal cancer from radiation can be compared to the natural incidence of fatal cancer in the US population, about 1 chance in 5. In other words, for any one person the risk of radiation-induced cancer is much smaller than the

Table 1.2. Common tests with estimated radiation exposures

Test	Radiation dose	
1 Stress MIBI	6 mSv	
1 LC spine	1.3 mSv	
1 Barium enema	7 mSv	
1 Upper GI	3 mSv	
1 Abdominal X-ray	1 mSv	
1 Dental X-ray	0.7 mSv	
1 Cardiac catheterization	2.5–10 mSv	
	Radiation dose for MDCT	**Radiation dose for EBCT**
Calcium scan	1–1.5 mSv	0.6 mSv
CT angiography	8–13 mSv	1–1.5 mSv
CTA dose modulation	5–8 mSv	–
Lung CT	8 mSv	1.5 mSv
Abdomen/Pelvis	10 mSv	2 mSv
Body scan	12 mSv	2.6 mSv
Virtual colon	8–14 mSv	2–3 mSv

natural risk of cancer. Nevertheless, this small increase in radiation-associated cancer risk for an individual can become a public health concern if large numbers of the population undergo increased numbers of CT procedures for screening purposes.

Since CT is the most important source of ionizing radiation for the general population, dose reduction and avoidance is of the utmost importance, especially for the asymptomatic person undergoing risk stratification, rather than diagnostic workup. Already, 50% of a person's lifetime radiation exposure is due to medical testing, and this is expected to go up with increased exposure to nuclear tests and CT scanning. Used as a tool in preventive cardiology, cardiac CT is increasingly being performed in the population of asymptomatic persons, a priori healthier individuals, where use of excessive radiation is of special concern.

The other variable involved in dose is the protocol used. EBCT protocols are fairly fixed; the only variable is the use, if any, of overlap. All data is acquired by prospective triggering; that is, the X-rays are only on during the acquisition of data that will be used for the image. MDCT, however, can use prospective triggering or retrospective gating, 120 or 140 kilovolts (kV) (with protocols possible with lower kV depending upon future research and tube current improvements), and a wide range of mA. Retrospective gating means that the X-rays are on throughout the heart cycle. One drawback of MDCT as compared to EBCT is the potential for higher radiation exposure to the patient, depending on the tube current selected for the examination. The X-ray photon flux expressed by the product of X-ray tube current and exposure time (mAs) is generally higher with MDCT. For example, 200 mA with 0.5 s exposure time yields 100 mAs in MDCT whereas 614 mA (fixed tube current) with 0.1 s exposure time yields 61.4 mAs in EBCT. In millisieverts, calcium scanning leads to an approximate dose of 1–1.5 mSv for MDCT, and 0.6 mSv for EBCT. This is in comparison to a conventional coronary angiogram, with effective doses of 2.1 and 2.5 mSv for men and women respectively.

There are primary three factors that go into radiation dosimetry. The X-ray energy (kV), tube current (mA), and exposure time. The distance of the X-ray source from the patient is a fourth source, but, unlike fluoroscopy, this distance is fixed in both MDCT and EBCT. Hunold et al. [24] recently performed a study of radiation doses during cardiac examinations. Cardiac scanning was performed with EBCT and four-slice multidetector CT (Siemens Volume Zoom, Ehrlangen, Germany), utilizing prospective triggering to assess patient effective radiation exposure, and compared to measurements made during cardiac catheterization. EBCT CAC protocols yielded effective doses of 1.0 and 1.3 mSv for men and women, while MDCT CAC protocols using 100 mA, 140 kV, and 500 ms rotation yielded 1.5 mSv for men and 1.8 mSv for women. In females, the effective radiation doses is another 25% higher than in males, raising the mean dose from 8 mSv in men to

10 mSv per study in women [25]. Since MDCT angiography utilizes retrospective imaging, and since radiation is continuously applied while only a fraction of the acquired data is utilized, high radiation doses (doses of 6–10 mSv/study) still play a role in decisions to utilize this modality [24,26]. In two studies of radiation dose comparing EBCT and four-slice MDCT, the first reported EBCT angiography doses of 1.5–2.0 mSv, MDCT angiography 8.1–13 mSv, and coronary angiography 2.1–2.3 mSv, while the other reported EBCT angiography doses of 1.1 mSv and MDCT doses of 9.3–11.3 mSv [23,24].

Theoretically, since narrow collimation (beam widths) causes "overbeaming," the dose efficiency is lower with four-slice scanners than with more detectors. Estimated efficiency goes from 67% with 4 slices (1.25 mm, 5 mm coverage) to 97% with 16 slices (at 1.25 mm, covering 20 mm). However, obtaining thinner slices will offset this gain, as obtaining more images will lead to higher radiation doses. Typical studies with four-slice MDCT scanners obtained 600 images, while 16-slice scanners typically produce about 1200 scans, and 64-detector scanners are reporting over 2000 images produced per study. Newer MDCT studies report that radiation doses are similar to four-slice studies with newer 16-level multidetector scanners [27].

The energy used can be altered in MDCT studies, and while typical imaging is done in the range of 120–140 kV, this can be varied with MDCT. The attenuation (densities) of calcium and iodine contrast agents increases with reduced X-ray energy (reduced kV settings). This can reduce the X-ray exposure, as the X-ray power emitted by the tube decreases considerably with reduced kV settings. To compensate for the lower power (and resultant increased noise of the image), the tube current (mA) can be increased. Scans with less than 120 kV tube voltage (i.e. 80 kV) can potentially maintain contrast-to-noise ratios that have been established for coronary calcium and CT angiography images, and significant lower radiation exposure. Preliminary experiments have demonstrated a reduction in radiation exposures of up to 50% with use of 80 kV. Jakobs et al. demonstrated that the radiation dose for CAC scoring with use of 80 kV may be as low as 0.6 mSv (similar to EBCT data) [28]. As the noise will go up with 80 kV imaging, this may be too low for CT angiography. CT angiography protocols may be possible with 100 kV protocols, providing a reduction in radiation of 30%. There is no research on the clinical diagnostic accuracy utilizing these radiation-dose-reducing options routinely. A lower kV is most often used for pediatric patients. Similarly, for obese patients, where penetration is important, a kV of 135 or 140 can be utilized. The power (mAs) used is directly proportional to the radiation dose. Higher mAs results in lower image noise, following the relationship: noise is inversely proportional to the square root of the mAs. Thus, limiting mAs can result in lower radiation, but higher noise. It is important to remember that reducing mAs too much to save radiation will increase noise to the point where the scan is non-diagnostic. Most centers use either an "automatic" mAs system, which adjusts the mAs based upon the image quality, or leave the mAs relatively fixed.

Prospective triggering or "sequential" mode is typically used and strongly recommended for coronary calcium assessment with MDCT, due to the lower radiation doses to which the patient is exposed. However, the drawback of using MDCT prospective triggering is the inability to perform overlapping images, and longer image acquisition times. Thus, all CT vendors currently recommend retrospective image acquisition in the "helical" mode for performance of MDCT angiography, despite the higher radiation doses. This is due to the requirement during retrospective imaging for slower table movement to allow for oversampling, for gap-less and motion-reduced imaging, as well as the possibility of multisegment reconstruction. Retrospective imaging allows the clinician to have multiple phases of the cardiac cycle available for reconstruction, to find the portion of the study with the least coronary motion. Many clinicians utilize multiple phases for reconstruction, with different phases used for different coronary arteries. However, constant irradiation is redundant, as most images are reconstructed during the diastolic phases of the heart cycle. Thus, a new method for reducing radiation dose with MDCT is to implement tube current modulation. Tube current is reduced during systole, when images are not utilized for reconstruction of images for MDCT angiography, by 80%, and then full dose is utilized during diastole. Depending upon the heart rate, this may reduce radiation exposure by as much as 47% [28], but with slower heart rates, this reduction will be less, as systole encompasses a shorter and shorter fraction of the cardiac cycle. Dose modulation protocols reduce radiation doses with MDCT by attempting to decrease beam current during systole, when images are not used for interpretation, and should be employed whenever possible [29]. Most of these protocols turn down the beam current (mA) during systole, so that diagnostic images are still available from roughly 40–80% of the R-R interval (cardiac cycle).

Dose modulation is not universally employed, as it is harder to use it with fast heart rates, as the time to ramp up and ramp down the radiation dose becomes significant, and the ever shortening diastole becomes a smaller target. The routine use of beta blockers makes even more sense in this setting, given the increased ability to use dose modulation with lower heart rates. Clinically, dose modulation is used less than expected, as many clinicians, nervous about not having a portion of the cardiac cycle available for analysis, choose to leave the dose modulation feature off. Another issue is the potential loss of wall motion and other functional data. If tube current modulation is used, there are no systolic images. Some investigators have reported that no functional information can be obtained while using dose modulation. This is probably not correct, as an image from end-systole (early diastole) and end-diastole can be compared to calculated wall thickening, ejection fraction, and cardiac motion. Due to these concerns, no studies of

CT angiography reported to date have utilized dose modulation routinely.

Another method to decrease radiation exposure is to increase the pitch. The pitch is usually very low, on the order of 0.25 to 0.4 for CT angiography cases, and usually 1 for coronary calcium scanning. This low pitch raises radiation exposure, but is partially compensated by the more efficient dose of using the larger collimation available with increased detectors. For individuals with different heart rates, different pitches can be used to obtain similar datasets. Thus, for those with slower heart rates, a faster pitch may allow for some reduction in cardiac exposure during these studies, and thus proportionally less radiation with dose modulation than for those with higher heart rates.

One must be careful and cognizant of the dose being given. In one study using 16-slice MDCT, the pitch was reduced based upon the patient being able to hold their breath for 20 seconds, so very high overlap was obtained (very small pitch). The mean irradiation dose received by the patients during this MDCT angiography study was 24.2 mSv [30]. Understanding the physics and implications of higher mAs and kV and thinner slices will help the clinician choose the necessary parameters, without over-irradiating the patient. This concept, called "information/milliSv," causes one to think about the benefit garnered from each mSv given.

Clinical Applications of Cardiovascular CT

Cardiac CT has several unique diagnostic capabilities applicable to the many facets of CAD, worth the radiation exposures and time needed to learn these applications. Each will be discussed at length in chapters throughout this book. The presence of coronary calcium is invariably an indicator of atherosclerosis [31,32]. Non-contrast studies can accurately identify and quantify coronary calcification (a marker of total plaque burden) [33], while contrast-enhanced studies can define ventricular volumes, ejection fraction, and wall motion and wall thickening with high accuracy [34]. Studies can be performed at rest, and during exercise can identify reversible ischemia [35].

Coronary angiography during cardiac catheterization is the clinical gold standard for definitive diagnosis and determination of coronary lesions. Pathologic studies have demonstrated that the severity of coronary stenoses is underestimated by visual analysis during clinical coronary angiography [36–39]. This may result from the limitations of resolution based upon fluoroscopy and the 2-D imaging inherent in coronary angiography, as well as the inability to see beyond the lumen with conventional angiography. The true promise of cardiovascular CT is to visualize the coronary artery, including the lumen and wall. Three-dimensional digital coronary images may provide more accurate representation of coronary artery anatomy and be more amenable to quantitation, thereby improving the

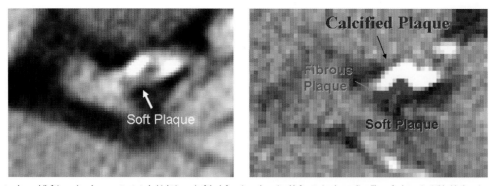

Figure 1.13. A contrast-enhanced (left image) and non-contrast study (right image) of the left main and proximal left anterior descending. The soft plaque is visible (dark region, representing fat density) with calcified plaque (white regions). A computer program can be applied (Acculmage, San Francisco, CA) to the individual pixels to measure lower density (fat density, pink squares), intermediate density (red squares, fibrous density) and high density (white squares, calcified plaque). This can theoretically quantitate the volume of soft plaque, fibrous plaque and calcified plaque in any given CT image.

diagnosis and treatment of CAD [40]. There is rapidly accumulating data with both MDCT and EBCT to visualize the coronary arteries accurately and reliably (CT angiography) [41–44]. Looking beyond the lumen by visualizing the wall and its constituents (including fat, calcium, and fibrous tissue) is now possible with cardiac CT (Figure 1.13). Coronary plaque composition evaluation is being actively investigated [45,46]. This so-called "soft plaque" evaluation may prove to have prognostic significance over coronary calcium or risk factors alone, as well as helping to target revascularization better than luminography alone.

Future of CT and MR

The strengths of magnetic resonance cardiovascular imaging include greater definition of tissue characteristics, perfusion, valvular function, lack of X-ray radiation, and lack of need for potentially nephrotoxic contrast media, compared to CT technologies. Several studies have been reported comparing this modality to coronary angiography [47–49]. Limited temporal and spatial resolution [50], partial volume artifacts (due to slice thickness limitations) [51], reliance on multiple breath-holds, and poor visualization of the left main coronary artery [52] all reduce the clinical applicability of MR angiography. Reported sensitivities for MR angiography range from 0% to 90% [47,53]. MR angiography remains a technically challenging technique with certain limitations hindering its clinical use. CT angiography offers advantages over MR angiography, including single breath-hold to reduce respiratory motion, higher spatial resolution, reduced slice thickness and overall study time of 35–50 seconds with CT techniques as compared to 45 to 90 minutes for MR angiography [53]. The rapidity and ease with which CT coronary angiography can be performed suggest possible cost advantages compared with MR angiography and selective coronary angiography [54]. Thus, for most applications (in the absence of renal insufficiency or contrast allergy), CT will be the preferred method to evaluate anatomy, be it coronary, renal, carotid or peripheral vascular beds (Figure

1.14). MR, in the foreseeable future, will remain a better test for intercranial imaging, as the bony structures cause some scatter with CT imaging.

For cardiovascular CT in general, better workstations (ease of use and diagnostic capabilities), as well as improvements in both spatial and temporal resolution will continue to push this diagnostic tool to the forefront of cardiology. For MDCT, increased numbers of detectors (64-slice systems are now available) will allow for better collimation and spatial reconstructions. Having more of the heart visualized simultaneously will also allow for reductions in the contrast requirements and breath-holding, further improving the methodology. Multisector reconstruction (combining images from consecutive heart beats) and dose modulation (to reduce radiation exposure

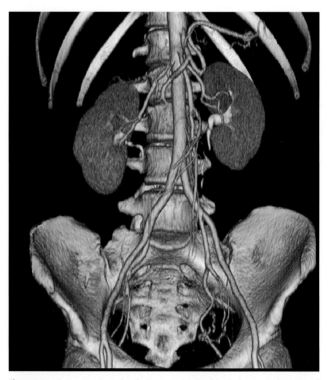

Figure 1.14. A contrast-enhanced study demonstrating the abdominal aorta, renal arteries and kidneys, and iliac circulation. This study can be done with 40 cc of iodinated contrast, taking between 5 and 10 seconds depending on the scanner used. Highly diagnostic vascular imaging is quite routine with EBCT and MDCT scanners.

during systole, when images are not used for reconstruction) are increasingly being applied, which will continue to improve the image quality and diagnostic rate of these machines.

References

1. Mao S, Budoff MJ, Oudiz RJ, Bakhsheshi H, Wang S, Brundage BH. A simple single slice method for measurement of left and right ventricular enlargement by electron beam tomography. Int J Card Imaging 2000;16:383–390.

2. Budoff MJ, Mao SS, Wang S, Bakhsheshi H, Brundage BH. A Simple single slice method for measurement of left and right atrial volume by electron beam computed tomography. Acad Radiol 1999;6:481–486.

3. Stuber M, Botnar RM, Fischer SE, et al. Preliminary report of in-vivo coronary MRA at 3 Tesla in humans. Magn Reson Med 2002;48:425–428.

4. Carr JJ, Nelson JC, Wong ND, et al. Calcified coronary artery plaque measurement with cardiac CT in population-based studies: standardized protocol of Multi-Ethnic Study of Atherosclerosis (MESA) and Coronary Artery Risk Development in Young Adults (CARDIA) study. Radiology 2005;234:35–43.

5. Nieman K, Rensing BJ, van Geuns RJ, et al. Non-invasive coronary angiography with multislice spiral computed tomography: impact of heart rate. Heart 200;88(5):470–474.

6. Ropers D, Baum U, Pohle K, et al. Detection of coronary artery stenosis with thin-slice multi-detector row spiral computed tomography and multiplanar reconstruction. Circulation 2003;107:664–666.

7. Nieman K, Cademartiri F, Lemos PA, Raaijmakers R, Pattynama PM, de Feyter PJ. Reliable noninvasive coronary angiography with fast submillimeter multislice spiral computed tomography. Circulation 2002;106:2051–2054.

8. Regenfus M, Ropers D, Achenbach S, et al. Noninvasive detection of coronary artery stenosis using contrast-enhanced three-dimensional breath-hold magnetic resonance coronary angiography. J Am Coll Cardiol 2000;36:44–50.

9. Kim WY, Danias PG, Stuber M, et al. Coronary magnetic resonance angiography for the detection of coronary stenoses. N Engl J Med 2001;345:1863–1869.

10. Blobel J, Baartman H, Rogalla P, Mews J, Lembcke A. Spatial and temporal resolution with 16-slice computed tomography for cardiac imaging. Fortschr Roentgenstr 2003;175:1264–1271.

11. Lembcke A, Rogalla P, Mews J, et al. Imaging of the coronary arteries by means of multislice helical CT: optimization of image quality with multisegmental reconstruction and variable gantry rotation time. Fortschr Roentgenstr 2003;175:780–785.

12. Wicky S, Rosol M, Hoffmann U, Graziano M, Yucel KE, Brady TJ. Comparative study with a moving heart phantom of the impact of temporal resolution on image quality with two multidetector electrocardiography-gated computed tomography units. J Comput Assist Tomogr 2003;27:392–398.

13. Dewey M, Laule M, Krug L et al. Multisegment and halfscan reconstruction of 16-slice computed tomography for detection of coronary artery stenosis. Invest Radiol 2004;39:223–229.

14. Mao S, Lu B, Oudiz RJ, Bakhsheshi H, Liu SCK, Budoff MJ. Coronary artery motion in electron beam tomography. J Comput Assist Tomogr 2000;24:253–258.

15. Baik HK, Budoff MJ, Lane KL, Bakhsheshi H, Brundage BH. Accurate measures of ejection fraction using electron beam tomography, radionuclide angiography, and catheterization angiography. Int J Card Imaging 2000;16:391–398.

16. Mao SS, Budoff MJ, Oudiz RJ, et al. Effect of exercise on left and right ventricular ejection fraction and wall motion in patients with coronary artery disease: an electron beam computed tomography study. Int J Cardiol 1999;71;23–31.

17. McKay CR, Brundage BH, Ullyot DJ, et al. Evaluation of early postoperative coronary artery bypass grafts patency by contrast-enhanced computed tomography. J Am Coll Cardiol 1983;2:312–317.

18. Nissen SE, Gurley GL. Assessment of coronary angioplasty results by intravascular ultrasound. In: Serruys PW, Straus BH, King SB III (eds) Restenosis after intervention with new mechanical devices. Dordrecht, Netherlands: Kluwer, 1992:73–96.

19. Ritchie CJ, Godwin, JD. Minimum scan speeds for suppression of motion artifacts in CT. Radiology 1992;185:37–42.

20. Wang Y, Vidan E. Cardiac motion of coronary arteries: variability in the rest period and implications for coronary MR angiography. Radiology 1999;213(3):751–758.

21. Hofman MB, Wickline SA. Quantification of in-plane motion of the coronary arteries during the cardiac cycle: implications for acquisition window duration for MR flow quantification. J Magn Reson Imaging 1998;8(3):568–576.

22. Marcus JT, Smeenk HG. Flow profiles in the left anterior descending and the right coronary artery assessed by MR velocity quantification: effects of through-plane and in-plane motion of the heart. J Comput Assist Tomogr 1999;23(4):567–576.

23. Morin RL, Gerber TC, McCollough CH. Radiation dose in computed tomography of the heart. Circulation 2003;107:917–922.

24. Hunold P, Vogt FM, Schmermund A, et al. Radiation exposure during cardiac CT: effective doses at multi-detector row CT and electron-beam CT. Radiology 2003;226:145–152.

25. International Commission on Radiological Protection. Recommendation of the ICRP. ICRP Publication 60. Oxford: Pergamon Press, 1990.

26. Knollmann FD, Hidajat N, Felix R. CTA of the coronary arteries: comparison of radiation exposure with EBCT and multi-slice detector CT. Radiology 2000;217(P):364.

27. Flohr TG, Schoepf UJ, Kuettner A, et al. Advances in cardiac imaging with 16-section CT systems. Acad Radiol 2003;10(4):386–401.

28. Jakobs TF, Becker CR, Ohnesorge B, et al. Multislice helical CT of the heart with retrospective ECG gating: reduction of radiation exposure by ECG-controlled tube current modulation. Eur Radiol 2002;12:1081–1086.

29. Trabold T, Buchgeister M, Kuttner A, et al. Estimation of radiation exposure in 16-detector row computed tomography of the heart with retrospective ECG-gating. Rofo 2003;175:1051–1055.

30. Leta R, Carreras F, Alomar X, et al. Non-invasive coronary angiography with 16 multidetector-row spiral computed tomography: a comparative study with invasive coronary angiography. Rev Esp Cardiol 2004;57:217–224.

31. Janowitz WR, Agatston AS, Viamonte M. Comparison of serial quantitative evaluation of calcified coronary artery plaque by ultrafast computed tomography in persons with and without obstructive coronary artery disease. Am J Cardiol 1991;68:1–6.

32. Blankenhorn DH. Coronary artery calcification: a review. Am J Med Sci 1961;242:1–9.

33. Breen JF, Sheedy PF, Schwartz RS, et al. Coronary artery calcification detected with ultrafast CT as an indication of coronary artery disease. Radiology 1992;185:435–439.

34. Lipton MJ, Higgins CB, Boyd DP. Computed tomography of the heart: evaluation of anatomy and function. J Am Coll Cardiol 1985;5:555–595.

35. Roig E, Chomka EV, Castaner A, et al. Exercise ultrafast computed tomography for the detection of coronary artery disease. J Am Coll Cardiol 1989;13:1073–1081.

36. Marcus ML, Armstrong MD, Heistad DD, Eastham CL, Mark AL. Comparison of three methods of evaluating coronary obstructive lesions: postmortem arteriography, pathologic examination and measurement of regional myocardial perfusion during maximal vasodilation. Am J Cardiol 1982;49:1688–1706.

37. Grondin CM, Dyrda I, Pasternac A, Campeau L, Bourassa MG, Lesperance J. Discrepancies between cineangiographic and postmortem findings in patients with coronary artery disease and recent myocardial revascularization. Circulation 1974;49:703–708.

38. Thomas AC, Daview MJ, Dilly S, Dilly N, Franc F. Potential errors in estimation of coronary arterial stenoses from clinical coronary arteriography with reference to the shape of the coronary arterial lumen. Br Heart J 1986;55:129–139.

39. Mintz GS, Painter JA, Pichard AD, et al. Atherosclerosis in angiographically normal coronary artery reference segments: an intravascular ultrasound study with clinical correlations. J Am Coll Cardiol 1995;25:1479–1485.

40. Van den Broek JGM, Slump CH, Storm CJ, Van Benthem AC, Buis B. Three-dimensional densitometric reconstruction and visualization of stenosed coronary artery segments. Comput Med Imaging Graph 1995;19:207–217.

41. Napel S, Rubin GD, Jeffrey RB Jr. STS-MIP: A new reconstruction technique for CT of the chest. J Comput Assist Tomogr 1993;17(5): 832–838.

42. Thomas PJ, McCollough CH, Ritman EL: An electron-beam CT approach for transvenous coronary angiography. J Comput Assist Tomogr 1995;19(3):383–389.

43. Achenbach S. Contrast enhanced electron beam tomography for the non-invasive 3-dimensional visualization of coronary arteries and detection of stenoses. Am J Card Imaging 1995;9(Suppl 1): A30.

44. Chernoff DM, Ritchie CJ, Higgins CB. Evaluation of electron beam CT coronary angiography in healthy subjects. AJR Am J Roentgenol 1997;169:93–99.

45. Schroeder S, Kopp AF, Baumbach A, et al. Noninvasive detection and evaluation of atherosclerotic coronary plaques with multislice computed tomography. J Am Coll Cardiol 2001;37:1430–1435.

46. Leber AW, Knez A, White CW, et al. Composition of coronary atherosclerotic plaques in patients with acute myocardial infarction and stable angina pectoris determined by contrast-enhanced multislice computed tomography. Am J Cardiol 2003;91:714–718.

47. Manning WJ, Li W, Edelman RR. A preliminary report comparing magnetic resonance imaging with conventional angiography. N Engl J Med 1993;328:828–832.

48. Pennell DJ, Keegan J, Firmin DN, Gatehouse PD, Underwood SR, Longmore DB. Magnetic resonance imaging of coronary arteries: technique and preliminary results. Br Heart J 1993;70:315–326.

49. Paschal CB, Haache EM, Adler LP. Coronary arteries: three-dimensional MR imaging of the coronary arteries: preliminary clinical experience. J Magn Reson Imaging 1993;3:491–501.

50. Duerinckx AJ, Urman MK. Two dimensional coronary MR angiography: analysis of initial clinical results. Radiology 1994;193:731–738.

51. Duerinckx AJ, Urman MK, Atkinson DJ, Simonetti OP, Sinha U, Lewis B. Limitations of MR coronary angiography. J Magn Reson Imaging 1994;4:81.

52. Duerinckx AJ, Atkinson DP, Mintorovitch J, Simonetti OP, Urman MK. Two-dimensional coronary MRA: limitations and artifacts. Eur Radiol 1996;6:312–325.

53. Kim WY, Danias PG, Stuber M, et al. Coronary magnetic resonance angiography for the detection of coronary stenoses. N Engl J Med 2001;345:1863–1869.

54. Chernoff DM, Ritchie CJ, Higgins CB. Evaluation of electron beam CT coronary angiography in healthy subjects. AJR Am J Roentgenol 1997;169:93–99.

2

Methodology for Image Acquisition

Songshou Mao and Jerold S. Shinbane

Introduction

Computed tomographic (CT) imaging is an important methodology for diagnosis, monitoring, and guidance to treatment of cardiovascular diseases. CT can assess cardiovascular pathology through characterization of gross anatomic abnormalities, assessment of tissue density changes associated with disease processes, and functional and hemodynamic abnormalities. Assessment of these characteristics requires the use of techniques to optimally capture images demonstrating cardiovascular structure and function. Cardiac structures are in constant motion, and possess low contrast within tissues and complex image characteristics [1]. Therefore, for most cardiac imaging, the correct localization of target structures, timing of imaging to capture images during the segment of the R-R interval with relatively slow cardiac motion [2], and injection of contrast media to improve contrast within structures throughout all slice levels must be performed. This chapter will focus on ECG triggering, contrast injection, and preview methods essential to obtaining diagnostic images for the assessment of cardiovascular pathology.

ECG Triggering

Several types of motion artifacts can significantly affect cardiovascular CT images. These artifacts can be caused by cardiac motion, chest motion induced by respiration, and heart rate variation during the imaging interval [3,4]. Advances in cardiac imaging have limited the role of respiratory artifact, as the newest generation of multidetector CT (MDCT) and electron beam CT (EBT, GE Imatron) techniques allow for cardiac imaging to be completed in a single breath-hold. Artifact due to cardiac motion and heart rate variation, though, remain significant challenges for cardiovascular CT imaging [3,4].

Cardiac motion during a single cardiac cycle is extremely complex. Multiple types of cardiac motion have

been noted: inward or outward motion of the endocardium with systole and diastole; rotation; torsion or wringing; translocation; and "accordion-like" base to apex motion [5]. Cardiac motion can be analyzed in the context of the -x, y-, and z-axis planes. There is greater x-y direction motion at the mid-portion of the left ventricle and greater z direction motion at the heart base [2]. Left ventricular contraction and relaxation are the main source of cardiac motion. Torsion or wringing of the left ventricle induces heart rotation along the left ventricular long axis during a cardiac cycle.

Specific motion issues relate to individual coronary arteries. Since the right coronary artery is further from the center of the left ventricle than the left coronary artery, this artery exhibits faster motion, especially in its mid-section [1]. Atrial systole and diastole are another important factor causing motion of the right coronary artery and left circumflex. The left main and proximal of left anterior descending coronary artery have greater z-plane motion [6], and therefore z-axis motion can induce left main motion abnormalities [2]. Quantitation of cardiac motion demonstrates the challenges of cardiac imaging. Left ventricular endocardial maximal motion speed has been reported at 41–100 mm/s [6,7]. The right coronary artery has 50 mm/s motion by angiography [8]. The motion speed of mid right coronary artery has been reported as 32.8–70.7 mm/s at rest and 56.9–108.6 mm/s on average during stress [1].

Given the imaging constraints caused by cardiac motion, appropriate collimation size and acquisition speed are factors important to the acquisition of images with less motion artifact. The collimation size for coronary artery calcium screening and angiography is 0.6–3 mm in current CT studies. The acquisition time per image is 50 to 250 ms [9–11]. This acquisition speed is insufficient to freeze heart motion. Therefore, cardiac triggering is essential in order to minimize cardiac and coronary artery motion speed during imaging and avoid image blurring. Studies have demonstrated that 19.1 ms per image is necessary to freeze left ventricular motion [7]. Additionally, studies have demonstrated that there is less cardiac motion at late systole to early diastole [1,12]. In this time interval, the coronary artery motion speed is ≤30 mm/s [1]. It is therefore possible to obtain adequate images with less than 100 ms temporal resolution in studies with ≤3 mm collimation.

In regard to variability of heart rate or rhythm, any change in heart rate or rhythm can alter chamber size, and therefore change in the spatial location of target structure in axial or 3-dimensional images, even if the individual axial image is not blurred [13]. All patients have some variability in heart rate, even those without atrial or ventricular ectopy [4]. In 118 cases with 30-slice coronary artery screening, the average difference between fastest and slowest heart rate was 20 beats/min. Assessment of cardiac timing intervals in reference to variability in heart rate has demonstrated that there is a relatively small change in the RT interval (systolic interval) compared to the TR interval (diastolic interval) [2,3,14]. Therefore, the artifact due to variation in heart rate can be decreased with an end-systolic trigger protocol.

Based on ventricular and atrial contraction and relaxation, there are six phases in a cardiac cycle (R-R interval). These are: isovolumic contraction time, ejection time, isovolumic relaxation time, left ventricular rapid filling, diastasis, and atrial contraction time. During ventricular systole, the motion of the right coronary artery and left circumflex mid-segment is in an anterior and inner direction, which reverses in diastole. At the end of isovolumic contraction and relaxation, the motion speed is close to zero, but the time interval for imaging is very short.

There are three relatively low speed motion segments: isovolumic contraction, isovolumic relaxation, and diastasis. Any choice of trigger point depends on the scan time. The isovolumic contraction time (after the R wave) and relaxation time (after the T wave) are approximately 50–140 ms [15–20], which correlate positively but weakly with heart rate [16]. Diastasis is the other slower motion segment, but the length is more variable following heart rate changes. In patient with heart rates of greater than 100 to 110 beats/min, diastasis is minimal [17]. The isovolumic contraction and relaxation segments are more optimal segments for imaging, but the time interval is too brief for 100 ms or 50 ms scan times in patients with rapid heart rates. Therefore, the scan time needs to cover late atrial or late ventricular contraction. Comparing both trigger times, end-systolic triggering is more optimal [2]. Since there is up to 200 ms temporal resolution per image in MDCT, the diastasis segment is the optimal scan time in patients with a lower heart rate.

Two ECG trigger techniques are used in current CT imaging, prospective [2,3] and retrospective triggering [21,22] for EBT and MDCT respectively. Prospective triggering can be performed with R wave triggering, end-systolic triggering, and both end-systolic and end-diastolic combined triggering (Figure 2.1). The R wave trigger is used for cine studies. End-systolic triggering is used for

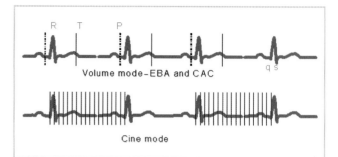

Figure 2.1. Schematics representing prospective ECG triggering. End-systolic triggering (solid black line) and end-diastolic trigger (broken line) are shown in the upper panel. The end-systolic trigger time is at 25 ms before the T wave. The end-diastolic trigger is at 25 ms before the R wave. Cardiac systolic function can be calculated using both end-systolic and end-diastolic triggered images. The R wave trigger is used for cine studies (lower panel). Each black line represents one image. EBA = electron beam angiography, CAC = coronary artery calcification.

volumetric and flow studies. End-systolic and end-diastolic combined triggering is used to measure chamber ejection fraction with e-Speed technology [23]. The R wave trigger can be performed automatically by any EBT computer. The end-systolic trigger can be calculated by a scanner computer or by an operator using the following formula:

$$\text{Scan delay time (from R wave to scan time)}$$
$$= RT - 0.5 \times \text{scan time/per image}$$
$$(\text{scan time 50 or 100 ms}).$$

The RT interval can be calculated by Mao's formulas [24]:

Male RT (millisecond) = 0.143 × RR + 224.2 or 8580/heart rate + 224.2; Female RT (millisecond) = 0.157 × RR + 221.2 or 9420/heart rate +221.2.

Today, these formulas can be used for automatic calculation by the e-Speed scanner computer. For C150 or C300 scanners, one needs to calculate the RT manually. Table 2.1 serves as a reference for trigger time based on heart rate.

Retrospective triggering is widely used with MDCT [21, 22]. The synchronized ECG signal is recorded simultaneously with images. Subsequently, image reconstruction can

Table 2.1. Scan delay time (from R wave peak to trigger time) in EBT volume study [7][21]

HR	R-R	RT	Imaging time 50 ms RS (ms)	Imaging time 50 ms RS (%)	Imaging time 100 ms RS (ms)	Imaging time 100 ms RS (%)
<40	1714	460	435	25	0.41	24
41–50	1333	408	383	29	0.358	27
51–60	1090	387	362	33	0.337	31
61–70	923	362	337	37	0.312	34
71–80	800	350	325	41	0.3	38
81–90	706	335	310	44	0.285	40
91–100	632	314	289	46	0.264	42
101–110	571	291	266	47	0.241	42
>110	522	282	257	49	0.232	44

R-R = R-R interval, RT = RT interval, RS = interval from R wave to scan start time, ms = millisecond, % = (RS ÷ R-R) × 100%.

be performed with single-sector and multisector (segmented) reconstruction. Using single-sector methodology, image sets are reconstructed in a specific time interval of the cardiac cycle. The reconstruction algorithm is a half revolution (usually 240° to 260° = 180° + detector angle) with a 190 to 250 ms interval. An optimal image can be found from these images sets in a given cardiac cycle. The sum of all cardiac cycle images can be used to obtain complete cardiac cycle images.

For scanning during rapid heart rates, temporal resolution can be improved through use of scan data from more than one cardiac cycle for reconstruction of an image (segmented reconstruction). The partial scan data set for reconstruction of one image then consists of projection sectors from multiple consecutive heart cycles. Depending on the relationship of rotation time and patient heart rate, a temporal resolution between rotation time/2 and rotation time/2M is present, where M equals the number of projection sectors and the number of used heart cycles [11] (Figure 2.2).

With any triggering technique, the greatest challenge to obtaining acceptable images is heart rate variation. Change in heart rate or rhythm can induce misregistration artifact of the target structure in both prospective or retrospective triggered images [11,13,14]. The overlap of structures is another important factor for any retrospective image trigger. Since pitch is based on couch rotation time and total collimator size, and the slice levels selected are based on the R-R interval, it is challenging to synchronize the slice thickness and the table movement in one beat. In most images, the slice thickness is larger than table increment. Therefore, overlap is an important tendency, especially using segmental trigger techniques, potentially leading to structure misregistration and misinterpretation. Advances in EBT and MDCT may decrease imaging time and therefore artifact induced by heart motion and heart rate change. Future MDCT technology will require greater synchronization of slice thickness and pitch, to decrease cardiac structure misregistration.

Contrast Media Injection

The aim of contrast media injection is increase the contrast between target structure and surrounding tissues, by increasing the CT Hounsfield units (CT HU) of the interest structure. Ideally, an injection protocol will achieve optimal enhancement through uniformity of contrast enhancement at all slice levels with optimal CT HU using as small a dose of contrast medium as possible. Important factors to consider in regard to contrast media injection are circulation time measurement and injection methodology.

The circulation time (scan delay time) is the time interval that it takes blood to transit from the access vein to the target area. Many factors influence circulation time, including age [25], cardiac out put [26], and venous anatomy and pathology. In the author's analysis of 1866 cases, the mean circulation time was 18.49 ± 5.16 (8–46) seconds (unpublished data). Data from these cases demonstrated a linear relationship between circulation time and left ventricular ejection fraction ($R = 0.35$, $P < 0.001$). No other factors demonstrated correlation with circulation time, including individual weight, height, age, gender, chamber volume, or heart rate. A delay time of 16–20 seconds would have resulted in optimal timing in only 40% of cases. Therefore, circulation time must be measured individually, rather than using empiric delay times.

The circulation time can be measured using a small contrast bolus injection with serial scanning of the same slice to obtain the peak enhancement time through time density curve analysis (Gamma variate curve) [27,28]. Another method utilizes an automatic bolus-triggering technique [29]. With this method, the first monitoring scan is obtained 10 to 12 seconds after the start of the contrast medium injection. When the CT HU reaches 120 HU, angiography imaging is activated.

Typically, our protocol uses 10–15 mL of contrast media injected at a rate of 3 to 5 mL/s to calculate the circulation time. It is important to use the same injection rate as the rate for the subsequent study. A 30-second scan time is necessary in most patients. For patients with left ventricular systolic dysfunction or venous issues, a 40-second scan time is often necessary.

Contrast medium is usually administered via an 18-gauge needle in the antecubital vein.

The use of low osmolar non-ionic contrast media significantly reduces adverse reactions to contrast media [30]. Optimal enhancement is very important for improvement of image quality. The optimal enhancement depends on the contrast media dose and injection rate. The dose of contrast media is dependent on multiple factors, such as patient size, scan time, and desired enhancement level (CT

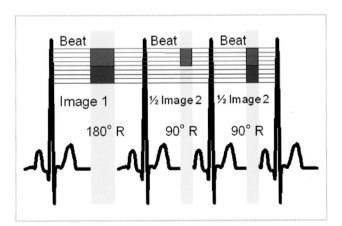

Figure 2.2. Schematic demonstrating retrospective triggering. Red and blue line represents the z-axis position of spiral signal data. The synchronized ECG signal is displayed. Beat 1 (segment 1) occurs at a slower hear rate than beats 2 and 3. Image 1 is reconstructed using a 180° rotation. When a heart rate increase occurs over a predefined threshold (beats 2 and 3), the segmental reconstruction uses 90° rotation data and uses two beats (beats 2 and 3) to complete the second image. If the heart rate increases continuously, four or more subsegments can be used to reconstruct images.

HU). The total dose for a procedure typically should not exceed 200 mL of high concentration contrast media for coronary arteriography and left ventriculography with EBT [14,31,32]. In current MDCT coronary arteriography studies, 80–150 mL contrast medium is commonly injected at a rate of 3–5 mL/s [11,21,22].

An important limitation of CT imaging of small vessels relates to volume effects. The purpose of contrast-enhanced studies is to increase contrast between coronary vessel lumen and surrounding tissues. Greater lumen enhancement (represented by increased CT HU) will create greater contrast between the vessel lumen and non-calcified vessel wall, which is especially important for visualization of small vessels. Luminal enhancement, though, will decrease the contrast between enhanced vessel lumen and calcified plaques. Our group analyzed CT coronary artery angiography quality in 1000 cases. In images with vessel enhancement less than 200 CT HU, it is rarely possible to display coronary arteries less than 2 mm in diameter, even with adjustment of the window level and threshold. In images with vessel enhancement greater than 300 HU, visualization of small vessels is better. With these 1000 cases, a formula representing contrast dose related CT HU and weight was developed.

$$\text{Dose/weight (kg)} = 0.0035 \times \text{CT HU} + 0.6772$$
$$(R = 0.62, P < 0.001), \text{for e-Speed scanner}$$
with a 30-second scan time.

$$\text{Dose/weight (kg)} = 0.0053 \times \text{CT HU} + 0.5826$$
$$(R = 0.6, P < 0.001), \text{for C150 or C300 scanners}$$
with a 47-second scan time.

In these formulas, the contrast media concentration is 370 mg I/mL. According to these formulas, one can roughly estimate the contrast dose which gives the desired CT HU at a defined scan time (30 and 47 seconds in e-Speed and C150 or/and C300 scanners respectively). For example, if the patient's weight is 80 kg, a target CT HU of 300 and 47-second scan time, then 174 cc (370 mg I/mL) non-ionic contrast media is necessary with C150 or C300 scanners. In cases with short scan times, the dose of contrast and injection time can be decreased. For scan times over 47 seconds, additional contrast media dose and injection time is not necessary due to the increased CT HU of the recirculating blood pool.

Injection Protocols

Venous blood flow occurs under low velocity and low pressure conditions. Under normal circumstances, blood flow depends on the pressure gradient between right atrium and antecubital vein, with a velocity of approximately 15–20 mm/s [33]. Following contrast injection, the pressure in the vein is increased by the injector. Single phase injection protocols result in non-uniformity of aortic enhancement as measured by CT HU, with a single peak value in the

mid-portion of the study and lower values at the beginning and end of the study [34–37]. The injection duration is 20–50 seconds for current CT technique. In order to increase vascular CT HU uniformity between slices, multiple phase injection protocols have been developed [35–37]. The injection rate needs to be decreased before the peak time, to assist with greater uniformity of enhancement of the later slices. A first injection stage with a high velocity, 5–6 mL/s for 10 seconds, is followed by a lower rate of injection, 2–4 mL/s, with subsequent saline injection to flush the remaining contrast out of the intravenous line and antecubital vein (50–70 mL). An injector with two syringes can perform this protocol (Medrad, Inc, Indianola, PA) (Figure 2.3). Using this injector, the total injection time for contrast and saline is equal to the scan delay time (circulation time) plus the scan time (Figure 2.4).

Certain clinical situations can limit the use of the above protocols. In patients with a history of allergy to iodinated contrast media, gadolinium contrast media can be used (50–70 mL, 2–3 mL injection rate and saline injection) [38]. The mean CT HU after enhancement by gadolinium can reach about 100 HU. With this protocol, only the large coronary artery can be displayed. Additionally, for patients with slow heart rates, the scan time can be too long for a single breath hold. In cases where breath hold would be too long

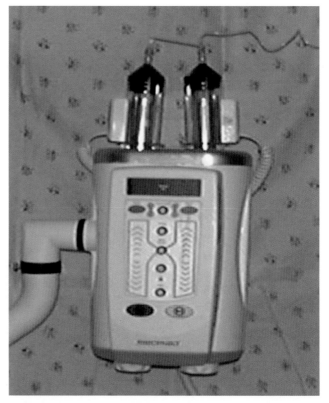

Figure 2.3. Injector set-up for multiphase contrast injection (Medrad, Inc, Indianola, PA). The left syringe is for injection of contrast media, which is followed by saline injection from the right syringe. A Y connector connects both syringes to the patient's intravenous access.

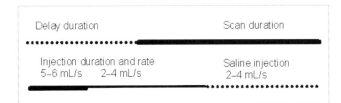

| Delay duration | Scan duration |
| Injection duration and rate
5–6 mL/s   2–4 mL/s | Saline injection
2–4 mL/s |

Figure 2.4. Schematic demonstrating a multiphase contrast injection protocol. The delay duration is equal to the peak value time of CT HU at the target structure after contrast injection. A first injection phase with a high velocity, 5–6 mL/s, is followed by a lower rate of injection, 2–4 mL/s. Subsequently, saline is injected at 2–4 mL/s in order to flush the remaining contrast out of the intravenous line and antecubital vein. The total injection time is equal to the delay time plus the scan time to help optimize vascular contrast enhancement and uniformity between slices.

due to slow heart rates, atropine can be used to increase heart rate and therefore reduce the scan time.

Preview Methods

The purpose of preview imaging is to delineate the *z*-axis location of a target object. Preview scans are performed in segments using a special scan path. The X-ray beam is directed off the scan path during the majority of the sweep and is directed onto the targets only briefly at the bottom and on the side of each path. The radiation dose for a preview scan is therefore much lower than that for a normal scan. A preview image provides a pair of projections (anteroposterior and lateral views) [39] (Figure 2.5). From these images, one can approximate the *z*-axis location of heart and great vessels. The most cranial structure of the heart is usually the left atrial appendage, and the most caudal structure is the ventricular apex. Therefore, a complete cardiac study requires scanning between these landmarks. The apex is usually easy to distinguish. It may be more challenging to define the most cranial aspect of

the heart. The carina has served as a marker to localize the most cranial aspect of the heart, with use of the carina plane, lower edge of the carina, or 1 to 2 cm caudal to the carina as the first slice level reported by various authors. The distance from carina to left main coronary artery is extremely variable, ranging from 15 to 66 mm [39]. Therefore, the carina is not an optimal anatomic marker for estimation of the most cranial aspect of the heart.

The left main coronary artery can be used as a landmark for definition of the most cranial aspect of the heart. In order to decrease image slice number, protocols have been devised to localize the left main coronary artery using a minimal number of axial images. Hamid et al. described localization of the left main coronary artery from six axial images [39]. The six axial images (3 mm in collimation with 9 mm table increment) were obtained with a starting point 8–10 cm above the xiphoid process or mid breast line (Figure 2.6). The most caudal aspect of the ventricles can be defined from these preview images. For complete cardiac imaging, scanning 10 mm cranial to the left main coronary artery and 10 mm caudal to the apex is subsequently performed with CT angiography [39]. In patients with coronary artery bypass grafts, the starting point of the scan is the top of the aortic arch or 10 mm higher than the surgical metal clips. The mid level of the right pulmonary artery can also be used as the beginning of the scan level, if it can be defined in preview images.

Summary

Cardiac CT imaging poses challenges due to the complex motion of the heart, variation in heart rate and rhythm, and tissue characteristics of cardiovascular structures. An understanding of these factors and meticulous attention

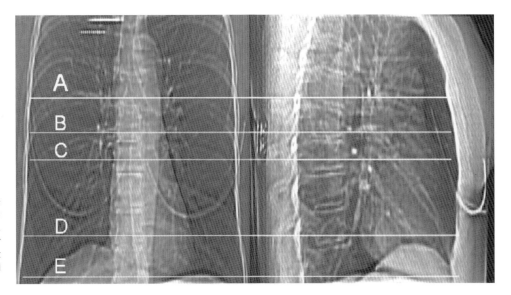

Figure 2.5. These images demonstrate preview scanning in the anteroposterior (AP) (left panel) and lateral views (right panel). Lines A, B, C, D, and E represent the lower border of the carina, mid-right pulmonary artery, left main coronary artery, mid-left ventricle and apex slice levels, respectively.

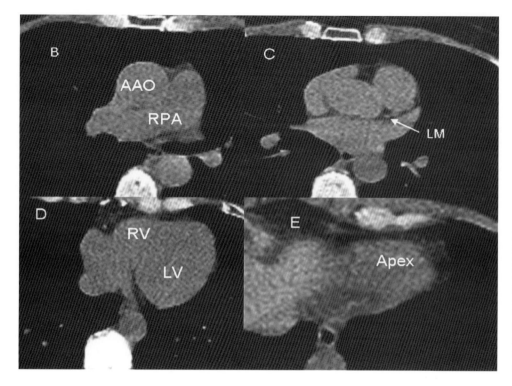

Figure 2.6. These axial images for a coronary artery calcium screen demonstrate axial images correlating with slice levels B, C, D, and E defined in Figure 2.5. The beginning slice level of the scan is at slice B representing the right pulmonary artery and the last slice is 10 mm below slice E. AAO = ascending aorta, RPA = right pulmonary artery, LM = left main coronary artery, RV = right ventricle, LV = left ventricle, Apex = most caudal level of left and right ventricle.

to triggering techniques, contrast injection methods, and preview methods can lead to images capable of visualization of anatomy and function critical to the diagnosis and treatment of patients with cardiovascular disease.

References

1. Mao SS, Lu B, Oudiz RJ, Bakhsheshi H, Liu SC, Budoff MJ. Coronary artery motion in electron beam tomography. J Comput Assist Tomogr 2000;24(2):253–258.
2. Mao SS, Budoff MJ, Bin L, Liu SC. Optimal ECG trigger point in electron-beam CT studies: three methods for minimizing motion artifacts. Acad Radiol 2001;8(11):1107–1115.
3. Mao SS, Bakhsheshi H, Lu B, Steve LS, Oudiz RJ, Budoff MJ. Effect of electrocardiogram triggering on reproducibility of coronary artery calcium scoring. Radiology 2001;220(3):707–711.
4. Mao SS, Oudiz RJ, Bakhsheshi H, Wang SJ, Brundage BH. Variation of heart rate and ECG trigger interval during ultrafast computed tomography. Am J Card Imaging 1996;10:1–7.
5. Marcus ML, Skorton DJ, Schelbert HR, Wolf GL. Cardiac Imaging: A Companion to Braunwald's Heart Disease. Philadelphia, PA: W.B. Saunders Company, 1991:671–731.
6. Rogers WJ Jr, Shapiro EP, Weiss JL, et al. Quantification of and correction for left ventricular systolic long-axis shortening by magnetic resonance tissue tagging and slice isolation. Circulation 1991;84(2):721–731.
7. Ritchie CJ, Godwin JD, Crawford CR, Stanford W, Anno H, Kim Y. Minimum scan speed for suppression of motion artifacts in CT. Radiology 1992;185:37–42.
8. Topol EJ, Nissen SE. Our preoccupation with coronary luminology: the dissociation between clinical and angiographic finding in ischemic heart disease. Circulation 1995;92:2333–2342.
9. Budoff MJ, Lu B, Shinbane JS, Chen L, Child J, Carson S, Mao S. Methodology for improved detection of coronary stenoses with computed tomographic angiography. Am Heart J 2004 Dec;148(6):1085–1090.
10. Budoff MJ, Achenbach S, Duerinckx A. Clinical utility of computed tomography and magnetic resonance techniques for non-invasive coronary angiography. J Am Coll Cardiol 2003;42(11):1867–1878.
11. Schoepf UJ, Becker CB, Ohnesorge BM, Yucel EK. CT of coronary artery disease. *Radiology* 2004;232:18–37.
12. Achenbach S, Ropers D, Holle J, Muschiol G, Daniel WG, Moshage W. In-plane coronary arterial motion velocity: measurement with electron-beam CT. Radiology 2000;216(2):457–463.
13. Mao SS, Budoff MJ, Bakhsheshi H, Steve L. Improved reproducibility of coronary artery scoring by electron beam tomography with a new electrocardiographic trigger method. Invest Radiol 2001;36:363–367.
14. Lu B, Zhuang N, Mao SS, Bakhsheshi H, Liu SC, Budoff MJ. Image quality of three-dimensional electron beam coronary angiography. J Comput Assist Tomogr 2002;26(2):202–209.
15. Tavel ME. Clinical phonocardiography and external pulse recording. Chicago, IL: Year Book Medical Publishers, 1985:279–299.
16. Poole-Wilson PA, Colucci WS, Massie BM, et al. Heart failure: Scientific principles and clinical practice. New York: Churchill Livingstone, 1997:339–343.
17. Weyman AE. Principles and practice of echocardiography, 2nd edn. Philadelphia: Lea & Febiger, 1994:721–741.
18. Chen W, Gibson D. Mechanisms of prolongation of pre-ejection period in patients with left ventricular disease. Br Heart J 1979;42(3):304–310.
19. Manolas J, Rutishauser W. Relation between apex cardiographic and internal indices of left ventricular relaxation in man. Br Heart J 1977;39(12):1324–1332.
20. Upton MT, Gibson DG, Brown DJ. Echocardiographic assessment of abnormal left ventricular relaxation in man. Br Heart J 1976;38(10):1001–1009.
21. Kopp AF, Küttner A, Trabold T, Heuschmid M, Schröder S, Claussen CD. Multislice CT in cardiac and coronary angiography. Br J Radiol 2004;77:87–97.

22. Schoenhagen P, Halliburton SS, Stillman AE, et al. Noninvasive imaging of coronary arteries: current and future role of multi-detector row CT. *Radiology* 2004;232:7–17.

23. Budoff MJ, Shinbane J, Child J, Carson C, Mao SS. Calculation of cardiac function by prospective adaptive triggering using e-Speed electron beam CT coronary angiography. RSNA 04; Radiological Society of North America scientific assembly and annual meeting program: p 481.

24. Mao S, Lu B, Takasu J, Oudiz RJ, Budoff MJ. Measurement of the RT interval on ECG records during electron-beam CT. Acad Radiol 2003; 10(6):638–643.

25. Hartmann IJ, Lo RT, Bakker J, de Monye W, van Waes PF, Pattynama PM. Optimal scan delay in spiral CT for the diagnosis of acute pulmonary embolism. Comput Assist Tomogr 2002;26(1):21–25.

26. Parvez Z, Moncada R, Sovak M. Contrast media: biologic effects and clinical application. Boca Raton, FL: CRC Press, 1987:61.

27. Mao S, Takasu J, Child J, Carson S, Oudiz R, Budoff MJ. Comparison of LV mass and volume measurements derived from electron beam tomography using cine imaging and angiographic imaging. Int J Cardiovasc Imaging 2003 Oct;19(5):439–445.

28. Mao S, Budoff MJ, Oudiz RJ, et al. Effect of exercise on left and right ventricular ejection fraction and wall motion. Int J Cardiol 1999;71:23–31.

29. Schlosser T, Konorza T, Hunold P, Kuhl H, Schmermund A, Barkhausen J. Noninvasive visualization of coronary artery bypass grafts using 16-detector row computed tomography. J Am Coll Cardiol 2004;44(6):1224–1229.

30. Katayama H, Yamaguchi K, Kozuka T, Takashima T, Seez P, Matsuura K. Adverse reactions to ionic and nonionic contrast media. A report from the Japanese Committee on the Safety of Contrast Media. Radiology 1990;175(3):621–628.

31. Budoff MJ, Oudiz RJ, Zalace CP, et al. Intravenous three-dimensional coronary angiography using contrast enhanced electron beam computed tomography. Am J Cardiol 1999;83(6):840–845.

32. Schmermund A, Rensing BJ, Sheedy PF, Bell MR, Rumberger JA. Intravenous electron-beam computed tomographic coronary angiography for segmental analysis of coronary artery stenoses. J Am Coll Cardiol 1998;31(7):1547–1554.

33. West JB. Best and Taylor's Physiological basis of medical practice. Baltimore,MD: Williams & Wilkins, 1991:119–139.

34. Bae KT, Tran HQ, Heiken JP. Multiphasic injection method for uniform prolonged vascular enhancement at CT angiography: pharmacokinetic analysis and experimental porcine model. Radiology 2000;216(3):872–880.

35. Fleischmann D, Rubin GD, Bankier AA, Hittmair K. Improved uniformity of aortic enhancement with customized contrast medium injection protocols at CT angiography. Radiology 2000; 214(2):363–371.

36. Hittmair K, Fleischmann D. Accuracy of predicting and controlling time-dependent aortic enhancement from a test bolus injection. J Comput Assist Tomogr 2001;25(2):287–294.

37. Fleischmann D, Hittmair K. Mathematical analysis of arterial enhancement and optimization of bolus geometry for CT angiography using the discrete Fourier transform. J Comput Assist Tomogr 1999;23(3):474–484.

38. Budoff MJ, Lu B, Mao S. Gadolinium-enhanced Three-dimensional electron beam coronary angiography. J Comput Assist Tomogr 2002; 26(6):879.

39. Bakhsheshi H, Mao SS, MD, Budoff MJ, Bin L, Brundage BH. Preview method for electron-beam CT scanning of the coronary arteries. Acad Radiol 2000;7:620–626.

3

Cardiac Anatomy by CT

Philip H. Tseng and Matthew J. Budoff

Introduction

Advances in spatial and temporal resolution, electrocardiographic triggering methodology, and image reconstruction software have helped in the evaluation of coronary artery anatomy and vessel patency, providing the ability to non-invasively diagnose or rule out significant epicardial coronary artery disease. This technique also allows the three-dimensional (3-D) simultaneous imaging of additional cardiac structures including coronary veins, pulmonary veins, atria, ventricles, aorta and thoracic arterial and venous structures, with definition of their spatial relationships for the comprehensive assessment of a variety of cardiovascular disease processes. This chapter will detail the two-dimensional (2-D) anatomy of the cardiac structures seen on typical cardiac CT studies. Figures 3.1 through 3.13 represent selected slices from a typical cardiac CT scan. These are carefully labeled to allow you to learn the anatomy in a systematic way.

Interpreting Cardiac CT Images

Reading cardiac CT scans in many ways is easier than interpreting cardiac angiography or echocardiography. The anatomy is always in the same orientation. For starters, we will use a convention that the sternum is 12 o'clock, and the spine is 6 o'clock. Since almost all imaging will be done with the patient supine, this will not change. Given these external landmarks, it is never confusing for physicians to orient themselves. For cardiac anatomy (and the same would apply to peripheral or carotid imaging), the easiest point of orientation is the aorta. On Figure 3.1, you can see the ascending aorta is in the center of the chest, and that provides easy identification of structures around them. Except for the rare adult congenital heart case (see Chapter 16), the landmarks described here will guide you through the typical cardiac anatomy as portrayed on CT scanning (axial cross-sectional imaging).

Starting with the aorta in the center of the image, the superior vena cava is usually just leftward (your left) on the image. The patient is on his back, usually oriented with his head in the scanner, so the feet of the patient are facing the technologist when scanning. Thus, all images are reversed on cardiac CT, with the left sided structures on the right, and the right sided structures on the left. The best way to keep your orientation in context to the patient is to equate reading the images with a handshake. If you are pointing with your right hand, you need to cross your body to get to right sided structures on the cardiac CT image. This is standard convention, and there should be no exceptions to demonstrating images in this way on the 2-D images (unless the patient was scanned prone). Some 3-D images are reconstructed differently, so this will apply to the true 2-D tomographic dataset only. Thus, the superior vena cava (SVC) is positioned just rightward (patient's right) of the aorta (at 11 o'clock). Throughout this chapter, we will be referring to the orientation in regard to the patient, so the SVC will be described as rightward, even though it is on your left as you are looking at the images. There is another easy way to identify the SVC on contrast images. The contrast is usually injected through an antecubital vein, so the structure that fills the brightest (with less admixture from non-contrast blood) is the SVC. This makes it the whitest structure of all the cardiac images, and thus, readily identifiable as compared to the other round structures on the superior levels.

Depending on how high the images start, the pulmonary artery (or right ventricular outflow tract) is always visible on the superior (cranial) images of a cardiac CT. Most datasets for cardiac CT should start at the level of the pulmonary artery, as the coronary arteries start just below. For studies of patients with bypass surgery or when more of the aorta is needed to be visualized (such as evaluating coarctations, dissections, and aneurysms), different starting levels will be needed. This chapter will mostly discuss the anatomy seen on the typical CT angiogram dataset, starting near the pulmonary artery and extending through the base of the heart. These datasets usually do not need to

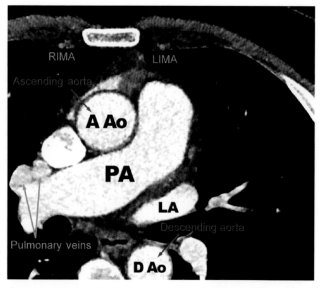

Figure 3.1. The typical top level of a CT angiogram, demonstrating the ascending aorta (A Ao), descending aorta (D Ao), left and right internal mammary arteries in the chest wall, and the pulmonary artery. LA = left atrium, LIMA = left internal mammary artery, PA = pulmonary artery, RIMA = right internal mammary artery.

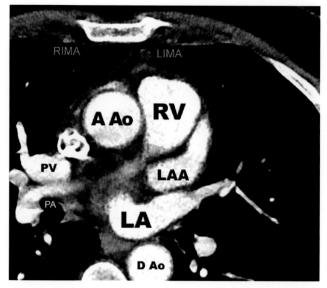

Figure 3.3. A level 1.5 mm caudal to Figure 3.2. The RV outflow tract is now present, in place of the pulmonary artery on the level above. A Ao = ascending aorta, D Ao = descending aorta, LA = left atrium, LAA = left atrial appendage, LIMA = left internal mammary artery, PA = pulmonary artery, PV = pulmonary vein, RV = right ventricle, RIMA = right internal mammary artery, SVC = superior vena cava.

include the transverse aorta, and to minimize radiation exposure, these extracardiac superior structures should only be imaged when necessary. Of course, for an aortic dissection, coarctation or imaging of the great vessels (to evaluate subclavian steal, carotid disease, etc.), different imaging sets will be necessary. However, this is outside the scope of the typical cardiac examination, and the anatomy

initially described will start with a typical dataset (starting below the aortic arch). Imaging of these other superior structures will be described later.

Top levels of the standard cardiac CT examination will either show the right ventricle (RV) outflow tract (Figure 3.3) or show the pulmonary artery as a sweeping structure from just left of the aortic root, extending posterior and rightward (Figures 3.1, 3.2). Using our clock descriptors, this will go from 1 o'clock and then sweep behind the aorta ending up at 9 o'clock. Behind the pulmonary artery is the

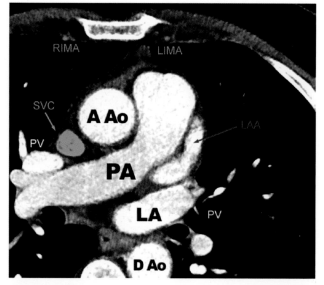

Figure 3.2. A level 6 mm lower than Figure 3.1. While all the structures seen in Figure 3.1 are still visible, the more caudal level now allows for visualization of the left atrial appendage. The superior vena cava is seen in blue to highlight this structure. A Ao = ascending aorta, D Ao = descending aorta, LA = left atrium, LAA = left atrial appendage, LIMA = left internal mammary artery, PA = pulmonary artery, PV = pulmonary vein, RIMA = right internal mammary artery, SVC = superior vena cava.

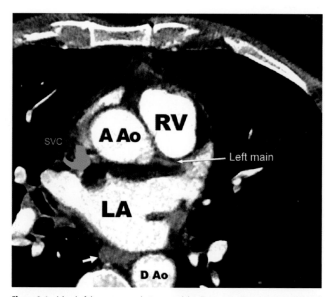

Figure 3.4. A level of the contrast study 9 mm caudal to Figure 3.3. Now, the origin of the left main coronary artery is seen. The esophagus is closed (white arrow). A Ao = ascending aorta, D Ao = descending aorta, LA = left atrium, RV = right ventricle, SVC = superior vena cava.

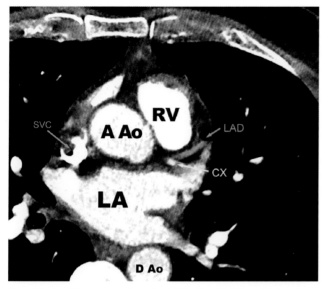

Figure 3.5. A level 3 mm caudal to Figure 3.4. The bifurcation of the left main into the left anterior descending and circumflex artery is now seen. A Ao = ascending aorta, CX = circumflex artery, D Ao = descending aorta, LA = left atrium, LAD = left anterior descending artery, RV = right ventricle, SVC = superior vena cava.

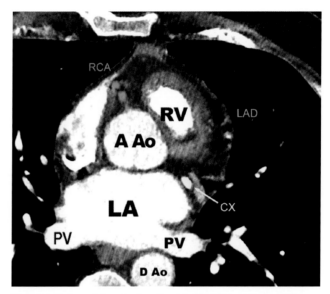

Figure 3.7. Moving caudally another 6 mm, the origin of the right coronary artery (RCA) is now visible. The right and left inferior pulmonary veins can be seen draining into the left atrium. A Ao = ascending aorta, CX = circumflex artery, D Ao = descending aorta, LA = left atrium, LAD = left anterior descending artery, PV = pulmonary vein, RCA = right coronary artery, RV = right ventricle.

left atrial appendage, usually a triangular structure at 2–3 o'clock (Figure 3.1). There have been several studies demonstrating that clot within the left atrial appendage can be visualized or excluded with similar accuracy to the transesophageal echocardiogram (TEE), and this is especially useful in cases of atrial fibrillation [1]. Atrial pathology such as atrial masses [2,3] and thrombi [1] have been

reported with cardiac CT. However, there is no randomized study (as there is with TEE) to demonstrate that patients have equal outcomes with TEE excluding clot as compared to weeks of anticoagulation with warfarin, so we would generally recommend that if CT is used for this purpose, it is done in patients unable or unwilling to undergo TEE to exclude clot.

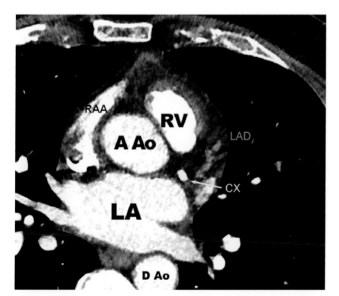

Figure 3.6. Another 6 mm caudal to the level in Figure 3.5, now the left anterior descending (blue) and circumflex (yellow) arteries are separate structures. The right atrial appendage (RAA) is also seen. A Ao = ascending aorta, CX = circumflex artery, D Ao = descending aorta, LA = left atrium, LAD = left anterior descending artery, RAA = right atrial appendage, RV = right ventricle.

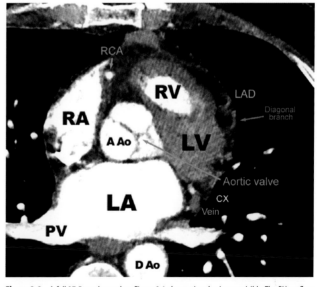

Figure 3.8. A full 37.5 mm lower than Figure 3.1, the aortic valve is now visible. The RV outflow tract is well seen at this level. The great cardiac vein (Vein) is seen, just posterior to the circumflex (CX). A Ao = ascending aorta, CX = circumflex artery, D Ao = descending aorta, LA = left atrium, LAD = left anterior descending artery, LV = left ventricle, PV = pulmonary vein, RA = right atrium, RCA = right coronary artery, RV = right ventricle.

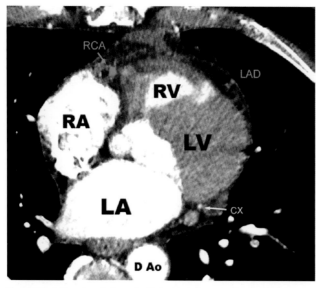

Figure 3.9. Halfway through the study, this level is similar to the "five-chamber" view seen with echocardiography, demonstrating the aortic outflow, left and right ventricles, and right and left atria. CX = circumflex artery, D Ao = descending aorta, LA = left atrium, LAD = left anterior descending artery, LV = left ventricle, RA = right atrium, RCA = right coronary artery, RV = right ventricle.

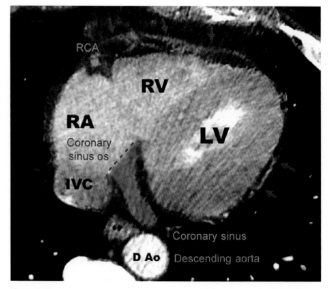

Figure 3.11. Approaching the bottom of the dataset, the coronary sinus is now visible, draining into the right atrium (RA). The inferior vena cava (IVC) is now seen, and the level is below the left atrium. The posterior wall of the left ventricle is now visualized. The normal pericardium in this case is well seen (red arrows) as a thin, non-calcified structure. D Ao = descending aorta, IVC = inferior vena cava, LV = left ventricle, RA = right atrium, RCA = right coronary artery, RV = right ventricle.

Many structures are hard to identify relative to other similar structures on any single image, and the best method to use is to scroll up and down through the dataset, following contiguous structures relative to known structures easily identified on the CT. For example, the aorta is almost always very easy to identify on any given image, so using this as a landmark to identify other structures as you move caudally through the dataset will be very helpful. In rare congenital cases (such as transposition), the aorta and pulmonary artery can be confused, and following the round structure into the left ventricle defines the aorta, and following the other round structure on caudal images to

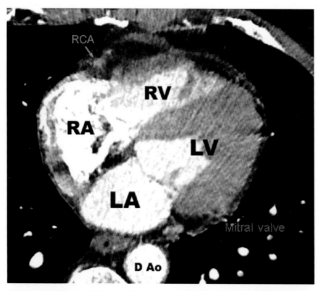

Figure 3.10. Now two-thirds through the coronary study, the four chambers of the heart are well seen. Since motion-free images are best obtained at end-systole for most heart rates, the left ventricular wall is thicker than end-diastolic imaging. The mitral valve is seen, however, due to incomplete contrast mixing between the superior vena cava (contrast enhanced) and inferior vena cava (non-enhanced blood), the tricuspid valve is most often not well visualized on cardiac CT. D Ao = descending aorta, LA = left atrium, LV = left ventricle, RA = right atrium, RCA = right coronary artery, RV = right ventricle.

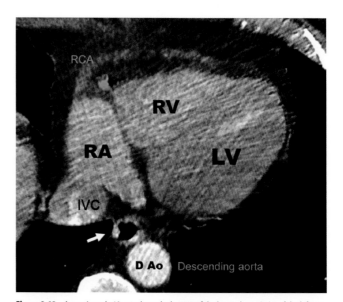

Figure 3.12. Approximately 10 mm above the bottom of the heart, the majority of the left ventricle (LV) visualized is the inferior wall. Only a small residual chamber is still visible. The esophagus (white arrow) is seen. D Ao = descending aorta, IVC = inferior vena cava, LV = left ventricle, RA = right atrium, RCA = right coronary artery, RV = right ventricle.

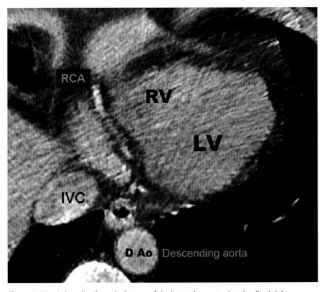

Figure 3.13. A data slice from the bottom of the heart, demonstrating the distal right coronary artery and the inferior wall of the left and right ventricles. D Ao = descending aorta, IVC = inferior vena cava, LV = left ventricle, RCA = right coronary artery, RV = right ventricle.

the right ventricle will easily and accurately define the appropriate structure. This scrolling technique is particularly useful in differentiating the left atrial appendage from other structures that are present on the patient's left, including the pulmonary artery, left ventricular outflow tract, and pulmonary veins. Also, when the rare persistent left SVC is present, it can be identified by following the structure on contiguous images down into the coronary sinus. An abnormally large coronary sinus is most often caused by this left sided SVC (Figure 3.14). By following structures that are familiar or obvious (such as the aortic root or left ventricle), you can sort out the different structures even in the most complex congenital case. With normal anatomy, you will find you will not need to do this often, as most cardiac structures are in the exact same place and same orientation on almost all patients. However,

when you are starting, and when you encounter the congenital anomaly, this technique will be most useful.

Again, considering the "non-congenital" patient, the most posterior structure is the descending aorta, sitting just next to the spine. In almost all cases, this is to the patient's left, except in cases of right sided aorta and situs invertus. The descending aorta should be of similar size to the ascending aorta at this level (just below the aortic arch, at the level of the pulmonary artery or RV outflow tract). The descending aorta is easy to follow on contiguous images throughout the cardiac examination, allowing for easy assessment of aneurysms, dissection, and coarctation (see Chapter 14). The pulmonary artery is usually slightly smaller than the ascending aorta, and this is an excellent modality to make exact measures of different cardiac structures. Because CT imaging is computerized, there are no magnification issues (the distance from the imaging tube to the patient is fixed, unlike fluoroscopy), and there is no need for calibration prior to making measurements. Enlarged pulmonary arteries do not always correlate with increased pulmonary pressures, but may reflect volume overload (such as tricuspid regurgitation, left to right shunts, etc.). Figure 3.15 demonstrates a markedly dilated pulmonary artery in a patient with a left to right shunt. Dilated chambers or vessels provide important clues that there is something wrong with that chamber, and echocardiography is usually adequate to further evaluate the pressures. It can also clue in the CT evaluator to pay more attention to things like: the presence of an atrial or ventricular septal defect, right ventricular hypertrophy, and enlargement of the right atrium or ventricle.

Just anterior to the spine is the esophagus, usually a thin opening with no air. The presence of air (air is black on the CT images) describes a lower esophageal sphincter that is open (it should be closed as patients lie on their back and hold their breath), and could represent esophageal disease (a cause of reflux esophagitis) or hiatal hernia (which would then be a large structure at the level of the base of the heart (Figure 3.16). Anterior to the esophagus is the left

Figure 3.14. Left sided superior vena cava (SVC). The left image demonstrates the persistent SVC (arrow), which is non-contrast enhanced due to injection of contrast in the right antecubital vein in this case. This can subsequently be followed, demonstrating a markedly dilated coronary sinus (due to the increased flow, right image). CS = coronary sinus, RA = right atrium.

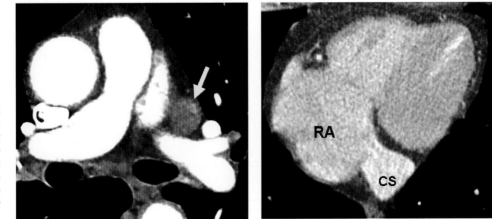

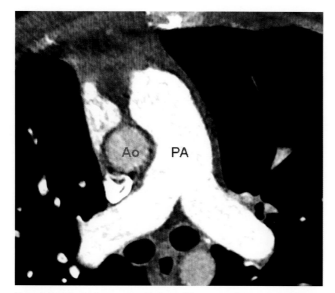

Figure 3.15. Dilated pulmonary artery. The inverted Y structure on this image is the pulmonary artery, which is clearly dilated and easy to measure on cardiac CT. Causes include both increased volume (shunts and regurgitation) as well as increased pulmonary pressure. It is difficult to discern the etiology of the pulmonary artery without further evaluation, as pressures cannot be measured with cardiac CT. Ao = ascending aorta; PA = pulmonary artery.

the top of which is usually visualized even at the superiormost images of the heart (Figure 3.1, just anterior to the descending aorta). Superior pulmonary veins are also seen on this superior level, found just lateral to the SVC. In Figure 3.1, there are two pulmonary veins, seen as gray circles anterior to the right pulmonary artery.

It is important to focus on the left atrium in several situations. The pulmonary veins are very well seen on cardiac CT, leading to a wider use of cardiac CT prior to, and following, atrial fibrillation ablation. The ability to visualize the pulmonary veins, either on 2-D images, 3-D images or endoscopically, is described in Chapter 18. It is difficult to differentiate the peripheral pulmonary veins from the pulmonary arteries, so using the method of scrolling to follow images up and down the dataset is necessary. If the structure eventually drains into the left atrium, it was a pulmonary vein. Following the four (or five) pulmonary veins into the atria to assess for left to right shunts (such as anomalous pulmonary venous return) should become a routine part of your evaluation on cardiac CT. Myxomas and clot will be easily seen on contrast cardiac CT, whether in the atria or ventricle (Figures 3.17–3.20). The only exception is the right atrium, where incomplete mixing of the SVC blood (contrast enhanced) and IVC (non-contrast blood) makes a swirling pattern (Figure 3.20). Myocardial tissue, blood and other soft tissues (such as thrombus or tumors) are all the same Hounsfield units (described in Chapter 1), and thus indistinguishable without contrast enhancement. While general chamber sizes, aortic size, and pericardium (both thickness, calcification and effusions) can all be well evaluated on non-contrast studies [4–6] (along with calcification due to the marked difference in Hounsfield intensity), contrast studies will be required for

atrium (the best structure visualized from the esophageal (TEE) probe is the left atrium). (Figure 3.4 demonstrates this best, with the esophagus closed as the gray structure between the spine and the left atrium, white arrow). The left atrium is the most posterior structure of the heart, so the TEE probe gets the best view of this structure. It should also be noted that the left atrium is a superior structure,

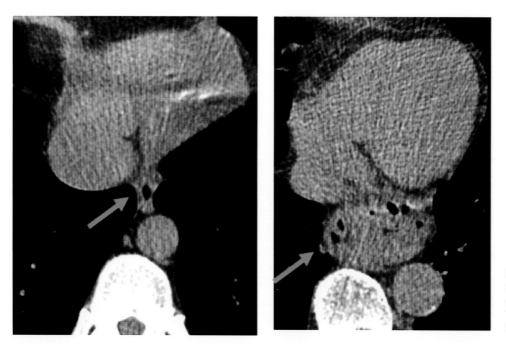

Figure 3.16. Hiatal hernia. The image on the left demonstrates a normal appearing esophagus at the level of the base of the heart (arrow). The right image demonstrates a large hiatal hernia between the heart and the spine.

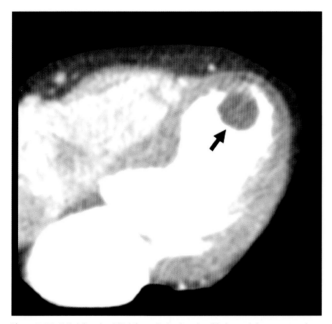

Figure 3.17. Apical thrombus. This left ventricular thrombus (black arrow) demonstrates a large pedunculated thrombus in the left ventricle.

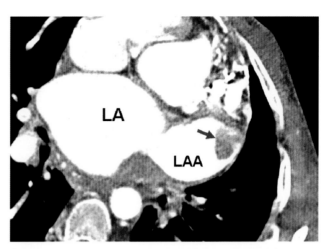

Figure 3.19. Left atrial thrombus. A person with atrial fibrillation with a large left atrium (LA) and left atrial appendage (LAA), demonstrating a thrombus on the lateral wall of the appendage (arrow). LA = left atrium, LAA = left atrial appendage.

most congenital evaluations and all evaluations of thrombus, tumors, shunts, and coronary stenosis.

Other structures seen on Figure 3.1 (a very superior cut) are the left internal and right internal mammary arteries, both well visualized just lateral to the sternum. This is useful for post-bypass patients; one can assess whether the arteries are utilized (if it is missing from the retrosternal region), or whether it is appropriate for utilization (it is easy to assess the "health" of the grafts) for an upcoming surgery. The slight contrast rim anterior to the ascending

aorta on Figure 3.1 is the left brachiocephalic vein draining toward the SVC.

Traversing down the images, new structures can be seen on Figure 3.3. These images are taken every 1.5 mm, so this is only 7.5 mm below the structures seen on Figure 3.1. This is one reason why cardiac CT offers a great advantage over magnetic resonance imaging (MRI), in that the nominal slice thickness is somewhere between 0.5 mm and 1.5 mm per slice on cardiac CT (depending on type of scanner and manufacturer), while most MRI studies are performed with 7 mm slice width. The aorta is still in the center of the image, and now we are at the level of the pulmonic valve and the right ventricular outflow tract is starting to be seen (labeled as RV on Figure 3.3). The pulmonic valve is the least well seen valve with cardiac CT. This may be due to

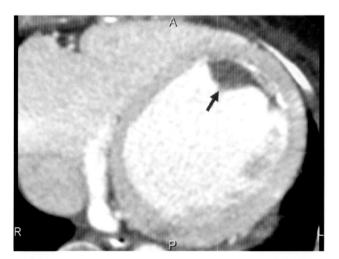

Figure 3.18. Apical thrombus. A markedly dilated heart (globular) with a large, laminar thrombus in the apex of the left ventricle (arrow).

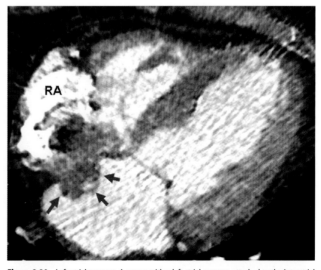

Figure 3.20. Left atrial myxoma. A person with a left atrial myxoma attached to the interatrial septum (arrows). The right atrium has a swirling contrast pattern, making distinction of mass or non-enhanced blood difficult. RA = right atrium.

its location parallel to the imaging plane or more likely because the leaflets are very thin. The SVC (just to the patient's right of the aorta) demonstrates a typical swirling pattern of contrast due to very high-resolution (bright white) contrast mixing with non-enhanced brachio-cephalic venous blood from the contralateral side of intra-venous injection. The left atrium is well visualized at this level, revealing no clot or filling defect. The left superior pulmonary vein can be seen draining into the left atrium at this level.

Moving caudally to Figure 3.4, the RV outflow tract is again well visualized, and the origin of the left main coro-nary artery is now present. The structure anterior to the ascending aorta is the right atrial appendage. Again, the only way you can be confident about cardiac structures is to follow them on sequential images to their origin. The left atrium is now well visualized, with the left atrial appendage (just lateral to the left main coronary artery) and two pul-monary veins draining. On the patient's right side (labeled R), the right superior pulmonary vein is draining, while below the letters LA on the figure, the left inferior pul-monary vein is seen entering the left atrium. While not well described in the literature, this is an excellent method to evaluate for partial anomalous pulmonary venous return, as you can obviously see the connection of the veins to the atria (see Chapter 16).

More caudally, we can see the left main on Figure 3.5, and the origin of the right coronary artery on Figure 3.7. The RV outflow tract at this level is thickened, and the diame-ter of the wall can be easily measured. The left atrium demonstrates the two inferior pulmonary veins entering at this level. Dropping down to Figure 3.8, the right inferior pulmonary vein can be better visualized, and the aortic valve is now visible. The circumflex (seen about 5 o'clock) is now visualized in cross-section, and on 2-D analysis this would appear as a fairly uniform and patent artery. Just lateral to the circumflex is the great cardiac vein, and on 3-D reconstruction, the circumflex is hard to visualize as the vein covers the artery. The 3-D images stack the data, but still only allow the outermost contrast structure to be seen well. If the great cardiac vein or coronary sinus covers the circumflex (positioned superior or lateral), the circumflex artery will be poorly seen unless editing is done to remove this structure. The complex relationship of the circumflex and great cardiac vein will be discussed in more detail in Chapters 4 and 18. The right coronary artery is also seen as a round circle in cross-section; again this would be rep-resented on a 3-D image as a patent artery. A small part of the right atrial appendage is still anterior to the right coro-nary artery (RCA). This is why editing of the images is nec-essary to completely visualize the coronary arteries. If one would make a 3-D object of this heart, the RA appendage would be covering this portion of the RCA, and it would be difficult to assess for patency on 3-D imaging without removing (either with computers or manually) the portion of the RA appendage covering this segment. An example of the need for editing is seen in Chapter 4, Figure 4.4. Con-

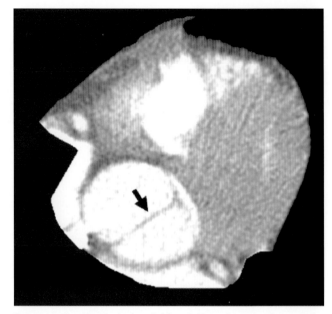

Figure 3.21. Bicuspid aortic valve. Instead of the typical inverted peace sign of a normal valve, this person has a thin line down the center of the ascending aorta (arrow), representing a bicuspid valve. The images are obtained during diastole, so the aortic valve is closed.

trast CT angiography allows for accurate assessment of aortic valve thickening and calcification [7]; however, movement and measures of regurgitation are better appre-ciated on echocardiography or MRI. One can easily visual-ize bicuspid aortic valves (Figure 3.21) and studies have demonstrated the accurate measurement of aortic valve area using cardiac CT.

Moving caudally, Figure 3.9 allows partial visualization of the mitral valve. The image was obtained during isovol-umetric relaxation, so the mitral and aortic valves were both closed at this time. On electron beam CT (EBCT), this has been shown to be the best time to image the coronary arteries without motion. The RCA and circumflex both again appear in cross-section as a round circle. The circumflex is giving rise to the obtuse marginal, as the branch is leaving the atrioventricular groove. The right atrium is well visualized, and the interatrial septum is seen. Atrial septal defects will be especially well visualized on CT, and the axial images will demonstrate the size and loca-tion of the defect most clearly (rather than relying on 3-D structures, Figure 3.22). Valve function cannot be discerned using cardiac CT, unlike MRI or echocardiography. How-ever, multiple thin cross-sectional images allow complete visualization of the mitral valve, including calcification (Figure 3.23), prolapse (Figures 3.24, 3.25), and prosthetic valves (Figure 3.26). The chordae tendineae can be seen on some images (Figure 3.23). Cardiac CT is not very useful in the detection of patent foramen ovale, as it is impractical to repeat scanning during different maneuvers due to radiation and contrast loads.

The aortic outflow tract is also seen at this level, again in the center of the image. Figure 3.10 now demonstrates a

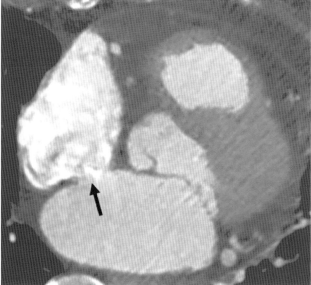

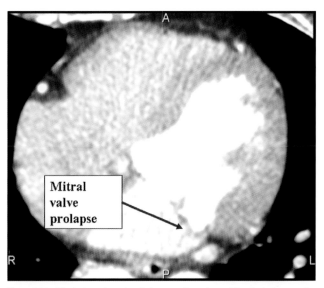

Figure 3.22. Atrial septal defect. The atrial septum can be well delineated and defects are quite readily apparent. Early studies suggest 100% sensitivity for atrial septal defects with cardiac CT. The size of the opening is easy to measure, yet exact flow rates/shunt fractions are not easy to quantitate.

Figure 3.24. Mitral valve prolapse. A study demonstrating prolapse of the mitral valve extending posteriorly into the left atrium. The magnitude of the prolapse can be measured on cardiac CT.

four-chamber view of the heart. The left ventricle looks thickened, but these are end-systolic images, so the normal 11 millimeters used to describe left ventricular hypertrophy (LVH) do not apply. Echocardiographic criteria for LVH of a wall thickness greater than 15 mm during diastole can be applied more accurately to these datasets. There are end-diastolic images also obtained (not as useful for coronary artery imaging due to increased motion) [8] which can be used to measure ejection fraction, wall thickening, and myocardial mass [9]. Figure 3.27 demonstrates an end-systolic and end-diastolic image from the same patient, demonstrating the marked difference in LV thickening. Also note the motion artifact in the right coronary artery with end-diastolic imaging. Figure 3.10 demonstrates the ability to visualize the interatrial septum and interventricular septum. The dark areas in the right atrium do not represent clot, but rather incomplete mixing of contrast (iodinated contrast from the SVC, mixing with

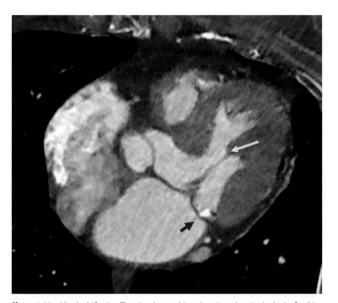

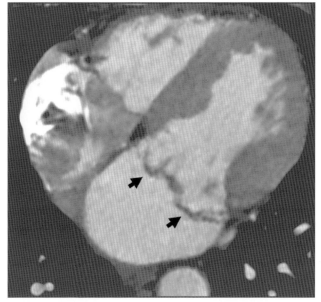

Figure 3.23. Mitral calcification. There is a dense calcium deposit on the mitral valve leaflet (blue arrow). This study demonstrates a well-visualized chordae tendineae (yellow arrow) extending from the anterolateral papillary muscle to the mitral valve.

Figure 3.25. Mitral valve prolapse. A more obvious case than in Figure 3.24, where there is more redundant tissue and both leaflets are involved. The presence or magnitude of mitral regurgitation cannot be measured.

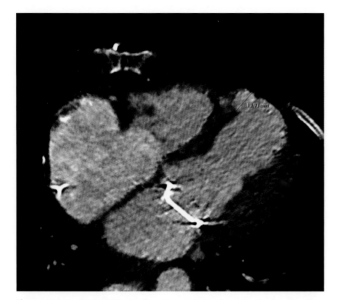

Figure 3.26. Prosthetic mitral valve. There is a prosthetic valve in the mitral position. These metallic valves do not inhibit the ability to visualize the coronary arteries or cardiac chambers on cardiac CT.

non-iodinated contrast from the inferior vena cava (IVC)). The mitral valve and leaflets are better visualized on this level, and the moderator band in the right ventricle is seen just next to the letter "V" in the right ventricle. The thin gray structure between the right ventricular free wall and the sternum is the pericardium, which is normal in this case.

Figure 3.11 demonstrates the base of the heart and the venous anatomy, including the coronary sinus (CS) os and a portion of the CS itself (in blue). The IVC (no contrast in this structure) is seen entering the RA. Because the contrast bolus timing was directed at the left ventricle to

enhance the coronary arteries and arterial structures, there is minimal to no contrast remaining in the right side at this time. Better contrast enhancement would demonstrate the tricuspid valve extending from the RCA to the anterior portion of the CS os. Figure 3.13 demonstrates the right coronary artery (dominant in this patient) extending along the bottom of the heart towards the interventricular septum. This particular study is not well contrast-enhanced at this level, but usually it is possible to follow the RCA to the crux, and in some cases, the length of the posterior descending artery.

Reviewing the 2-D Images

There are a number of reasons to carefully evaluate the 2-D images prior to looking at the 3-D datasets. One can evaluate the relationships of the cardiac structures, and the size and condition of the chambers of the heart, pericardium, and extracardiac structures of interest. Papillary muscles are quite easily seen on cardiac CT, and the chordae tendineae are usually well visualized (Figure 3.23). The pericardium is also easy to depict on cardiac CT, reported by some to be the reference standard technique for pericardial thickening or calcification. A normal pericardium can be seen in Figure 3.24. Pericardial thickening (Figure 3.28), calcification (Figure 3.29), and effusions (Figure 3.30) can all be seen and quantified. It is important to note that to evaluate the pericardium, no contrast is necessary.

Other pathologies can also be identified on review of the axial images. Myocardial infarctions, seen either as a dark area (rarefaction, as fatty replacement of the dead myocardium occurs) or as a thinned out area (or both), can easily be identified and the extent of myocardial involvement is easily noted (Figure 3.31). These types of findings should also trigger more careful evaluation of the coronary

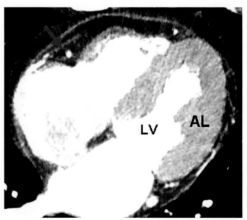

Figure 3.27. Cardiac phases. Images can be obtained at different phases of the cardiac cycle. On the left is an image at late-diastole. This gives a good representation of the thickness of the myocardium (LV). However, it is not as useful in determining the caliber of the right coronary artery (arrow), as there is a marked motion artifact. The artery should look round, not cashew-shaped. On the right is end-systole, demonstrating the real (without motion artifact) appearance of the cross-

section of the right coronary artery at this level. The LV walls are thicker, and the anterolateral (AL) papillary muscle is easily discerned. Wall thickness, stroke volume, and ejection fraction can be accurately depicted by measuring the LV at these two phases. AL = anterolateral papillary muscle, LV = left ventricle.

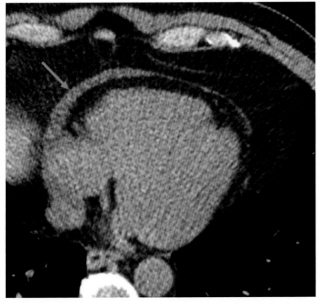

Figure 3.28. Pericardial thickening. The anterior portion of the pericardium is thickened (arrow). There is no associated pericardial effusion in this case.

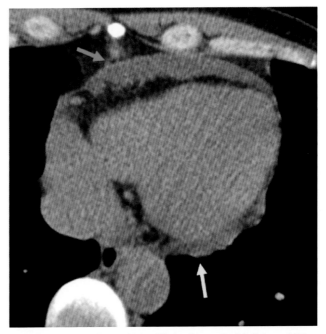

Figure 3.30. Pericardial effusion. While it is difficult to discern pericardial effusions and thickening based upon Hounsfield units, the presence of a dependent filling that fills the space between the heart and the pericardium (yellow arrow) strongly suggests that this is a pericardial effusion and not pericardial thickening. The presence of the effusion both posteriorly (yellow arrow) and anteriorly (green arrow) would classify this effusion as at least moderate.

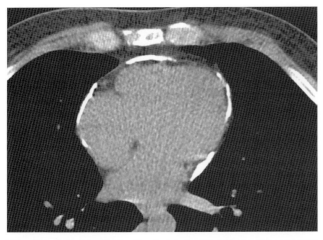

Figure 3.29. Pericardial calcification. There is circumferential calcification of the pericardium (seen as bright white areas), seen anteriorly, laterally, and posteriorly on this image.

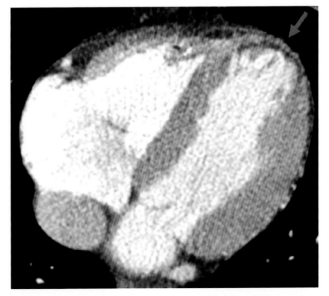

Figure 3.31. Myocardial infarction. Rarefaction of the apex of the left ventricle is present due to a prior myocardial infarction. The subendocardial dark area represents the area and extent of the myocardial infarction (arrow).

tree in the distribution of the infarct. While not as well validated as the viability studies of MRI or positron emission tomography (PET) scanning, it is clear that this can give at least some qualitative (and possibly quantitative) evaluation of the myocardium.

Non-cardiac Structures of Interest on Cardiac CT

The superior- and inferior-most cuts have several noncardiac structures worth commenting on. The superiormost images will cut through the bronchi (seen on Figure 3.15 as two very black circles). Air density on the Hounsfield scale approaches –1000, so this is black on cardiac CT. The brightness and width of each image can be changed to see different structures (called windows). The extreme imaging windows are for bone (where everything is black except for bony structures, not useful in cardiac

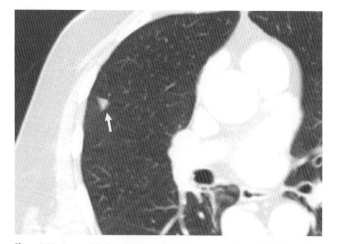

Figure 3.32. Lung nodule. Resetting the windows demonstrates a lung nodule in the periphery of the right lung field.

imaging), and lung windows (where the soft tissue densities are more easily seen), mostly applied to screening for lung cancer and evaluation of lung parenchyma (Figure 3.32). This window level is not useful for evaluating cardiac structures, since the denser tissues of the heart become very white. It should be noted that it is possible to change the window levels on obtained datasets, so lung or bone windows can be visualized separately. This raises a medical-legal question as to whether non-coronary pathology should be routinely overread by a radiologist, to evaluate for tumors and other potential abnormalities.

The inferior-most cuts usually include the liver (Figure 3.13), the inferior vena cava as well as the esophagus and hiatal hernias, if present (another cause of chest pain) (Figure 3.16). There have been many cases of normal coronary arteries by CT angiography in which the finding of a hiatal hernia explained the patient's symptoms and directed treatment. Other common findings outside the heart include old granulomatous disease (Figure 3.33). These densely calcified lymph nodes are easily seen, and easily discerned to be outside the pericardium. In general, these findings have no prognostic significance and can be ignored.

Pulmonary Embolism

One important finding is that of pulmonary embolism. There have been several cases of patients presenting with shortness of breath found to have multiple pulmonary emboli as the etiology during non-invasive angiography. While a rare presentation of this disease, this is an important possible application of cardiac CT, most easily seen on 2-D images (Figure 3.34). Thin slice imaging, with 3-D reconstructions have made multislice CT the preferred evaluation for patients with possible pulmonary emboli (Figure 3.34) [10]. The improved resolution and ability to

gate the study allows routine evaluation of the fourth and perhaps even fifth generation branches of the pulmonary vasculature (Figure 3.35). CT has become the primary approach to evaluating for pulmonary embolism at many centers, surpassing or completely replacing nuclear imaging. Some experts suggest that the 3-D imaging now available (especially with gated acquisition) may surpass invasive pulmonary angiography [11]. By freezing the motion (similar to the need in cardiac CT) and looking at the pulmonary arteries sequentially or in 3-D images), the sensitivity and specificity of pulmonary emboli should continue to rise with newer CT scanners. It is interesting to note that pulmonary motion is greater than cardiac motion even with breath holding (due to the "accordion" motion from being next to the heart, and being pulled in during ventricular systole) [12]. It was carefully described in the study by Ritchie and Godwin [12] that imaging times of 35 milliseconds would be necessary to totally obviate all cardiac motion, and imaging times of 18 milliseconds would be necessary to stop motion in the pulmonary vasculature.

CT Imaging of Chest Pain

The differential diagnosis of patients presenting to the emergency department with chest pain – coronary artery disease, aortic dissection, and pulmonary embolism – can all be well discerned on the 2-D images. It is possible that this may become a standard test in the emergency department for patients presenting with certain chest pain syndromes, allowing rapid evaluation of coronary artery disease (CAD), dissection, and pulmonary embolism in one test [13]. Aortic dissection is quite easily evaluated with

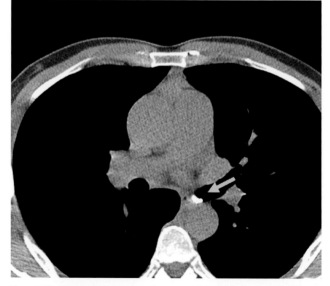

Figure 3.33. Old granulomatous disease. A common and benign finding on cardiac CT representing calcified lymph nodes (arrow).

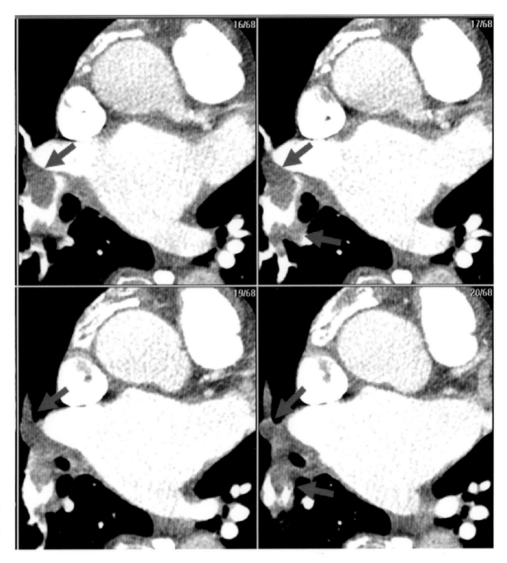

Figure 3.34. Pulmonary emboli. This was an elderly woman with progressive shortness of breath referred for CT angiography to evaluate both the coronary arteries and myocardial function. The heart was found to be normal; however, multiple pulmonary emboli were detected (red arrows demonstrating multiple filling defects in the pulmonary arteries).

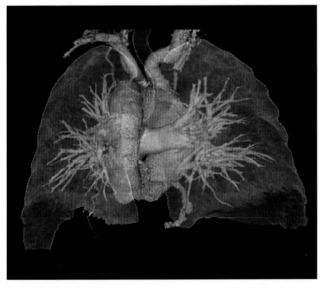

Figure 3.35. Three-dimensional chest. The pulmonary arteries are depicted in blue, demonstrating third and fourth generation branches.

cardiac CT. The ability to scan the entire aorta in one breath hold has produced nearly 100% sensitivity [14]. The modality allows for visualization of extension proximally into the carotid artery and great vessels of the head, as well as distally into the renals, mesenterics, and celiac axis (see also Chapter 14) [15]. Studies evaluating cardiac CT during acute myocardial infarction have been reported [16]. Advances in cardiac CT have significantly improved our ability to evaluate these multiple thoracic areas in one scan. The development of 64-detector CT, with the ability to gate the entire thoracic study, will continue to improve the detection of pulmonary emboli, aortic dissection, and acute coronary syndromes.

Summary

Two-dimensional images are the basis for interpretation of all CT imaging, including CT angiography. Understanding the anatomy, being able to track the structures on consecutive slices, and ultimately diagnosing these studies accurately will be dependent on the CT user's understanding of the axial images and corresponding anatomy. This is probably the most important skill to learn, as virtually all diagnoses can be made based solely on the original axial image set. Analysis of the 2-D images has been shown to be as accurate for the diagnosis of obstructive CAD as 3-D imaging, and superior to some reconstruction methods (see Chapter 4).

References

1. Tani T, Yamakami S, Matsushita T, et al. Usefulness of electron beam tomography in the prone position for detecting atrial thrombi in chronic atrial fibrillation. J Comput Assist Tomogr 2003;27:78–84.
2. Burri H, Bloch A, Hauser H. Characterization of an unusual right atrial mass by echocardiography, magnetic resonance imaging, computed tomography, and angiography. Echocardiography 1999; 16:393–396.
3. Rothenberg DM, Brandt TD, D'Cruz I. Computed tomography of renal angiomyolipoma presenting as right atrial mass. J Comput Assist Tomogr 1986;10:1054–1056.
4. Budoff MJ, Mao SS, Wang S, Bakhsheshi H, Brundage BH. A simple single slice method for measurement of left and right atrial volume by electron beam computed tomography. Acad Radiol 1999;6: 481–486.
5. Mao S, Budoff MJ, Oudiz RJ, Bakhsheshi H, Wang S, Brundage BH. A simple single slice method for measurement of left and right ventricular enlargement by electron beam tomography. Int J Card Imaging 2000;16;383–390.
6. Budoff MJ, Lu B, Mao SS, et al. Evaluation of fluid collection in the pericardial sinuses and recesses: noncontrast-enhanced electron beam tomography. Invest Radiol 2000;35(6):359–365.
7. Shavelle DM, Takasu J, Budoff MJ, Mao SS, Zhao QX, O'Brien KD. HMG CoA reductase inhibitor (statin) and aortic valve calcium. Lancet 2002;359(9312):1125–1126.
8. Mao SS, Budoff MJ, Bin L, Liu SCK. The optimal ECG trigger point in electron beam volumetric studies: 3 electrocardiographic trigger methods for minimizing motion artifacts. Acad Radiol 2001;8(11): 1107–1115.
9. Baik HK, Budoff MJ, Lane KL, Bakhsheshi H, Brundage BH. Accurate measures of left ventricular ejection fraction using electron beam tomography: a comparison with radionuclide angiography, and cine angiography. Int J Card Imaging 2000;16:391–398.
10. Schoepf UJ, Costello P. CT angiography for diagnosis of pulmonary embolism: state of the art. Radiology 2004;230:329–337.
11. Patel S, Kazerooni EA, Cascade PN, et al. Pulmonary embolism: optimization of small pulmonary artery visualization at multi-row detector CT. Radiology 2003;227:455–460.
12. Ritchie CJ, Godwin JD. Minimum scan speeds for suppression of motion artifacts in CT. Radiology 1992;185:37–42.
13. Novelline RA, Rhea JT, Rao PM, et al. Helical CT in emergency radiology. Radiology 1999;213:321–339.
14. Goldman CK, Deitelzweig SB. CT angiography of aortic dissection and left renal artery stenosis. Vasc Med 2004;9:69.
15. Suzuki S, Furui S, Kotahake H, et al. Isolated dissection of the superior mesenteric artery: CT findings in six cases. Abdom Imaging 2004;29:153–157.
16. Gosalia A, Haramati LB, Sheth MP, Spindola-Franco H. CT detection of acute myocardial infarction. Am J Roentgenol 2004;182:1563–1566.

4

Interpreting CT Angiography: Three-Dimensional Reconstruction Techniques

Matthew J. Budoff

This chapter will take you through the performance and evaluation of the non-invasive coronary angiogram. Using the skills you developed looking at two-dimensional images in Chapter 3, this chapter will help you understand how to perform and create three-dimensional images on cardiac CT. The exact methods used for reconstruction by any given workstation may be different, and those skills will need to be acquired through live training. However, this chapter will help you understand the steps to performing a CT angiogram, and then understand the different image reconstruction methods commonly utilized to interpret and evaluate non-invasive coronary angiography.

Performing the Cardiac CT Angiogram

Performing the cardiac CT examination is performed in three or four steps. The sequence is always similar, with some variations dependent upon the equipment used. First, scout images are taken to know where to obtain the non-contrast (heart) scan. Then a flow study is performed; with administration of minimal contrast (10–20 mL), one can determine the time from antecubital vein (or other venous access) to aortic root (the circulation time). Finally, using the non-contrast scan to determine how high and low one must go to cover the appropriate anatomy, and the flow study to determine the waiting time prior to scanning, the non-invasive angiogram can be performed. Each step will be described in detail below.

Simply, the steps are as follows:

1. one or more planar scout images,
2. non-contrast cardiac gated CT,
3. a timing scan (can be avoided with certain new scanners), and
4. a contrast-enhanced CT angiogram.

Scout Images

Scout images are unenhanced planar tomograms (a chest X-ray-like, anteroposterior projection of the entire chest), landmarked to the patient by a laser alignment system (Figure 4.1). This can be projected in both an anteroposterior and lateral view, with images similar to chest X-rays. The CT operator uses the scout images to prescribe subsequent scan volumes. This gives the user some idea of the anatomy, with either the tracheal bifurcation or the origin of the left main coronary artery used as a landmark to start the non-contrast (heart) scan [1]. Typically, 10–15 unenhanced scout images are obtained during inspiration breath-hold. Patients need to be instructed to take the same degree of breath-hold to allow for consistent imaging. From a review of these images, the scan volume can be selected to place the vasculature of interest within the center of the scanning volume.

Choosing the Top Levels for the Coronary Calcium Evaluation

The technologist should start well above the origin of the left main when imaging; however, changes in breathing will alter the cardiac images. If the person breathes deeper than expected, the heart will be lower, and the dataset will start higher. This is not a problem to see the top of the heart, but often this will lead to missing the distal right and posterior descending artery. Similarly, if the person takes a more shallow breath during the cardiac CT examination, the heart will be higher than anticipated, and the top of the heart will be missed. Another source of error on the part of the technologist is the belief that the left main coronary artery is the superior-most structure in the coronary tree. While this is mostly true, there are a percentage of cases where the left anterior descending artery will arc upwards and can be seen as much as 6–8 mm above the origin of the

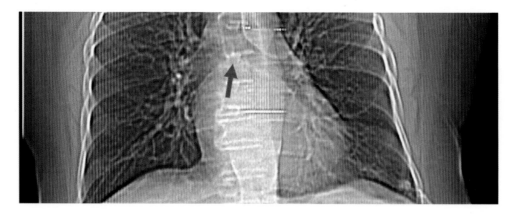

Figure 4.1. Scout image obtained with cardiac CT. This allows the user to visualize the location of the heart, estimating the location for high-resolution imaging for all cardiac applications. The red arrow depicts the tracheal bifurcation, which is the most common landmark used to define the superior aspect of the heart.

left main. Thus, we recommend starting the imaging at least 10 mm above the origin of the left main [1].

Calcium Scan

The second step is the calcium scan. This non-enhanced scan gives a lot of information about the cardiac anatomy, and is underused by users who do not understand the potential of this non-invasive scan. There are several distinct advantages of having a high-resolution scan of the coronary arteries without contrast that will complement the contrast scan. For example, on a contrast scan, calcium, metal, and contrast are all white. Thus, it is sometimes difficult to differentiate calcium from the contrast density. It is useful, when reviewing the contrast studies, to have a non-enhanced scan to evaluate these differences. Calcium appears very white relative to non-enhanced coronaries, and is not easily mistaken for anything else on a non-contrast scan (see Chapter 6). Similarly, these scans are very useful for evaluating the exact placement of stents or metal clips (after bypass). This non-contrast cardiac gated CT (heart scan) is used to identify the location of coronary calcium, stents, catheters, foreign bodies, or other findings which partially obscure the contrast agent. The additive radiation dose is very small, as relatively few gated images are obtained during this scan (Chapter 1).

There is perhaps a better reason to obtain a heart scan on every non-invasive angiogram. As with all imaging modalities, the image quality of CT angiograms is not always what you see in the journals. There are artifacts, problems with obese patients (increased image noise), difficulties with breath-hold and arrhythmias that will affect the quality of the image in some cases (examples will be shown later in this chapter). The pretest probability of finding obstructive disease is important in any test, perhaps more so in a test such as non-invasive angiography, where missing disease may have more significant ramifications. The pretest and posttest probabilities can be altered dramatically by the calcium score [2]. Hundreds of studies have been performed on the relationship between calcification of the coronary arteries and atherosclerosis and luminal obstruction. Calcification does not occur in a normal vessel wall, and its presence signifies atherosclerosis. While this will be discussed in much greater detail in Chapter 6, it is worth mentioning at this point.

Simply, there are four uses of the calcium scan as part of the non-invasive angiogram that make it invaluable in the accurate depiction of the CT angiogram. The most common use among CT angiographers is to carefully define the top and bottom of the image set, to ensure complete coverage of the coronary anatomy. While there is a radiation dose associated with the calcium scan (Chapter 1), this can actually decrease the overall radiation of the entire study. By only scanning the area of interest, and knowing exactly where to stop scanning at the bottom of the heart, one can obtain less volume with the CT angiogram, saving the high radiation exposure by cutting down on the area of interest. This can only be done well by defining the exact anatomy on two-dimensional axial images (such as the calcium scan), as the scout image (an X-ray equivalent) will only show the diaphragm and not the exact bottom of the coronary vasculature.

Second, there is a very high negative predictive value of the coronary calcium scan (a score of zero has up to a 99% chance of being associated with normal or non-obstructive disease in the coronary arteries) [3]. In the study by Haberl et al. [3], none of the 220 women with a normal coronary arteriogram had detectable coronary artery calcium (CAC), yielding a negative predictive value of 100%. Thus, if the calcium score is very low or zero, one must have more skepticism at the finding of high-grade obstructive disease, especially on a suboptimal study. The general exception is the younger patient or the young smoker, who have a higher prevalence of false-negative calcium scans. Nonetheless, this adds quite a bit to the pretest probability of obstructive coronary artery disease, and can help in the interpretation.

Third, high calcium scores can make interpretation of the obstructive plaque more difficult. Calcium can obscure the visualization of the lumen, and higher scores have been linked with a lower sensitivity on CT angiography [4].

Some studies have used strict calcium score cutoffs to determine that there is a higher chance of missing a significant stenosis. Some studies have suggested scores of >1000 as being non-diagnostic [3,5], while others have suggested that even lower burdens of coronary calcium may reduce sensitivity [6,7]. Schmermund et al. [8] reported that if two continuous levels demonstrate dense calcification that obscure more than half the lumen, that is a non-diagnostic segment of the coronary artery. Thus, there is probably no specific cutoff of calcium score, but rather dense calcifications in any specific area will cause some problems. This remains a problem with the 16-slice MDCT systems [6,9], and most likely will not be solved by the current generations of EBCT (e-Speed) or MDCT (64-slice) scanners, as these do not improve the spatial resolution sufficiently to exclude coronary calcium. The problem may be fixed with image manipulation, but no computer workstation has reported the ability to extract calcification without demeaning the diagnostic value of the study. Again, the non-contrast scan may demonstrate the calcific regions better than the contrast study, aiding in interpretation.

Finally, there is a relationship between increasing calcium burdens and atherosclerosis and angiographic disease. Rumberger and colleagues examined randomly selected autopsy hearts and compared measures of coronary calcium using EBCT with direct histologic plaque areas, and percent luminal stenosis [10,11]. These studies determined that the total area of coronary artery calcification quantified by EBCT is linearly correlated ($r = 0.90$) with the total area of histologic coronary artery plaque, and increasing calcification levels are associated with increasing levels of obstructive disease on angiography. There are large studies demonstrating that increasing calcium scores can increase the probability of obstructive disease in a linear fashion [2,3]. While calcified plaque burden parallels overall plaque burden, CAC testing is not always appropriate as a surrogate for angiographic disease detection because of the modest relationship between CAC and obstructive coronary artery disease. Keep in mind that a positive calcium test implies atherosclerosis and increased cardiovascular risk, so even if the CT angiogram fails to show luminal disease, you may want to interpret the study in this context. In these cases (where the CT angiogram looks normal, but the calcium scan shows disease), it may be appropriate to state "atherosclerosis without significant stenosis present." This will avoid false reassurance with a CT angiogram, something that physicians and patients are very concerned about. Thus, the calcium scan to the CT angiogram will be worthwhile for many reasons, and worth the time and the slight increase in radiation exposure required to add this to the study.

Administering Intravenous Contrast

The goal of CT angiography is to image the coronary arteries during arterial enhancement following the intravenous (IV) injection of contrast material. An 18- or 20-gauge 3 cm IV catheter is usually inserted into the antecubital vein. Other injection sites include external jugular and other veins in the hands or forearm. Hand veins are not routinely utilized because the flow rates can cause extravasation more commonly in smaller veins, and the delay times can be significantly longer than the typical 15–18 seconds. Newer MDCT systems do not alter the need for good timing of scans. Obtaining more simultaneous levels will decrease the scan times (see Table 4.1). However, regardless of the breath-hold or scan times, the appropriate delay is very important. Remember that the contrast must flow from the IV site, through the right-sided (pulmonary) circulation, and then into the left ventricle and to the coronary arteries. Imaging must take place when contrast has reached the left side, so no matter how fast the image can be performed, the delay must be appropriate. Early studies for coronary arteries and renal artery CT angiography utilized an empiric delay (assuming that patients would have filling of the arterial segments by 20 seconds) [12]. These studies found that there is a wide range of transit times through the pulmonary vasculature to the central aorta.

The timing scan or flow study is used to accurately determine the transit time of contrast from the injection site to the ascending aorta. This sequence typically consists of a single slice repeated at some time interval (every 1–2 seconds) using a low radiation dose technique. Scans are obtained at the same point in the ascending aorta to determine the transit time of contrast. A region of interest is then placed in the ascending aorta, resulting in a time–density curve with which delay times can be predicted from the time to peak opacification (Figure 4.2). The measured transit time is then used as the delay time from the start of the contrast injection to imaging start for the CT coronary angiogram. Typical "transit times" are on the order of 15–18 seconds. In one small study, delay times ranged from 12 to 25 seconds [12], in another, delay times were seen as late as 40 seconds [13]. Of course, low ejection fractions, poor cardiac outputs, and pulmonary disease will all play a role. We have seen delays as long as 40 seconds for contrast to get from the IV site in the antecubital vein to the central aorta, and as short as 10 seconds in patients with tachycardias and high cardiac output states.

The patient-specific delay time (transit time) ensures that images are obtained in conjunction with the arrival of the intravenous contrast at the coronary circulation. Newer systems with bolus tracking software do not require this timing scan, as the scanner can acquire images every second, and when the contrast density increases to a specific cutoff, the scanner starts the final scan. Bolus tracking software (SureStart, Toshiba as one example) is used to determine the scan start timing after the start of contrast medium injection. These types of automated systems may be useful to save both radiation exposure (very slightly, as they still require additional scans to check on the timing) and contrast, but being automated, may not work accurately in every case.

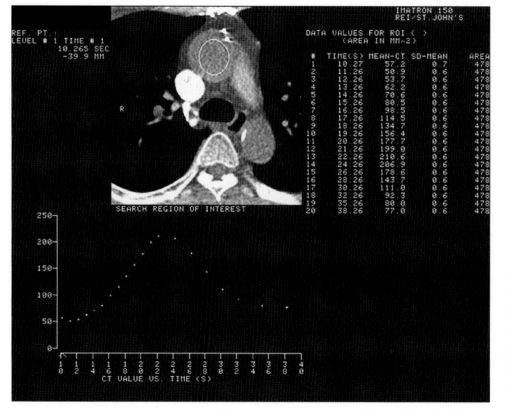

Figure 4.2. Flow study on an electron beam scan, demonstrating a rise and fall of the contrast density during the timing study. With a bolus of 10 mL of contrast, the time from the intravenous catheter to the aortic root can be measured. The white circle in the ascending aorta represents the area of interest for the study. The rise and peak at 22 seconds represents the time needed to wait prior to imaging during the CT angiogram.

Contrast Injectors

In most instances, the test can be performed on an outpatient basis in 20 minutes of patient time. At Harbor-UCLA, we routinely schedule patients every 30 minutes for CT angiography, to allow for any problems that might arise. These are typically very rare, but inability to start an IV injection, allergic reactions, and venous extravasation are possible complications.

Several advances with contrast protocols and injectors have improved utilization and decreased time needed to perform the non-invasive angiogram. Non-ionic contrast agents are preferably used because they are better tolerated by patients [14,15]; and extravasation of non-ionic contrast agents tends to cause less serious complications [16]. Compared with dynamic incremental CT, smaller amounts of contrast agent are required [14]. Due to cost issues, as well as possible decreased nephrotoxicity with lower contrast amounts, a double power injector can be used to facilitate the examination procedure and to avoid mixing contrast material with the saline solution. The use of dual-headed injectors (with one filled with contrast and one filled with saline) allows for reduced contrast requirements and improved uniform opacification of the coronary tree.

Several factors contribute to non-uniformity of vascular enhancement. Venous circulation blood flow is a low pressure and low velocity system, with significant variation in blood flow velocity due to heart rate, right atrial pressure, left ventricular diastolic pressure, and patient postural position. An additional factor contributing to variation of vessel opacification is laminar blood flow characteristics. When blood flows through a vessel, there is a higher velocity in the center of the vessel as compared to the lumen wall [17]. This non-uniformity of blood velocity due to laminar flow results in increasing or decreasing opacification with different injection rates.

Due to the loss of venous pressure after injection, as well as the issue of wasted contrast media present in the tubing and arm vein of the patient during imaging, most centers now utilize a saline injection to maximize distal contrast opacification without increasing contrast dose to the patient. Injection of contrast material followed by a saline solution bolus using a double power injector when performing cardiac CT allows for more uniform opacification of the cardiac study (more uniform HU from top of aorta to base of heart) as well as a 20% reduction of contrast material volume to 60 mL with a similar degree of enhancement [18]. In addition, perivenous artifacts in the superior vena cava (SVC) are significantly reduced. This refers to a over-enhancement of the SVC, which causes a star artifact as the MDCT X-ray beam reflects off the denser contrast material. This should be less problematic with saline mixing (decreasing the brightness at the time of the scanning, so there is no artifact in structures near the SVC – such as the pulmonary artery or right coronary artery).

New Contrast Injectors

As with all invasive procedures, safety is a key concern. There are few dangers or procedural complications from non-ionic contrast enhancement, mostly allergic reactions (including anaphylactoid reactions to contrast) and extravasation from the vein. Cardiac CT uses contrast flow rates from 3.5 to 5 mL/s, so extravasation, while very rare, is possible. In the last 5000 CT angiography cases in our laboratory, we have had a handful of cases of significant extravasation (with arm swelling or significant pain at the injection site). Some units are now equipped with extravasation alarms that automatically turn off the injector prior to the large bolus of contrast being injected. Several safety features of the injectors are common. Operator alerts beyond those typical for use include: contrast empty; used syringe warning; pressure limits reached; and scan delay time expired. In addition to these standard alerts, contrast media injectors may also offer any of the three following safety features:

- Embolism detection: Occurs if air is accidentally injected, resulting in a possible fatal air embolism. Most manufactures also provide a procedure for inspecting and purging the syringe.
- Extravasation detection: The movement of contrast media (medium) back into the injector or surrounding tissue.
- Overpressure protection: Limits the pressure of contrast media into the catheter to ensure the safety of low-pressure catheters and also avoid over-infusion.

One manufacturer offers a patented technology, EDA, to detect contrast media extravasation before it becomes clinically significant, thereby minimizing the risk of severe skin and subcutaneous tissue damage and the potential need for skin grafts or plastic surgery.

Another manufacturer also addresses the issue of contrast administration with pre-filled syringes. According to a study conducted by the American Society of

Table 4.1. Typical scan times for CT angiography (based upon Available Scanners)	
EBCT (C-150 or C-300)	30 seconds
MDCT (4 Slice)	30 Seconds
e-Speed EBCT	15 seconds
8- or 16-slice MDCT	15 seconds
32- or 40-slice MDCT	12 seconds
64-slice MDCT	5–10 seconds

Radiologic Technologists, the use of pre-filled syringes was based upon four factors: saving time; improving cost-effectiveness; enhancing healthcare quality; and improving patient safety. The report also states, "both user and nonusers believed that pre-filled syringes result in a faster procedure, thereby freeing up time to perform other tasks" (www.reillycomm.com/it_archive/it_to0303_2.htm).

Breath-hold

The breath-hold during the study is most important, regardless of equipment. The breath-hold times have dropped dramatically with the advent of the 64-slice MDCT, down to 10–12 seconds. Scanning times of 5 seconds still require breath-hold times slightly longer, as the patient must be at end-inspiration by the time the scan begins, and usually a 1–2-second delay is inherent in the scanner from when the technologist starts the scan and the first images are obtained. Faster image acquisition allows for more adequate imaging, with less problems due to breathing artifacts. A typical breathing artifact on a scan will look like an accordion, with the image going in and out during the breath (Figure 4.1). Typical scan times are listed in Table 4.1.

Thus, the contrast study needs to take into account the delay from the IV site to the aortic root, as well as the time it will take to perform the non-invasive angiogram. Let's take an example (Figure 4.3) of a "transit" time of 20 seconds, and a scan time of 12 seconds. The actual injection of contrast needs only to be 12–15 seconds long, but

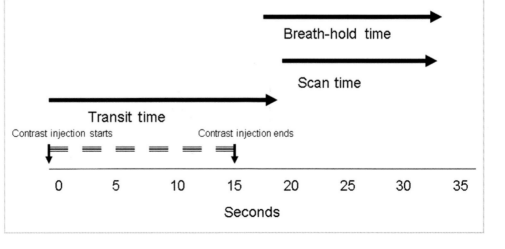

Figure 4.3. A typical MDCT angiogram timescale demonstrating the timing and relationships between the contrast injection (dashed line), the scan time, and breath-hold time. The study takes 30 seconds, even though the scanning only takes 12 seconds. Breath-holding is typically a few seconds longer than the scan time, so the patient would have to hold his breath for about 15 seconds for this study.

the timing is critical, and not totally intuitive. The contrast is injected in this case (with a long transit time and a short scan time) completely before breath-holding or scanning begins. Figure 4.3 is an example of the proper timing and the relationship between the breath-hold, the injection of contrast, and the scan.

"Obtaining the Study": MDCT Angiogram High-resolution Axial Images

While these vary with manufacturer and number of detectors, the principles are the same. Retrospective gating is utilized, with continuous images obtained throughout the study. As discussed in Chapter 1, the scan parameters for coronary CT angiography require retrospective gating, in which continuous images are obtained (sometimes up to 1600 images are obtained for one CT angiography study) and then the reconstructions are possible at different times in the cardiac cycle. When these systems were first available, the user had to choose the optimal trigger point on each cardiac cycle, taking up to 2 hours just to derive the images that were useful for analysis. Now, the computer workstations can do this in seconds, allowing for evaluation of the images at any point in the cardiac cycle. By evaluating end-diastolic and end-systolic images, one can derive the stroke volume, wall motion, and ejection fraction (see Chapter 5 for more details).

Because the scanner is moving at a standard speed (table feed, somewhere in the range of 2–3 mm per rotation), the heart rate must be regular throughout the imaging to allow for alignment of different levels of the heart to reconstruct a 3-D image (see Chapter 1). The advantage to retrospective triggering is the ability to reconstruct at different times (for example, one could do a reconstruction at 40%, 50%, and 60% of the R-R interval). Hong et al. reported that when still images are to be obtained using MDCT, the trigger delay differs: R-R 50% for the right coronary artery and R-R 60% for the left coronary artery [19]. Thus, one gets more than one phase of the cardiac cycle, and can reconstruct accordingly. However, the downside of this is the very large dataset generated, as well as the excessive radiation dose still necessary to obtain such images [20]. Thus, the process for obtaining MDCT angiograms is fairly straightforward and reproducible from study to study. However, the reconstruction techniques differ.

Typical MDCT Study

Because reliable electrocardiographic (ECG) triggering is crucial for diagnostic image quality in MDCT angiography (due to retrospective gating), patients must be in stable sinus rhythm for the investigation. Patients with significant arrhythmias (including atrial fibrillation, as well as frequent premature atrial or ventricular beats) are typically excluded from these evaluations. These arrhythmias are especially problematic, as slice gaps between adjacent images (since retrospectively gated images are no longer reconstructed in the same point in the cardiac cycle) are inevitable and cause severe image degradation. For EBCT studies, the heart rate will not critically influence image quality, but in MDCT the heart rate should be below 60 beats per minute; many authors have suggested routine premedication with beta blocking agents. Multisector reconstruction has improved the temporal resolution by utilizing portions of multiple heartbeats to create an image (Chapter 1), so higher heart rates can be utilized. Best image quality will still be with the lower heart rates, as multisector reconstruction is not always possible or successful.

Beta Blockade

As temporal resolution is still somewhat limited with current generation MDCT scanners, most CT angiography studies are performed with beta blockade. Two different approaches have been widely used. One approach is to premedicate every patient. Typically, a beta blocker (metoprolol 50–100 mg) is administered to every patient unless contraindicated. If resting heart rate immediately before the scan was >75 beats/min, an additional intravenous beta blocker (esmolol 500 μg/kg or metoprolol 5 mg) is given [21]. Alternatively, patients who have a resting heart rate above 70 beats/min can receive an oral beta blocker. Interestingly, some studies have reported that the dose used is atenolol, 50–75 mg, given 24 hours prior to scan in order to reduce their heart rate. Pharmacology would suggest this would be highly ineffective, as the half-life of atenolol is 6–7 hours, and although FDA approved as a once a day beta blocker, it has little 24-hour coverage. Thus, giving metoprolol orally 30–60 minutes prior to the study makes more sense physiologically, or use of a longer half-life beta blocker, such as metoprolol XL or betaxolol, would be prudent for this purpose. Newer scanners, by using portions of each cardiac cycle to create the image (multisector reconstruction, Chapter 1), can somewhat obviate the need for beta blockade, but will still have heart rate limitations. The exact heart rate cutoffs for the 32, 40, and 64 level scanners will need to be determined.

First, the calcium score is performed (prospective ECG-gated mode). Typical values are: collimation 2.5 mm, scan time 250 ms, tube voltage 120 kV, tube current 165 mAs. Thereafter, the circulation time is measured using a small test bolus and time lapse imaging: the time density within a region of interest of the ascending aorta was determined in consecutive steps of one second after administration of a contrast bolus (15 mL with 3 mL/s). For high-resolution MDCT angiography, the scanner is operated in spiral mode retrospective ECG tagged mode. Typical values are: collimation 0.5 to 1.0 mm, scan time 180–250 ms, table feed 1.5 mm/rotation, tube voltage 120 kV, tube current 260–

300 mAs. The scan parameters used for most studies are: 0.375 pitch, 333–500 ms rotation time, 120 kV, and 300 mAs. Pitch is calculated as table speed divided by collimator width. With the older four-slice scanners, typical values were a table speed of 3 mm/s, with collimation of 3 mm, resulting in a pitch of 1. Overlapping images will allow for oversampling, which will permit multisector reconstruction; thus the use of 0.25 to 0.5 pitch is a 2-fold to 4-fold overlap of images. Newer systems have thinner slice thickness and collimation, allowing for even smaller pitch. This results in more images, thinner reconstruction intervals, and better visualization of the coronary anatomy. The visualization of non-calcified (soft) plaque (discussed in Chapter 12) has become more promising with improvements in spatial and contrast resolution with newer CT scanners.

Injection of X-ray contrast agent is necessary, which leads to the usual contraindications and side effects of iodinated contrast. The patients should be fasting for at least a few hours (although nausea and vomiting is much less common with non-ionic contrast agents currently employed). We routinely ask patients to come in well hydrated, to minimize potential renal complications and make starting the IV injection easier. Most authors have suggested the use of sublingual nitroglycerin immediately before the scan to achieve vasodilation of the coronary arteries. Patients are given either 0.4 mg sublingually or 0.2 mg of intravenous nitroglycerin for coronary vasodilatation just prior to the CT angiogram. This has been shown to objectively improve visualization of stenosis for both MR and CT angiography. The scan is started after application of 80–140 mL of contrast agent (3–4 mL/s) with a temporal delay equal to the circulation time plus 2–4 seconds (offset due to scanner initialization).

All patients are trained to hold their breath and informed about the heat sensation during contrast administration. Up to a total of 140 mL of non-ionic iodinated contrast (300–370 mg of iodine per mL) is administered intravenously in the antecubital vein using a power injector at 3–4 mL/s and starting some time (transit time, usually 12–20 s) before onset of image acquisition. Newer scanners, with increased numbers of detectors, have reduced contrast requirements, down to 60–80 mL with 40- or 64-detector systems. The scan is performed craniocaudally starting at the carina (field of view 220 mm). An ECG is recorded simultaneously with the scan and used for retrospective gating after completion of the scan. The average radiation exposure of calcium scoring according to the specifications of the scanner amounts to 1.2–1.8 mSv. For CT angiography the equivalent values are 5.8 to 7.4 mSv in men and 7.6 to 9.8 mSv in women [20,22,23].

With MDCT, ECG waveforms are recorded simultaneously during the acquisition. All acquired data are sent to a workstation where they are reviewed and analyzed. Retrospectively gated axial images are reconstructed at multiple diastolic phases. Routinely, phase reconstructions are performed at several phases of the cardiac cycle. Most commonly, 40%, 50%, and 80% of the cardiac cycle are chosen. Additional phase reconstructions are used, if necessary [19]. For each individual artery, the dataset with the fewest motion artifacts is chosen for analysis. The datasets are reconstructed with contiguous images using a thin (typical value = 0.7 mm) increment.

"Obtaining the Study": EBCT Angiogram High-resolution Axial Images

Contrast-enhanced EBCT of the coronary arteries typically uses a sequential scan mode with prospective ECG triggering. This is the cardinal difference between EBCT and MDCT. Prospective imaging only obtains 50–60 images, rather than hundreds with MDCT retrospective gating, and thus the radiation profile of this technique is much lower. Another advantage of this technique is that it can be gated to the R wave, enabling imaging of patients with arrhythmia, as it tracks the R wave similar to a pacemaker, and fires appropriately after the R wave, regardless of atrial fibrillation, irregular heart rates, or premature beats (Figure 4.4). However, usually only one set of images is obtained, and if there are motion artifacts on this dataset, there are no other phases to look at. The newer scanners (e-Speed) allow for flex-phase imaging, letting the user choose their image timing, and obtaining up to seven phases of the cardiac cycle (depending upon the heart rate). Since each image is obtained in 50 milliseconds, slower heart rates will allow for more imaging. Of course, the radiation exposure goes

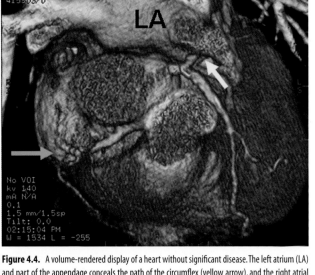

Figure 4.4. A volume-rendered display of a heart without significant disease. The left atrium (LA) and part of the appendage conceals the path of the circumflex (yellow arrow), and the right atrial appendage conceal the right coronary artery (green arrow). Further editing would need to be done to fully evaluate the coronary arteries in this case.

up proportionally with more phases imaged. Using this adaptive triggering technique, several metrics of global cardiac function and 3-D coronary artery image can be obtained simultaneously with EBCT angiography using the e-Speed scanner.

Non-overlapping 1.5 mm slices are usually obtained. This produces 50–60 images (depending on the length of the coronary tree in the individual). This type of prospective gating minimizes radiation (as there are only 60 images produced by the scan), and this is seen as a strength of EBCT for this application. The trigger must be chosen prospectively, so choosing the optimal trigger point within the R-R interval is important. Much work has been done to determine that the end-systolic image has the least coronary motion for CT imaging, and this is increasingly being used for both calcium imaging and CT angiography [24–26].

EBCT Patient Scanning Protocol

The EBCT studies are performed in the high-resolution volume mode using either 50 or 100 ms exposure times. Electrocardiographic triggering is employed, so that each image will be obtained at the same point in diastole. Dependent upon the results of the ECG gating substudy, this will correspond to a fixed point of the R-R interval. Previous studies have gated to 80% of the R-R interval [4,7,8]; now gating is done at end-systole to minimize coronary motion [27]. The subject is positioned head first into the scanner aperture with no couch angulation. All patients will be scanned by EBCT in the supine position without table tilt or slew. Three ECG leads will be attached so that data acquisitions can be triggered to a constant phase in diastole of the cardiac cycle. The subject is instructed to take a few deep breaths and then hold his breath (at end inspiration) while an 11 cm localization scan is performed, beginning 180 mm below the sternal notch. This produces an anteroposterior view of the chest on the image monitor at the operator console (similar in appearance to an antero-posterior chest X-ray). From this the patient centering will be checked and the position for the highest scan will be chosen by the technician (1 cm below the bifurcation of the main pulmonary artery). The couch will be automatically moved to this start position.

A 512 × 512 matrix with the smallest possible field of view will be employed, not to exceed 18 cm, as previously described [4]. The field of view will determine the pixel size, and the smaller the field of view utilized, the smaller the pixel size. The technologist will choose the smallest field of view that allows for imaging of the entire cardiac silhouette on each scan. With smaller pixel sizes, the number of pixels that encompass each portion of the coronary arteries will be greater, possibly increasing spatial resolution. A field of view of 15 cm results in a pixel size of 0.08 mm², while an 18 cm field of view results in a pixel size

of 0.12 mm². Images will be acquired in 100 ms acquisition times during breath-holding at end-inspiration. The slice thickness is typically 1.5 mm with table increments of 1.5 mm, to maximize resolution of the coronary tree. Non-ionic contrast is administered through an 18- or 20-gauge IV catheter placed percutaneously in an antecubital vein. The contrast flow rate and total contrast dose will be determined on an individual basis by the technologist or physician based upon the weight, length of the coronary tree to be covered, and heart rate.

Interpreting Cardiac CT Images

CT angiography, with either EBCT or MDCT is performed in two stages: data acquisition and post-processing. The typical time for the patient (data acquisition) is 20 minutes. Post-processing includes interpolation of the spiral data into axial sections, segmentation to exclude any unnecessary structures, then rendering. Initial segmentation on an off-line workstation with use of 3-D analysis requires less than 10 minutes of user interaction in most cases. However, for complex cases or cases with large venous structures or atrial appendages, editing the entire dataset may take up to 20–30 minutes. Interpretation times are variable, usually dependent upon the image quality and how experienced the user is with cardiac CT and the individual workstation. Experienced users usually spend no more than 10 minutes segmenting and interpreting most cardiac CT studies.

Now that you understand the anatomy as it is displayed on axial tomographic images (Chapter 3) and how to obtain the images on contrast CT, it is important as an evaluator that you spend the first minute of each interpretation making sure the dataset is adequate. That implies that the entire coronary tree is visualized. Thus, the left main and superior portions of the left anterior descending (LAD) artery should be seen in their entirety. While this seems obvious, it is important to concentrate on this.

Besides including the entire coronary tree, the contrast must be fairly uniform throughout the study. The methods of reconstruction rely on Hounsfield units (HU) to make images, and if the contrast-enhanced proximal right coronary artery (RCA) is 300 HU, and the distal is 80 HU, the distal portion of the RCA may not be visible on the 3-D reconstruction. Figure 3.13 demonstrates this problem, as the contrast in the distal right (and the LV cavity) is almost gone by the end of the imaging cycle. This problem is much more likely on EBCT than MDCT, as it takes more time to do the imaging with EBCT (1–2 detectors per heartbeat, time to complete a study on the order of 20–40 seconds), as compared to MDCT (currently up to 64 simultaneous images, so the time to finish a study is only 5–15 seconds on MDCT). This will cause the appearance of a distal stenosis, when in fact it is just poorly filled due to contrast timing issues. The best way to visually assess the adequacy of the contrast is to look at the descending aorta. It should be equally (or almost as) bright on the first image and the last. Figure 3.1 demonstrates a well-enhanced descending aorta, and Figure 3.12 (near the bottom of the heart) still shows good contrast enhancement. However, Figure 3.13 shows a decrease in enhancement of the descending aorta (now it appears gray), so you should be cautious when evaluating the very distal RCA in this case.

Preliminary Observations from Non-invasive Coronary Angiography

We performed a pilot study of 48 patients who underwent both EBCT coronary angiography and cardiac catheterization [4]. In this study done in the mid-1990s, the overall scan time for the acquisition of the EBCT images was 30–40 seconds, dependent primarily upon the patient's heart rate. With patient instruction, most patients were able to hold their breath throughout the entire scanning time. The total contrast amount per patient was 175 ± 53 mL. Studies of our first 48 patients have provided substantial insight into the current limitations and difficulties of developing this new technology. Since that time, the MDCT was developed, and EBCT has advanced. Currently, the contrast requirements for these studies is between 60 and 100 mL (usually between 300 and 370 mg/mL of non-ionic, iodinated contrast medium), and studies can be performed in a third to a half of the original time.

Good delineation of structures on CT requires a differential CT number (Hounsfield unit measure) from surrounding structures. Myocardial contrast enhancement during non-invasive CT coronary angiography has been shown to be an important factor in image quality [28]. The difference in CT values (peak Hounsfield units) between the myocardium and the blood pool has been shown to be a contributing factor in CT study quality and resolution. In a pilot study performed early in the CT angiography experience, we have demonstrated that myocardial contrast uptake, expressed as a peak CT number, as compared to peak contrast enhancement of the coronary arteries, is the most important factor in improving resolution of the coronary arteries on CT angiography [29]. The number of detectors (and associated resolution) has increased exponentially in both EBCT and MDCT over the last 5 years, markedly improving image resolution. Improved gating software improves scan registration, critical to 3-D reconstructions, making the investigation of 3-D minimally-invasive coronary arteriography feasible. With less cardiac motion occurring during imaging, visualization of the coronary arteries can be maximized. The success rate is now in the low 90% range for diagnostic images in all vessels, including problems with breath-holding, motion artifacts, severe calcification, and arrhythmias causing misregistration [30,31]. Higher calcification scores and more regions of significant calcification will also add significant time to the interpretation. An experienced user can inter-

pret datasets and generate reports for cardiac CT studies in as little as 10 minutes. However evaluating studies with dense calcifications may double or triple this interpretation period.

Three-dimensional Imaging of the Heart

In the foreseeable future, neither CT nor MRI will reach the same image quality as invasive, selective coronary angiography nor provide means for interventional treatment. Nevertheless these methods may gain a valuable place in the clinical workup of coronary artery disease if sufficiently large studies show that significant coronary stenoses could be reliably ruled out in those segments of the coronary arteries that would be potential targets of revascularization therapy. One intrinsic advantage of cardiac CT angiography is that conventional invasive angiography is a projectional technique that displays vessels through only a limited number of viewing angles. If a certain angle is not adequately obtained, there is no post-processing to develop that image. With CT angiography, projections can be rendered from any viewing angle. However, since images are not isotropic (lower image quality than coronary angiography), the resolution of CT angiography is dependent upon the viewing angle. The best image resolution of the CT angiographic images is rendering through the craniocaudal axis, a view not possible with conventional invasive angiography.

While the utilization and application of cardiac CT angiography should increase dramatically over the upcoming years, clear visualization of the coronary arteries in a method that is not too time-consuming and is convenient for interpretation will require reconstruction methods to allow clinicians easy interpretation of the 2-D images. This is the biggest divergence in the need for training between cardiologists and radiologists. Radiologists have learned tomographic imaging from day 1 of their residency. Some radiologists may have never performed 3-D analysis of any structure, just relying on the 2-D images to make interpretations. They would "create" a 3-D object in their mind, to follow structures up and down their length. Cardiologists have traditionally not spent much time with axial imaging, especially computed tomography of the heart. Thus, the ability to make 3-D images can allow approximation of the coronary tree, in a method that can look more and more like images from coronary angiography (Figure 4.5). This requires the use of a computer workstation, and different reconstruction methods. There are a number of different reconstruction methods used in current practice for non-invasive CT imaging. The four methods most commonly used are volume and shaded surface rendering, maximum intensity projection, and multiplanar reformatting. The accuracy of CT angiography is dependent upon the rendering technique used. Table 4.2 depicts the strengths and weaknesses of each reconstruction method.

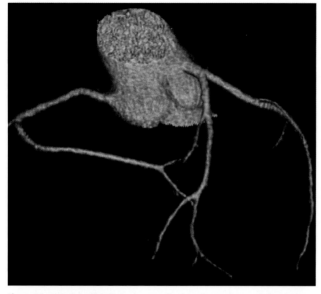

Figure 4.5. A shaded surface display demonstrating the entire coronary tree similar to coronary angiography. With careful editing, the heart and soft tissues can be excluded, leaving only the aortic root and coronary arteries.

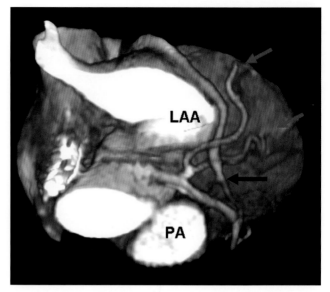

Figure 4.6. A volume-rendered image demonstrating the circumflex and obtuse marginals (red arrows) and the great cardiac vein becoming the anterior interventricular vein (black arrow). To visualize these structures, the left atrial appendage (LAA) needed to be edited out, and the pulmonary artery (PA) was removed to better visualize the left anterior descending and left main arteries.

Shaded Surface Display

This was one of the first methods employed [12]. The shaded-surface rendering technique discards all pixels below a certain HU threshold, and the remaining pixels are shaded according to depth and lighting from a computer observer. This is done by transferring the original 2-D images from the scanner to an off-line computer workstation for analysis. To create 3-D shaded surface display reconstructions requires manual segmentation of the original images. To generate 3-D reconstructions, the atrial appendages and pulmonary trunk need to be removed, to expose the circumflex (under the left atrial appendage) and the left main (under the pulmonary artery, see Figure 4.6).

Specifically, thresholds are established based upon a review of the individual sections to maximize contrast material-filled vascular structures while eliminating partially enhanced viscera and unenhanced vascular structures. The window width is set (usually a default of 1 is used) and then the level (brightness) adjusted to a point at which approximately 90% of pixels corresponding to non-vascular structures disappear. This allows for visualization of the entire surface of the heart, including the inner vessel lumens of the epicardial vessels while excluding the walls and other non-contrast structures (see Figure 4.7). While review of edited and unedited structures can be done with this technique, the osseous structures, as well as venous and other contrast-filled cavities, often need to be edited first. Since bony structures are brighter than contrast, they will not be eliminated by this technique, so the bones need to be removed prior to image analysis. Typical shaded surface display reconstructions are produced using a lower threshold of 80–100 HU. There is no "upper limit" or threshold, so everything brighter than the cutoff value chosen (often done manually depending on the brightness of the dataset) is depicted. This is done to visualize selectively the contrast-enhanced lumens of the coronary

Table 4.2. Relative strengths of common reconstruction methods

Method	Anatomically correct 3-D reconstruction (assess 3-D relationships)	Ability to discern calcium or metal from contrast	Ability to visualize thrombus	High sensitivity and specificity	Accurate measurements of structures or lumens	Entire coronary artery in one image
Two-dimensional Images	↔	↑↑↑	↑↑↑	↑↑↑	↑↑	↔
Shaded surface	↑↑↑	↔	↔	↔	↔	↔
Maximal intensity	↑	↑↑↑	↑↑↑	↑↑↑	↑↑	↑↑
Volume rendering	↑↑↑	↑	↑	↑	↔	↑
Curved multiplanar	↔	↑↑↑	↑↑↑	↑↑↑	↑↑↑	↑↑↑

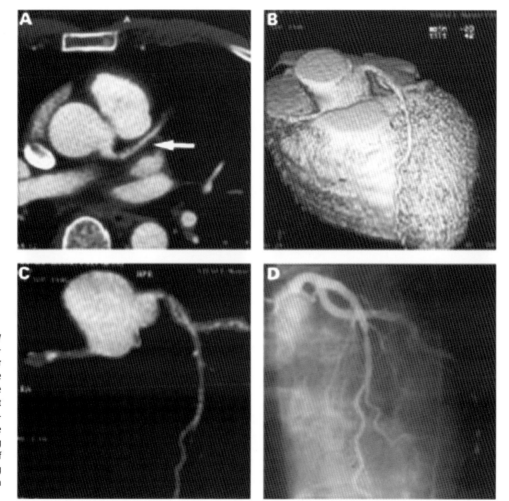

Figure 4.7. Contrast-enhanced EBCT study in a 36-year-old man. **A** Axial image demonstrating the left main and left anterior coronary artery (arrow). **B** Shaded surface display demonstrating reconstruction of the left anterior descending artery without significant disease. **C** Maximal intensity projection of the coronary arteries showing the left anterior descending. **D** Corresponding invasive angiogram demonstrating absence of significant stenosis in left anterior descending distribution. (Reprinted with permission from the BMJ Publishing Group [32].)

arteries, while automatically deleting the vessel wall and surrounding connective tissue. Thus, the resulting image is not depicting the vessel walls and perivascular connective tissue [32]. After a threshold is chosen and editing is done, 3-D surface reconstructions are rendered in various angles to depict all parts of the coronary arteries. The picture looks much like a plaster cast of the heart (Figure 4.7B).

Most of the early EBCT angiography studies utilized this methodology, as this was the predominant method available in the mid and late 1990s for image reconstruction. Further depiction of the coronary tree can be performed to make the images appear more like conventional coronary angiography. With further editing, only the aortic root and coronary epicardial arteries can be included in the 3-D representation (Figures 4.5, 4.7C). This requires much time and effort, but the coronary arteries can then be displayed in a form more similar to a coronary angiogram (a luminogram, without the walls of the arteries, the heart or other cardiac structures in the image). Careful editing of each level of the coronary arteries (50–60 different tomographic images) is required, by circling manually each portion of each coronary artery that is to be included in the image. Thus, one literally has to circle the portion of

the LAD, diagonal, RCA, and circumflex on every single image (such as how the coloring was done on Figure 3.7). The results are often determined by how carefully the reconstructionist did the work, rather than the true anatomy. This can also be automated, but is prone to errors due to similar contrast brightness in the veins and arteries. The computer starts to track the venous structures, and leaves the center of the artery of interest, creating a false stenosis.

As the interpretation of shaded surface 3-D rendering relies on gray scale (density) values above the preset threshold, it has been previously speculated that calcium may be difficult to differentiate from contrast opacification owing to the overlap in density values [8]. This technique, more so than others employed, is especially prone to not properly interpreting the coronary arteries due to calcifications and other high-density structures. In several studies, the sensitivity for obstructive disease was markedly lower with this technique than with maximum-intensity projection [12,33]. This is because the attenuation of calcium (130–1500 HU) and intravascular contrast material (80–300 HU) are within the threshold ranges for shaded surface display (SSD) CT angiography, and demonstrated with the same gray scale value. Typically, in the presence of calcium, the vessel lumen is overestimated with SSD CT angiography because of the misleading appearance that the calcium is intravascular contrast material.

The overestimation of luminal patency in the presence of calcium within the artery lumen is the single greatest reason for SSD CT angiography to be less accurate than other methods of evaluating CT angiography. SSD is especially prone to underestimation of luminal narrowing, due to a more general problem of cardiac CT (relative to invasive angiography), which is partial volume effects. This is due to the anisotropic imaging (voxel size larger than coronary angiography), causing volumes of only a portion of the depth of the image being demonstrated as if they were present throughout the dataset. Partial volume effects reflect the problem that a 3-D volume is displayed as a 2-D dataset. So, if only a 0.5 mm calcification existed on a 1.5 mm thick slice, this may not show up on the final image, as "most" of the image had no calcification. Conversely, a calcification that took up 0.4 mm of a 0.7 mm deep image may appear to be taking up the entire slice, potentially worsening the apparent stenosis. The inaccuracy is more

prevalent with SSD than with other forms of reconstructions (such as maximal intensity projection – MIP) [12], as the partial volume effect is accentuated by the threshold cutoff about the margin of the stenosis.

The two biggest problems with interpretation of both MDCT and EBCT angiography are dense calcifications of the coronary arteries and stents [9]. Coronary artery calcium and metal are much brighter than contrast (Hounsfield units for contrast can go from 130 HU to >500, and metal is often close to 1000 HU in brightness). Metal is often so bright, that a scatter artifact (sunburst) is seen surrounding larger metal objects (such as bypass clips and wires). Coronary stents have become one of the mainstays of interventional cardiology. Cardiac gated CT can accurately describe stent location. Flow through stents can be evaluated and occlusion assessed (Figure 4.8) [34]. However, the metal intrinsic to current generation stents prevents CT from imaging the stent interior accurately in most cases. Stents do not usually cause a starburst, but still can reflect some of the X-ray beam and cause some local scatter, making interpretation of the center of the stent difficult (Figures 4.9, 4.10). Since shaded surface display has

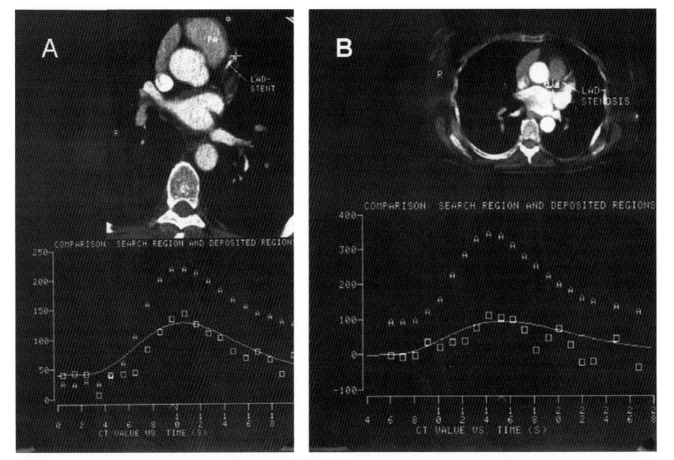

Figure 4.8. Flow studies, with the region of interest (x) in the left anterior descending (LAD) artery just after a proximal stent. Image **A** is a demonstration of a patent stent, with flow approximating the aortic root flow (marked with A's), both in peak and height. The flow is not quite as bold in the LAD (boxes), but follows both timing and pattern. Image **B** demonstrates a stent that has a high-grade stenosis present. The LAD flow distal to the stent (represented as boxes) does not follow the pattern of the corresponding aorta (marked with A's), and is both delayed and blunted. This shows the flow at any region of interest over time, and can be used to demonstrate stent patency (or stenosis).

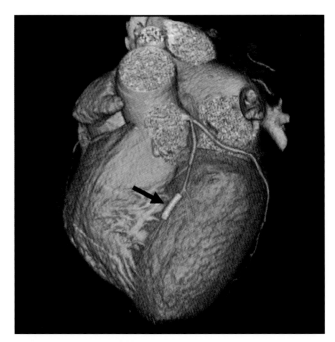

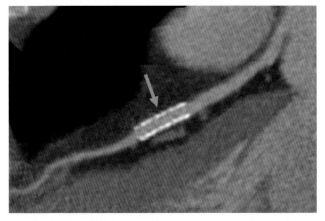

Figure 4.11. A maximal intensity projection demonstrating a patent stent. This e-Speed electron beam CT image does depict the lumen of the stent quite well, and the stent struts do not impede the image. This is a relatively rare image, and in general, not the typical presentation of stents on any current cardiac CT scanner.

Figure 4.9. A stent in the mid-left anterior descending artery (black arrow) on a volume-rendered image. There is filling distal to the stent, but within the stent cannot be reliably imaged. This demonstrates the problem of stent visualization currently with cardiac CT.

no upper limit, the resulting image displays everything as one density (white) and does not allow for the differences between coronary artery calcification and contrast. If a densely calcified plaque was present obstructing the artery,

the artery would look complete and unobstructed on shaded surface images. Maximal intensity projection can depict the stent better (Figure 4.11), but consistent and reliable in-stent imaging is not yet possible with any reconstruction technique or scanner. Maximal intensity projection imaging also overcomes some of the calcification imaging by differentiating calcifications from lumen (Figure 4.12).

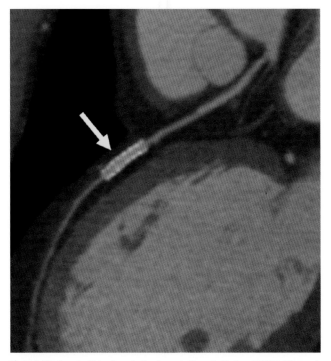

Figure 4.10. A maximal intensity projection demonstrating a stent in the mid-LAD (white arrow). Stent patency cannot be determined reliably on this study due to scatter artifacts from the stent struts, despite imaging with 0.625 mm slice width on a 64-slice scanner.

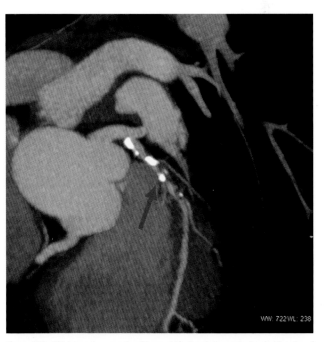

Figure 4.12. This image shows a series of dense calcifications in the proximal and mid portion of the left anterior descending artery, with both calcified and non-calcified plaque forming a significant stenosis just distal to the diagonal takeoff (arrow).

Volume Rendering

The volume rendering technique relies on identifying all pixels above a certain threshold. The pixels are assigned a value (Hounsfield unit, HU) that correlates with their attenuation. The results are most similar to conventional coronary angiography, in that there is no change in the true anatomic course or relationship with other structures, and the coronary arteries are seen as relatively smooth structures with 3-D landmarks present. This methodology allows for measurement of the stenosis, although the same limits as any measure of small structures, such as quantitative coronary angiography exist, including identification of the leading edge of the stenotic segment, and proper comparison to a "normal" segment (Figures 4.12, 4.13). The image can be rotated to different views, allowing the interpreter some flexibility in seeing the segment from multiple angles.

Since all pixels above the threshold are shown on the reproduced image, it has some of the same limitations of shaded surface display, which include showing the structures as fairly uniform in appearance. There is a lot more variation in the final image than the "plaster of Paris" appearance of shaded surface display, and brightness does help identify stenosis with volume rendering, but nowhere near as much as with maximal intensity projection (see below). A stenotic region will look darker as well as narrowed on volume-rendered images (Figures 4.14–4.16). The "smoothing" that takes place will make smaller arteries disappear, so it is not as good as maximal intensity projection to see small vessels and distal arteries (Figure 4.14).

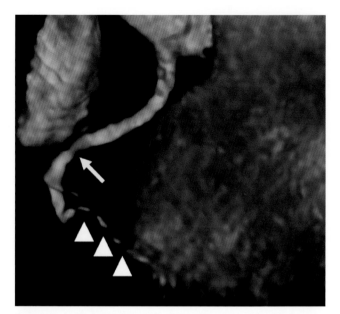

Figure 4.14. A volume-rendered image with mild to moderate disease of the mid right coronary artery (arrow). The right ventricular marginal branch (white arrowheads) is not well seen due to its small diameter. It is not diseased, but rather demonstrates drop out. The smoothing technique of volume rendering causes smaller arteries to be visualized in this way. Maximal intensity projection would demonstrate this small branch vessel more clearly.

Another condition encountered on volume-rendered or shaded surface images, not seen well with invasive angiography, is myocardial bridging, where the artery goes under the myocardium. While rarely a condition with any significant clinical sequelae, it is commonly seen on cardiac CT. Figure 4.17 demonstrates a person with bridging as it appears on 3-D images with cardiac CT. A typical appearance is a "normal" artery (very smooth and of uniform diameter) that "dives" into the myocardium, then reappears more distally as a normal appearing non-stenosed vessel. The only way to truly differentiate bridging from a 100%

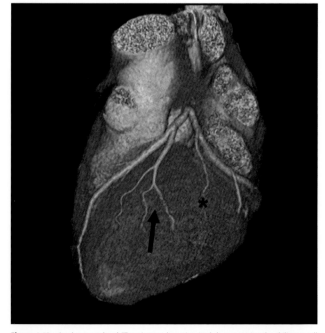

Figure 4.13. A volume-rendered CT angiogram (superior view) demonstrating the ability to well visualize both side branches including diagonals (black arrow) and obtuse marginal branches (asterisk).

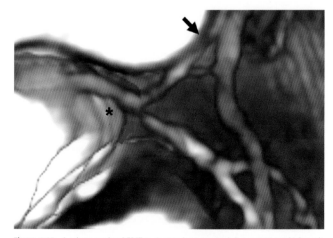

Figure 4.15. A volume-rendered EBCT angiogram (superior view) demonstrating a high-grade stenosis of the left anterior descending artery (red arrow), as well as a high-grade stenosis of the circumflex (black arrow) and a mild stenosis of the left main coronary artery (asterisk).

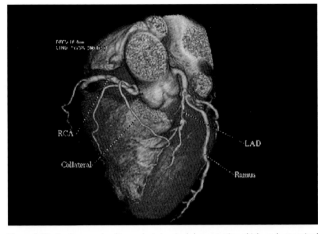

Figure 4.16. A volume-rendered image (anterior view) demonstrating a high-grade stenosis of the left anterior descending artery (LAD) and a collateral branch from the right coronary artery (RCA) inserting distally into the left anterior descending artery.

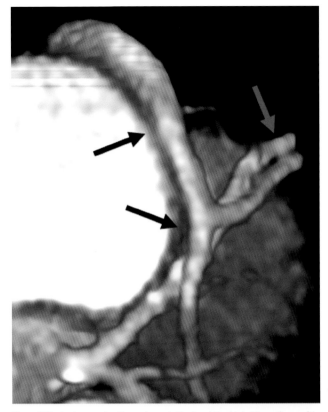

Figure 4.18. A volume-rendered image demonstrating the relationship in this specific case of the circumflex and great cardiac vein. The vein (black arrows) completely overlies the circumflex artery (red arrow) in this case, making the interpretation of the circumflex difficult using this projection without further editing the image to "remove" the great cardiac vein from the image.

stenosis is to look at the 2-D images, where the vessel in question will be seen as a normal, round segment, covered by myocardium. Since the myocardium has contrast enhancement that exceeds the HU threshold set for volume rendering, the myocardium overlying the vessel is seen, but the vessel cannot be seen on the external surface. Since the brightness of the artery lumen is greater than the myocardium, maximal intensity projections may be of more use in this situation (described below), as the brighter lumen will be seen better through the less enhanced myocardium.

Calcification still obstructs view of the lumen with this (and all) reconstruction modalities, as seen with maximal intensity projections in Figure 4.12. Editing of the image needs to be done (as in SSD), whereby the left atria appendage, pulmonary artery, and coronary sinus/great cardiac vein need to be edited prior to reconstruction (as these venous structures overlap the circumflex – Figure 4.18). Figure 4.19 shows a person with mild LAD disease

with volume rendering using multiple different angles. There is no limit to the number of angles or views possible with these datasets.

The left internal mammary is easily seen when the diameter is greater than 1 mm and there are no (or few) surgical clips (Figure 4.20). Obviously, this is not always the case, and this can be the most challenging of the vessels to visualize, due to the small diameter of the mammary arteries

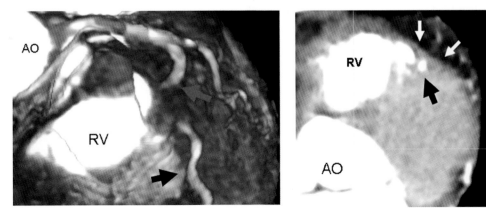

Figure 4.17. On the left is a volume-rendered image of the left anterior descending, demonstrating "bridging" of the mid-LAD. The artery is very smooth and of normal diameter (red arrow) until it "dives" into the myocardium, then reappears (black arrow) as a normal appearing non-stenosed vessel. The only way to truly differentiate bridging from a 100% stenosis is to look at the 2-D images (right). This axial image demonstrates a normal, round LAD segment (black arrow), covered by myocardium (white arrows).

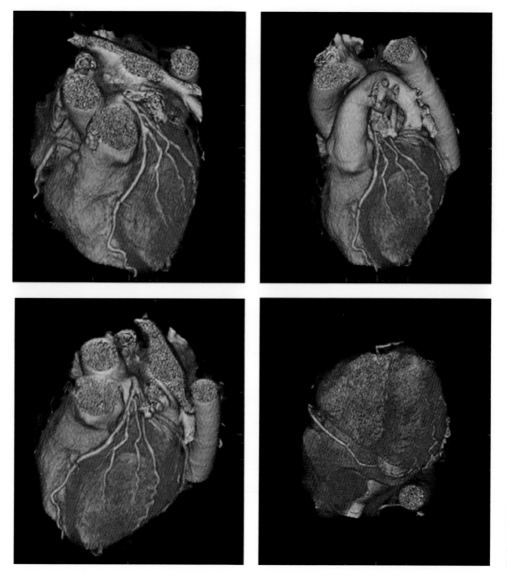

Figure 4.19. A volume-rendered dataset demonstrating the coronary anatomy from multiple views. It is important to evaluate these images from multiple views, as any given artery cannot be fully visualized from any one angle.

(and arterial conduits in general), as well as the use of surgical clips. Rotating the heart helps visualize the coronary arteries from multiple views, alleviating some of the problems of these clips obscuring the lumen (Figure 4.21). Since the metal clips are usually extraluminal (used to close off side branches from the mammary artery), they can usually be excluded by obtaining the proper view, using either MIP or volume rendering techniques (Figure 4.22). Saphenous vein grafts are very well seen using this method, and since there is minimal or no calcification of the saphenous vein grafts, the issues relating to calcification obscuring the lumen are less problematic (Figure 4.23).

Maximal Intensity Projections

In this reconstruction method, only the maximal density values at each point in the 3-D volume are displayed, and the final picture is similar to a conventional (arterial)

angiogram in that structures are projected over one another. To generate maximum intensity projections, a cross-sectional projectional display is created in which every pixel is assigned a gray scale value corresponding to its actual attenuation. Usually some editing needs to be performed to remove at least the left atrial appendage and pulmonary artery (as these structures overlap the left main and left anterior descending arteries), and most of the time, the great cardiac vein and coronary sinus. Osseous structures are also removed, so that the ribs, spine, and sternum do not obscure visualization of the coronary arteries. Newer workstations automatically remove external non-cardiac structures with high accuracy in only seconds. If one wanted to obtain images more consistent with invasive coronary angiography (in which only the lumen of the arteries is present, and the myocardium and other cardiac structures are not present on the image), the original datasets can be segmented further to remove everything but the coronary arteries. Maximal intensity

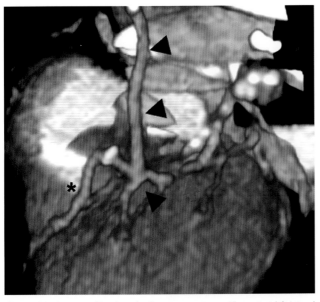

Figure 4.20. A 64-year-old patient after bypass surgery, now with a patent left internal mammary artery (black arrows). The graft first inserts into a totally occluded diagonal branch (red arrow), then acts as a "skip graft" to the left anterior descending (asterisk). This would be difficult to follow on 2-D axial images, and much easier with a 3-D image such as this volume rendering.

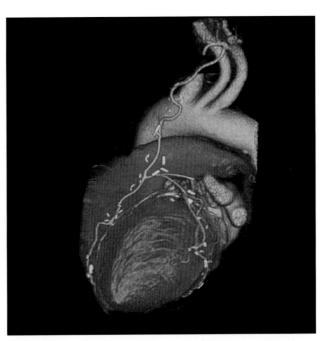

Figure 4.22. A 3-D volume-rendered image of the heart obtained on a 64-slice MDCT scanner. The mammary artery can be seen from the origin, followed to the insertion site. The yellow objects are the metal clips used for side branches of the mammary artery during surgery.

projections are then rendered in multiple views to depict all parts of the coronary arteries (Figures 4.24, 4.25). Maximal intensity projections have been used to help differentiate structures within the coronary artery. Because the structures are displayed based upon their brightness, calcium and metal are easily distinguished from the contrast-enhanced lumen (Figures 4.11, 4.12). This is very useful to detect calcium in the lumen (unlike the problems seen with volume rendering or shaded surface reformatting, Figure 4.26), but they may not always permit reliable detection of stenoses because of the overlap of different structures in the planar projection format. SSD images cannot display X-ray attenuation values for structures within the threshold range (80+ HU). The advantage of MIP

Figure 4.21. A demonstration of a typical image of the left internal mammary artery using maximal intensity projection imaging. The small diameter (here <1.5 mm) and multiple surgical clips (arrows on left image) make interpretation of patency more difficult. Using multiple views, one can discern that this graft is actually patent.

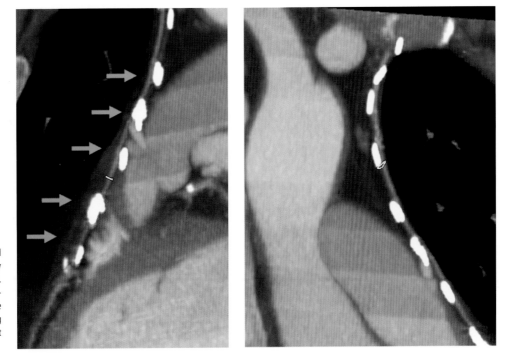

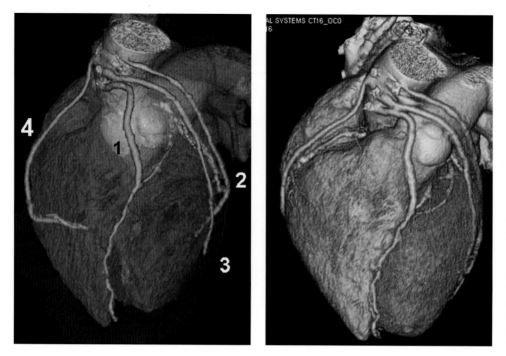

Figure 4.23. A 78-year-old woman who had bypass surgery 10 years previously, now presenting with shortness of breath. All four saphenous vein grafts are patent. Graft 1 inserts to the left anterior descending, graft 2 to the circumflex, graft 3 to the obtuse marginal branch, and graft 4 to the right coronary artery. Two different volume-rendered projection techniques are shown (one more transparent on the left, more opaque on the right).

is that the gray scale reflects CT attenuation rather than simulating light reflections as in SSD, thus distinguishing between materials with different attenuation, such as intra-arterial iodinated contrast material, vascular calcification and differentially perfused myocardium. MIP is closer to a thick 2-D slab than a 3-D object. Maximum intensity projection, by relying on density differences and avoiding image smoothing, allows the visualization of smaller vessels and better visualization of the left internal mammary artery (Figure 4.21). MIP does not convey depth relationships nor does it depict overlapping vessels (Figure

4.24) [12,33]. The lack of 3-D information inherent in a single MIP is minimized by displaying multiple MIPs through a single axis.

Multiple MIP images can be obtained, and reviewed in a cine loop (Figure 4.27). Typically, images every 6–12° around a rotation will be taken, creating a cine of 30–60 images with equal spacing around the 360° object. This is possible with all reconstruction methods, allowing for multiple angle assessment of any segment of the coronary tree. Furthermore, "soft" (better described as non-calcified) plaque is visible by this methodology. This is better

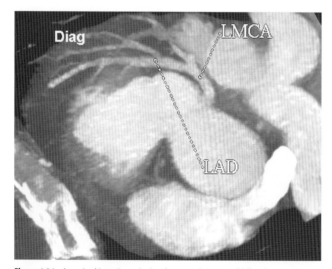

Figure 4.24. A maximal intensity projection demonstrating a normal left main coronary artery (LMCA), left anterior descending (LAD), and several diagonal branches (diag).

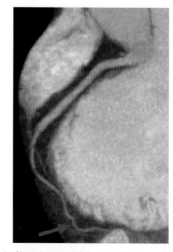

Figure 4.25. A maximal intensity projection demonstrating a normal right coronary artery. This e-Speed electron beam image demonstrates a normal posterior descending artery (arrow). This reconstruction technique allows for better visualization of smaller vessels.

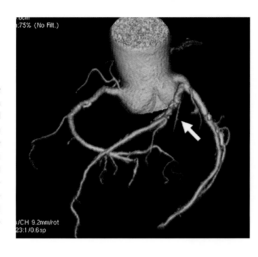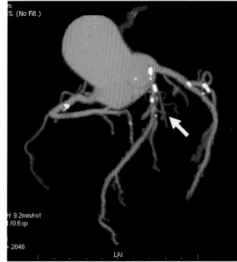

Figure 4.26. Two reconstructions of the same patient. The left image demonstrates a volume-rendered image, which does not well distinguish the calcification from the lumen in the left anterior descending artery (white arrow). The right image demonstrates a maximal intensity projection, displaying the sequential calcifications in the LAD distribution. Since MIP is more transparent, the overlapping vessels (particularly the septal perforators in this image) become more problematic.

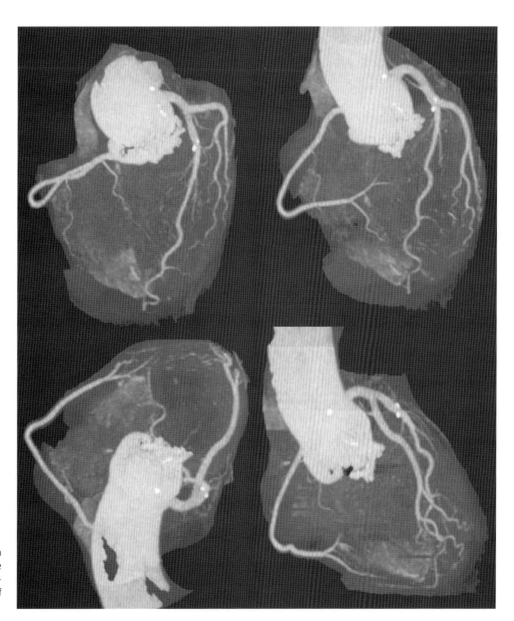

Figure 4.27. Multiple projections of a person with normal coronary arteries using the maximal intensity projection rendering technique. This allows for complete visualization of the coronary arteries.

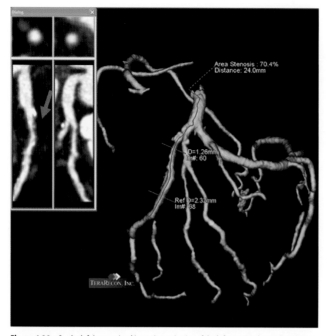

Figure 4.28. On the left is a maximal intensity projection of the left anterior descending demonstrating a severe luminal stenosis (non-calcific or "soft") of the proximal LAD (arrow). On the right is the volume-rendered image, without the myocardium, giving a much more "traditional angiographic" view of the coronaries. Measurement tools are easily applied to the dataset, and semi-quantitation of diameters and stenoses is possible.

described in Chapter 12. While metal and calcium are much brighter than contrast-enhanced lumens, fibrous tissue, thrombus, and fat are lower density, thus looking like a filling defect or dark region in the lumen of the artery (Figure 4.28). MIP imaging has been shown to provide a superior accuracy in detecting significant obstructions in the coronary arteries as compared to other techniques (Figure 4.26) [35].

An example of a maximal intensity projection image demonstrating a stenosis can be seen in Figure 4.12. This image shows a stenosis in the left anterior descending (white arrow), consisting of both calcification (bright white) and non-calcified plaque (gray or black). The non-calcified plaque is sometimes called "soft plaque" but in reality it may be fibrous; thus the term soft is being utilized less often to describe this non-calcified atherosclerosis. The stenosis is probably at least 70%; however, the calcified section makes the exact measurement difficult. There is no current method of reconstruction that can eliminate the calcium without eliminating the entire lumen. In contrast to the underestimation of luminal stenosis with SSD or volume rendering due to dense calcifications, stenosis can be overestimated with MIP if an eccentrically located or very large calcification overlies the luminal contrast material on a given MIP image. In a study of renal CT angiography, calcium was detected and visualized 5 times as frequently with MIP CT compared to SSD imaging and invasive angiography [12]. Thus, interpreting these areas of dense calcification is not yet ideal with cardiac CT.

Multiplanar Reformatting (MPR)

Otherwise known as "curved surface reformation," multiplanar reformatting (Figures 4.29, 4.30) can be used to evaluate the entire coronary tree in one view. In this technique, the plane of a specific artery is chosen to be displayed as a 2-D image. This then represents a "curved surface" from within the 3-D volume, following the curved trajectory of the respective artery. Retrospectively gated axial images are reconstructed at three diastolic phases (usually between 40% and 80%). After initial review, the phase with the least amount of motion artifacts is used for analysis. Using a

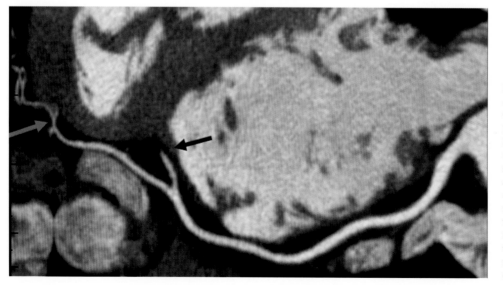

Figure 4.29. A Toshiba 64-MDCT image demonstrating a multiplanar reconstruction of the entire right coronary artery, including a long segment of a posterolateral marginal branch (red arrow). The posterior descending (black arrow) would require a second reconstruction to follow that artery. Side branches are not well seen in this projection, as only one course of the artery can be shown with each reconstruction. For an artery such as the RCA, this usually proves adequate without multiple reconstructions. The left anterior descending, with multiple diagonal branches, often needs multiple reconstructions to demonstrate its entire course.

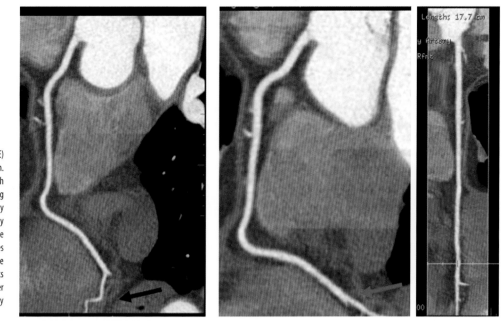

Figure 4.30. This 64-slice image (GE) demonstrates a multiplanar reconstruction. The vessel can be seen in long lengths with this technique. However, the surrounding anatomy can get quite distorted. The artery appears to leave the pericardium and go away from the heart, obviously just an artifact of the reconstruction. The black arrow demonstrates the posterior descending (left image), and the red arrow is another reconstruction that tracks the posterolateral marginal branch (center image). The artery can be displayed as a very straight line (right image).

dedicated manual vessel tracking algorithm, the centerline of the coronary artery can be traced. The application then provides multiplanar reconstructions (Figures 4.29, 4.30) that are orthogonal to the vessel centerline, thus creating cross-sectional cuts of each coronary arterial segment. Multiple cross-sectional images are generated at 10 mm increments from the coronary ostia to the most distal segments with a diameter equal to or greater than 2 mm. With some basic knowledge of the cardiac anatomy, these images can be rendered in approximately 10–15 minutes, with fairly low variability of the reconstructions.

The artery plane can be chosen, and the computer then uses this centerpoint as the focus of the reconstruction. All other structures are automatically eliminated that are any distance from this centerpoint, possibly decreasing problems seen with other reconstruction methods from tortuosity and overlap. One center reported superior results for CT angiography of the renal arteries with this technique as compared to MIP and SSD [36]. Curved multiplanar reconstructions with CT coronary angiography has also been reported, with high sensitivity and specificity [37]. This permits visualization of the complete course of the coronary arteries within one image, and significant stenosis and occlusions of the coronary arteries can be visualized with an accuracy that exceeds 90%. One reason is that the CT value is preserved, making it fairly easy to delineate calcifications from the lumen. Recognition of calcifications with either higher or lower density than inner lumen contrast is very difficult with 3-D SSD, somewhat better with MIP, and best with MPR.

The biggest reason this technique is popular is that compared with other reconstruction techniques (volume rendering, MIP, and SSD), curved multiplanar reconstructions can be rendered quickly and accurately, without the need for manual segmentation. By identifying the centerpoint of the artery, there is no reason to manually exclude the pulmonary veins or arteries, or even the atria or other contrast-enhanced structures. In contrast to all other reconstruction techniques, distance measurements in the curved MPR images represent the true distances and are not subject to shortening due to projection (Figure 4.30).

The reason many centers do not employ this methodology exclusively is that with multiplanar reformation, uncertainties as to the true center of the vessel may be of concern, causing the computer to "create" stenosis by following the vein instead of the artery, or just missing the centerpoint of the artery, making the image completely non-diagnostic. The biggest drawback is that only one vessel can be visualized in one image and that side branches are not depicted unless separate reconstructions are rendered for every side branch [37]. Since the computer relies on the user tracing the centerpoint from beginning to end, each branch must be re-traced as a new reconstruction. Evaluating multiple diagonal branches or obtuse marginals becomes more difficult and time-consuming with this method, and is much easier with either volume rendering or maximal intensity projection (Figure 4.26). Severe calcifications are still problematic with this technique [37]. Respiration and motion artifacts cannot be recognized on the curved MPR image, a disadvantage not present with volume rendering or SSD techniques. The landmarks are taken away, so a curved or tortuous right coronary artery is displayed as a fairly straight image, making estimating which segment the stenosis is present in more difficult. Also, the anatomy gets quite distorted, and the arteries can appear to leave the heart, obviously just an artifact of the reconstruction technique (Figure 4.30). Overall, curved multiplanar reconstructions, because they can be rendered quickly and convey all the information about the different CT densities within the vessel, are an extremely useful tool to evaluate contrast-enhanced CT angiography data.

Other Reconstruction Techniques

There are a few other less used or less well-developed reconstruction techniques available with different workstations. One that we utilize from time to time is the "radiograph projection," which shows the images as if they were images with fluoroscopy. This is useful when evaluating pacemaker wires and other metal objects and their relationship (Figure 4.31). We will sometimes use this when we are evaluating patients not doing as well as anticipated post bi-ventricular pacing, to see how far the pacemaker leads are and if they are in optimal position. The arteries can be displayed with the contrast black instead of white (by inverting the image) (Figure 4.32), similar to the black blood technique of MRI. Similar to images in the catheterization laboratory, sometimes inverting the image makes the lumen easier to visualize.

Another technique is virtual endoscopy. Extracting the contrast-enhanced blood pool from the image datasets allows for virtual viewing of the inner vessel wall. This technique generates a view as if you were "flying through" the vessel itself, in place of the blood. This technique is highly user dependent and time-consuming, and has not been demonstrated to improve the visualization of plaque or anatomy. However, as improvements in spatial resolution continue, flying through a stent or densely calcified segment may be possible.

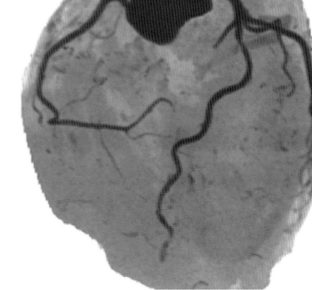

Figure 4.32. An inverted image demonstrating the blood as black and the surrounding myocardium as white. This can assist in the visualization of the lumen in some cases.

Recent Advances in Computer Workstations

An automated program is now possible to track the coronary arteries. Using placement of a single point in the proximal, middle, and distal segments of each artery, the computer can trace the artery and extract the images in seconds, obviating the need for sequential editing (which takes 10–20 minutes per case to fully examine the circumflex, right and left anterior descending). This automated program (now available with some workstations) tracks a given coronary vessel departing proximally and distally from the point chosen. Since the quality and ability of the computer workstation for tracking the vessel depends on border definition and overall image quality, this may very well require some editing in most cases. It is doubtful that this will produce perfect images of the entire coronary tree with each application, but computer workstations are developing at a faster rate than the hardware and CT systems, so anything may be possible in the next few years. When we first started doing computer reconstructions and 3-D imaging of the coronary anatomy in 1995, it took 3 weeks to finalize a reconstruction for evaluation. Now we can complete reconstruction in seconds, and interpretation of the coronary tree in minutes. Keep in mind, when performing interpretations, that the most

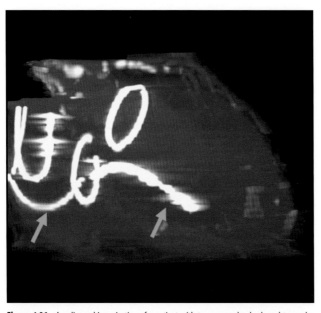

Figure 4.31. A radiographic projection of a patient with two pacemaker leads and two valve rings. The right ventricular lead (arrows) can be seen going through the tricuspid valve ring.

important aspect of cardiac CT is the 2-D images, as these are what are used to create these beautiful 3-D datasets.

Interpreting Three-dimensional Images

Realizing from the outset that no single method of analysis is without limitations, we always incorporate review of the 2-D images, including the calcium scans, and the different 3-D renderings into final consensus opinions. Significant lesions should be seen by at least two methods to confirm they are not an imaging artifact or editing error. If the editor were to remove part of the circumflex when editing out the coronary sinus or great cardiac vein, this would "create" a stenosis that is not real. Using the original 2-D dataset can confirm that there is a stenosis at this level. Some investigators only use the 2-D datasets to read the studies, and Dr Achenbach demonstrated that this provides as sensitive a methodology to read studies as relying on the 3-D reconstructions as well. However, the drawback of this technique (utilizing only 2-D images) is that the coronary arteries are often tortuous and following each segment on each level (over 50–80 contiguous images) may be difficult. Since the 3-D reconstructions are only as good as the data obtained on the true cross-sectional axial images (garbage in = garbage out), authors emphasize the importance of careful observation of true cross-sectional images [38].

Practically, we start with a 3-D image set – usually volume rendering – to provide an overview of the coronary tree and look for segments of stenosis. This provides a highly specific way of looking for stenosis, and will also identify obvious problems with gating or breathing artifact, as the 3-D image will look deformed or have an obvious triggering error in which the heart does not properly align to form a uniform image (Figures 4.33–4.35). Also, more complex anatomy (such as congenital heart disease or bypass grafts) are easily seen as a 3-D dataset (Figures 4.21, 4.23), and the reader is better oriented when approaching the 2-D axial images. Three-dimensional reconstructions are especially helpful with skip grafts, as the vessel often goes up and down between 2-D images, making this very difficult to follow on axial images only (Figure 4.20). However, the downside of this methodology is that calcification can "fill in" gaps, making the artery look non-stenotic, despite significant abnormalities (Figure 4.26). Classic appearance of a stenosis on volume rendering can be seen in Figures 4.14, 4.15, and 4.16. Figure 4.14 demonstrates a mid-RCA lesion, with the stenotic segment being both a little darker and narrower than the other segments. The overall artery looks smooth from top to bottom, so there is no breathing, motion, or triggering artifacts. One drawback of volume rendering is that because it smoothes the image, the smaller vessels are not seen as well, and there is a right ventricle marginal branch that is not well visualized, appearing as highly stenotic, when in fact it is probably just too small to be reli-

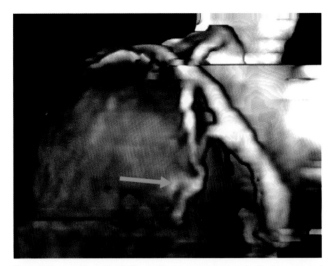

Figure 4.33. A motion artifact (white streaking) is seen at the arrow in this obtuse marginal branch. While this is not a dramatic artifact in this case, accurately diagnosing stenosis in these areas is not possible.

ably visualized. Important to note, small vessels will "drop out," looking like high-grade disease, especially when the artery diameter is less than 1 mm. Do not interpret small arteries as highly diseased, or every patient's study you

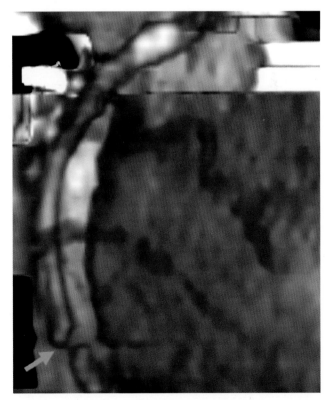

Figure 4.34. A premature beat causing an artifact on the volume-rendered image of a right coronary artery. The arrow demonstrates where gating after a premature ventricular beat caused that particular level to the imaged at a different time in the cardiac cycle, leading to an apparent artifact. This person had normal coronary arteries, and only by interpreting the axial images (seeing a round circle demonstrating a normal lumen on every image) could the proper diagnosis be made.

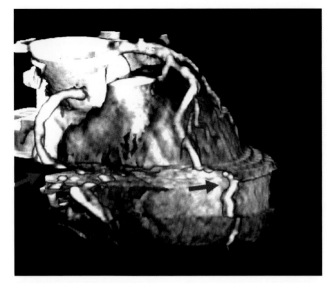

Figure 4.35. A breath-holding artifact during a cardiac CT scan. The arrows point to the area where breathing caused the heart to move caudally, "stretching" out the heart, causing pseudo-stenosis and marked distortion. This artifact makes the study uninterpretable, at least in the areas affected at the time of the breathing artifact.

evaluate will have significant disease if the smaller vessels are taken into account by 3-D methods.

Figure 4.15 is a volume-rendered EBCT angiogram (superior view) demonstrating a high-grade stenosis of the left anterior descending (white arrow), as well as a high-grade stenosis of the circumflex (black arrow) artery. Figure 4.16 shows a volume-rendered image (anterior view) demonstrating a high-grade stenosis of the left anterior descending and a collateral vessel from the RCA. Collaterals are usually not well visualized by cardiac CT due to their small diameter. Keep in mind that all volume-rendered images (and all reconstructions) are 3-D objects that can be rotated.

Thus, after volume rendering, it is important to look at the original images, making note of densely calcific regions, as well as confirming the stenosis seen with the volume-rendered set, or if the artery is just of small diameter and not diseased. Finally, maximal intensity images are used as needed to evaluate segments that have questionable findings. Maximal intensity will show smaller diameter vessels, useful to see smaller arteries and side branches (Figure 4.12). Vessel segments which show extensive calcification in the original images and maximal intensity projections (calcification covering more than half of the artery diameter in at least two consecutive images) need to be excluded from further analysis, as do vessels with artifacts caused by motion, triggering, or inconsistent breath-holding. These segments can be mentioned in the conclusions as questionable due to the aforementioned problem.

We typically describe segments as: normal, mild disease (<50% stenosis), moderate (implying 40–60% stenosis), significant (>70% stenosis), and severe or complete (>95%

stenosis). It must be noted that subtotal stenosis or complete stenosis are not well differentiated on cardiac CT. Partial volume effects tend to result in vessel discontinuity at a point of high-grade stenosis, rather than depiction of an extreme narrowing seen with invasive angiography. The opposite problem also exists. Bridging collaterals are small diameter vessels, they are either hard or impossible to see well on cardiac CT. Thus, what appears to be a high-grade stenosis with good filling of the distal vessel on reconstructed CT images is actually a 100% stenosis on invasive angiography. This can sometimes lead the interventionist to anticipate the wrong treatment path, but usually does not misdiagnose patients as having (or not having) obstructive coronary artery disease.

Other experienced physicians use other sequences to examine the coronary arteries. Some investigators start by evaluating the 2-D axial images. Dr Achenbach describes methodology used in his study by stating:

The cross-sectional images were screened for artifacts caused by motion and for calcifications of the coronary arteries. Calcifications were rated as too severe to permit further evaluation if a calcified plaque occupied more than half the diameter of the artery in two consecutive images. Manual segmentation of the images was performed on an image-by-image basis to eliminate all structures that would obstruct the view of the coronary arteries, such as the chest wall, pulmonary vessels, and atrial appendages. Three-dimensional reconstructions were rendered interactively from at least six angles (equivalent to posteroanterior, left anterior oblique, and right anterior oblique projections, each in at least two craniocaudal angulations). If necessary, reconstructions were rendered from additional angles to visualize the entire coronary tree. [32]

Summary

Presently, CT angiography has advantages over MR angiography, with a higher resolution examination (with pixel sizes down to 0.25×0.25 mm, using a 512×512 matrix, increasing to a higher resolution matrix of 1024×1024 in some scanners), compared with pixel sizes of 1×2 mm in the MR angiographic acquisition plane (matrix size of 256×128). There are no ill effects for claustrophobic patients or patients with cardiac pacemakers or other factors that are contraindicated for magnetic resonance or MR angiography. Additionally, cardiac CT can demonstrate mural and atherosclerotic calcifications, MR cannot. However, the advantages of MR include well-quantified and validated perfusion imaging to supplement anatomic information. The advent of PET/CT allows for coupling of good perfusion imaging with anatomic information, and the diagnostic accuracy of this technique will be described in Chapter 17. Some of the current limitations of CT angiography are listed in Table 4.3. These include the inability to adequately image patients weighing more than 325 pounds because of the unacceptable noise levels. Additionally, significant

Table 4.3. Current limitations of CT angiography

Need for iodinated contrast
Radiation dose
Stent evaluations
Visualizing vessels less than 1 to 1.5 mm in diameter
Morbid obesity (weight >325–350 pounds)
Dense calcifications

amounts of iodinated contrast are generally required to create diagnostic images, and this is obviously unacceptable in patients with severe azotemia. As tube currents and number of detectors increase, the required dose of contrast material will continue to diminish. MR has a distinct advantage in this regard, obtaining images without need for radiation or iodinated contrast.

The recent introduction of 16-detector (and greater) systems has resulted in several significant improvements and the potential to further improve image quality is significant [39,40,41]. The possibility of acquiring data with thinner slice collimation has improved spatial resolution. Higher tube outputs allow thinner collimation settings, which leads to the ability to obtain thin slices without increased noise. Faster rotation times (now as low as 330 milliseconds in some systems) lead to higher temporal resolution and, along with the larger coverage, substantially reduce the overall duration of the scan (from approximately 35 to as low as 6–10 seconds). This reduces the amount of contrast agent that is necessary and greatly facilitates the breath-hold for the patient. Currently, limitations in X-ray tube outputs lead to increased image noise and preclude even thinner slices. X-ray tubes with greater heat capacities will allow for smaller collimation widths and improved spatial resolution.

The increased channel MDCT systems (32-, 40-, and 64-detector systems) now use the additional detector rows to improve temporal resolution, reduce breath-hold time, and reduce contrast dose. Higher numbers of detectors allow the study to be done in even fewer heart beats. The newer applications of the MDCT angiogram utilize multisector reconstruction to decrease temporal resolution. The increased detector arrays will allow for less heart-rate variability during studies, improving the diagnostic accuracy and decreasing the number of non-diagnostic tests. The continued rapid technologic advancement of MDCT and EBCT suggests that there will be further improvements in CT coronary angiography. In the near term, the development and introduction of MDCT systems with more than 64 channels is likely. The e-Speed EBCT system (GE, San Francisco, CA) now is limited to two channels, but possibly will be used to create a hybrid scanner (utilizing the temporal resolution of the EBCT at 50 milliseconds, and either flat panel or MDCT detectors to improve spatial resolution). We shall see continued rapid advancement in CT for coronary angiography and a series of comparative studies evaluating these new CT techniques against existing measures of coronary heart disease.

References

1. Bakhsheshi H, Mao SS, Budoff MJ, Lu B, Brundage BH. Preview method for electron beam scanning of the coronary arteries. Acad Radiol 2000;7:620–626.
2. Budoff MJ, Raggi P, Berman D, et al. Continuous probabilistic prediction of angiographically significant coronary artery disease using electron beam tomography. Circulation. 2002;105(15):1791–1796.
3. Haberl R, Becker A, Leber A, et al. Correlation of coronary calcification and angiographically documented stenoses in patients with suspected coronary artery disease: results of 1,764 patients. J Am Coll Cardiol 2001;37:451–457.
4. Budoff MJ, Oudiz RJ, Zalace CP, et al. Intravenous three dimensional coronary angiography using contrast enhanced electron beam computed tomography. Am J Cardiol 1999;83:840–845.
5. Kuettner A, Trabold T, Schroeder S, et al. Noninvasive detection of coronary lesions using 16-detector multislice spiral computed tomography technology: initial clinical results. J Am Coll Cardiol 2004;44(6):1230–1237.
6. Kuettner A, Kopp AF, Schroeder S, et al. Diagnostic accuracy of multidetector computed tomography coronary angiography in patients with angiographically proven coronary artery disease. J Am Coll Cardiol 2004;43(5):840–841.
7. Achenbach S, Moshage W, Ropers D, Nossen J, Daniel WG. Value of electron-beam computed tomography for the noninvasive detection of high-grade coronary-artery stenoses and occlusions. N Engl J Med 1998;339:1964–1971.
8. Schmermund A, Rensing BJ, Sheedy PF, Bell MR, Rumberger JA. Intravenous electron-beam computed tomographic coronary angiography for segmental analysis of coronary artery stenoses. J Am Coll Cardiol 1998;31(7):1547–1554.
9. Hoffmann U, Moselewski F, Cury RC, et al. Predictive value of 16-slice multidetector spiral computed tomography to detect significant obstructive coronary artery disease in patients at high risk for coronary artery disease: patient-versus segment-based analysis. Circulation 2004;110(17):2638–2643.
10. Rumberger JA, Schwartz RS, Simons DB, et al: Relations of coronary calcium determined by electron beam computed tomography and lumen narrowing determined at autopsy. Am J Cardiol 1994;73:1169–1173.
11. Rumberger JA, Simons DB, Fitzpatrick LA, et al: Coronary artery calcium areas by electron beam computed tomography and coronary atherosclerotic plaque area: a histopathologic correlative study. Circulation 1995;92:2157–2162.
12. Rubin GD, Dake MD, Napel S, et al. Spiral CT of renal artery stenosis: comparison of three-dimensional rendering techniques. Radiology 1994;190:181–189.
13. Lu B, Dai RP, Jing BL, et al. Evaluation of coronary artery bypass graft patency using three-dimensional reconstruction and flow study on electron beam angiography. J Comput Assist Tomogr 2000;24:663–670.
14. Hopper KD. With helical CT, is nonionic contrast a better choice than ionic contrast for rapid and large IV bolus injections (answer to question)? AJR Am J Roentgenol 1996;166:715.
15. Debatin J, Cohan RH, Leder RA, Zakrzewski CB, Dunnick NR. Selective use of low-osmolar contrast media. Invest Radiol 1991;26:17–21.
16. Cohan RH, Dunnick NR, Leder RA, et al. Extravasation of nonionic contrast media: efficacy of conservative treatment. Radiology 1990;176:65–67.
17. West JB. Best and Taylor's Physiological basis of medical practice. Baltimore, MD: Williams & Wilkins, 1991:139.
18. Haage P, Schmitz-Rode T, Hübner D, et al. Reduction of contrast material dose and artifacts by a saline flush using a double power injector in helical CT of the thorax. AJR Am J Roentgenol 2000;174:1049–1053.
19. Hong C, Becker CR, Huber A, et al. ECG-gated reconstructed multidetector row CT coronary angiography: Effect of varying trigger delay on image quality. Radiology 2001;220:712–717.

20. Hunold P, Vogt FM, Schmermund A, et al. Radiation exposure during cardiac CT: effective doses at multi-detector row CT and electron-beam CT. Radiology 2003;226:145–152.

21. Schroeder S, Kopp AF, Kuettner A, et al. Influence of heart rate on vessel visibility in noninvasive coronary angiography using new multislice computed tomography: experience in 94 patients. Clin Imaging 2002;26(2):106–111.

22. Jakobs TF, Becker CR, Ohnesorge B, et al. Multislice helical CT of the heart with retrospective ECG gating: reduction of radiation exposure by ECG-controlled tube current modulation. Eur Radiol 2002; 12(5):1081–1086.

23. Poll LW, Cohnen M, Brachten S, Ewen K, Modder U. Dose reduction in multi-slice CT of the heart by use of ECG-controlled tube current modulation ("ECG pulsing"): phantom measurements. Rofo Fortschr Geb Rontgenstr Neuen Bildgeb Verfahr 2002;174(12):1500–1505.

24. Lu B, Mao SS, Zhuang N, et al. Coronary artery motion during the cardiac cycle and optimal ECG triggering for coronary artery imaging. Invest Radiol 2001;36:250–256.

25. Achenbach S, Ropers D, Holle J, et al. In-plane coronary arterial motion velocity: measurement with electron-beam CT. Radiology 2000;216:457–463.

26. He S, Dai R, Chen Y, et al. Optimal electrocardiographically triggered phase for reducing motion artifact at electron-beam CT in the coronary artery. Acad Radiol 2001;8: 48–56.

27. Mao SS, Budoff MJ, Bin L, Liu SCK. The optimal ECG trigger point in electron beam volumetric studies: 3 electrocardiographic trigger methods for minimizing motion artifacts. Acad Rad 2001;8(11): 1107–1015.

28. Baumgartner C, Rienmueller R, Bongaerts A, Keru R, Harb S, Weihs W. Measurements of myocardial perfusion using electron beam computed tomography. Am J Card Imaging 1996;10(2) Suppl 1:8.

29. Lu B, Dai R, Bai H, et al. The effects of scanning and reconstruction parameters on image quality of three-dimensional electron-beam tomographic angiography: coronary artery phantom study. Acad Rad 2000;7:927–933.

30. Lu B, Shavelle DM, Mao SS, et al. Improved accuracy of noninvasive electron beam coronary angiography. Invest Radiol 2004;39(2):73–79.

31. Budoff MJ, Achenbach S, Duerinckx A. Clinical utility of computed tomography and magnetic resonance techniques for noninvasive coronary angiography. J Am Coll Cardiol 2003;42;1867–1878.

32. Achenbach S, Ropers D, Regenfus M, Muschiol G, Daniel WG, Moshage W. Contrast enhanced electron beam computed tomography to analyse the coronary arteries in patients after acute myocardial infarction. Heart 2000;84(5):489–493.

33. Napel S, Marks MP, Ruben GD, et al. CT angiography with spiral CT and maximum intensity projection. Radiology 1992;195:607–610.

34. Lu B, Dai RP, Bai H, et al. Detection and analysis of intracoronary artery stent after PTCA using contrast-enhanced three-dimensional electron beam tomography. J Invasive Cardiol 2000;12:1–6.

35. Moshage WE, Achenbach S, Seese B, et al. Coronary artery stenosis: Three-dimensional imaging with electrocardiographically triggered, contrast agent enhanced, electron-beam CT. Radiology 1995;196:707–714.

36. Galanski M, Prokop M, Chavan A, et al. Renal arterial stenosis: spiral CT angiography. Radiology 1993;189:185–192.

37. Achenbach S, Moshage W, Ropers D, Bachmann K. Curved multiplanar reconstructions for the evaluation of contrast-enhanced electron beam CT of the coronary arteries. AJR Am J Roentgenol 1998;170: 895–899.

38. Ota H, Takase K, Igarashi K, et al. MDCT compared with digital subtraction angiography for assessment of lower extremity arterial occlusive disease: importance of reviewing cross-sectional images. AJR Am J Roentgenol 2004;182:201–209.

39. Hoffmann U, Moselewski F, Cury RC, et al. Predictive value of 16-slice multidetector spiral computed tomography to detect significant obstructive coronary artery disease in patients at high risk for coronary artery disease: patient-versus segment-based analysis. Circulation 2004;110(17):2638–2643. Epub 2004 Oct 18.

40. Ropers D, Baum U, Pohle K, et al. Detection of coronary artery stenoses with thin-slice multi-detector row spiral computed tomography and multiplanar reconstruction. Circulation 2003;107:664–666.

41. Nieman K, Cademartiri F, Lemos PA, Raaijmakers R, Pattynama PM, de Feyter PJ. Reliable noninvasive coronary angiography with fast submillimeter multislice spiral computed tomography. Circulation 2002;106:2051–2054.

5

Assessment of Cardiac Structure and Function by X-ray Computed Tomography

John A. Rumberger

Introduction

Contrast ventriculography has long been the standard for assessment of cardiac performance and from knowledge of ejection fraction [1], absolute ventricular volumes [2,3], and definition of the location and extent of regional wall motion abnormalities has provided diagnostic and prognostic information of significant benefit to the clinician. However, non-invasive cardiac imaging has emerged as an alternative which, in many circumstances, has obviated and even replaced traditional contrast left and right ventriculography. In the 1960s ultrasonic imaging of the heart was introduced. Today, two-dimensional echocardiography and Doppler ultrasound are mainstays in clinical practice, and three- and four-dimensional imaging is now feasible. Nuclear medicine techniques followed with multigated imaging of the left ventricle soon after the introduction of clinical ultrasound imaging. Now modern nuclear cardiology studies include not only imaging of the left and right ventricle, but assessments of myocardial perfusion, infarct size, and viability. The technique of NMR (nuclear magnetic resonance) was developing as early as the 1950s and is now widely known as MRI (magnetic resonance imaging). MRI has been established as an important clinical tool in assessing cardiac function and valvular abnormalities.

X-ray computed tomography (CT) of the chest was introduced in the early 1970s with imaging times as long as 30 minutes and image reconstruction times of comparable length. Today, X-ray CT imaging can be done using either a scanning electron beam (EBCT) or validated multidetector CT (MDCT) with rapid acquisition and reconstruction, to facilitate detailed studies of the heart and coronary arteries. The rapid development of computer-assisted imaging, image reconstruction, and three-dimensional registration and rendering of the cardiac, myocardial, and coronary surfaces promises novel methods of looking at the heart which have the potential to extend the boundaries of all other non-invasive cardiac imaging methods.

EBCT is discussed in detail in Chapter 1. It was introduced into clinical imaging in 1984 and validation of its application to define cardiac size, shape, and function followed rapidly. The initial methods involved defining multiple tomographic images, acquired during the cardiac cycle, into specific end-diastolic and end-systolic images at each ventricular level (Figure 5.1). The perimeters of each end-diastolic and end-systolic frame were then defined using a modified Simpson's rule method to quantify global left ventricular (and eventually right ventricular) end-diastolic (EDV) and end-systolic (ESV) volumes and left ventricular muscle mass (Figure 5.2) [4–6]. From this, ejection fraction (EF) was then a straightforward calculation as EF(%) = (EDV – ESV)/EDV × 100.

More modern methods have obviated the need to "trace" each tomographic level and have allowed three-dimensional calculations of volumes and EF using image manipulation performed post acquisition on the computer workstation.

EBCT dominated the field of cardiac CT from 1984 until 2002, when high-resolution MDCT scanners (8–16 channels or greater) came into full production. These scanners allow for gated imaging at multiple tomographic planes with calculations then done using the same computer algorithms used to validate current state-of-the-art EBCT. This chapter is intended to discuss the use of both EBCT and MDCT for assessment of cardiac size and function, additionally imaging of the pericardium will be discussed.

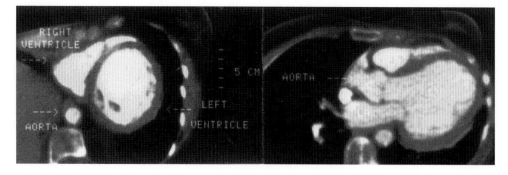

Figure 5.1. Short axis (left) and vertical long axis (right) end-diastolic images from an early EBCT study.

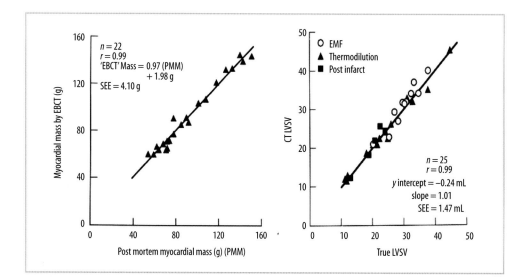

Figure 5.2. Validation studies done using EBCT in quantifying left ventricular muscle mass and left ventricular stroke volume (LVSV). EMF = electromagnetic flow probe, SEE = standard error of the estimate. (Adapted from data presented in Reiter et al. [4] and Feiring et al. [5].)

Nomenclature

Nuclear medicine, echocardiography, cardiac MRI, positron emission tomography (PET), conventional coronary angiography, and cardiac computed tomography have all been used to measure cardiac chamber sizes, muscle mass, wall thicknesses, cardiac chamber function, and for some, myocardial perfusion. Although all of these imaging methods are somewhat different, a major objective in communicating information is consistency and standardization of reporting and nomenclature as it relates to left ventricular viewing and function. Rees et al. proposed as early as 1986 that CT adopt standardized "short" and "long" axis images for CT [7].

The American Heart Association in 2002 [8] published a set of standards for myocardial segmentation and nomenclature for tomographic imaging of the heart for all cardiac imaging modalities. Whenever possible, it is recommended that this be followed for cardiac function as discussed in that publication. Digital cross-sectional or tomographic

imaging by CT as practiced by radiologists has traditionally oriented and displayed the body using planes that were parallel or at 90° degree angle to the long axis of the body, called transaxial or body-plane orthogonal views. The cardiac planes generated by using the long axis of the body do not satisfy the prior standards of cardiac imaging as they do not cleanly transect the ventricles, atria, or myocardial regions as supplied by the major coronary arteries. The two most widely used cardiac imaging methods, single photon emission computed tomography (SPECT) and two-dimensional echocardiography, have defined and oriented the heart for display at 90° relative to the long axis of the left ventricle that transects the apex and the center of the mitral valve plane. This approach then maintains the integrity of the cardiac chambers and the distribution of coronary arterial blood flow. For these reasons, it has been suggested that this approach is optimal for use in research and for clinical patient management involving assessment of cardiac size and function.

The nomenclature suggested is: the short axis, vertical long axis, and horizontal long axis, as shown in Figure 5.3.

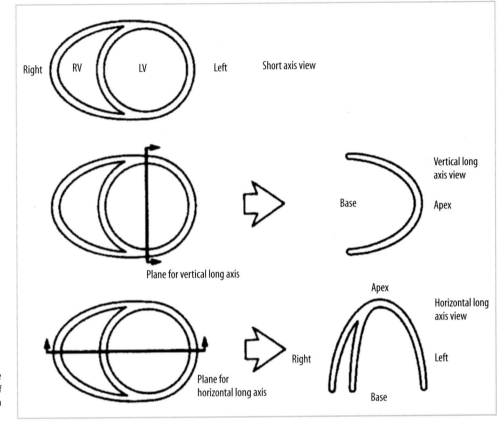

Figure 5.3. Recommended nomenclature and scanning axis for presentation of CT of the left ventricle (LV). (Adapted from Cerqueira et al. [8].)

For those familiar with two-dimensional echocardiography, these correspond to the short axis, apical two-chamber, and apical four-chamber views. These planes are oriented at 90° angles relative to each other.

Methods

EBCT and MDCT acquire CT images using different methods, the former with a scanning electron beam and the latter with a rotating mechanical X-ray source. However, the actual differences are related to potential frame rates and slice thicknesses. EBCT is capable of prospective triggering image rates of 17 frames per second in the 50 ms mode with slice thicknesses ranging from 1.5 mm to 8 mm. MDCT is capable of retrospective gating image rates that nominally are on the order of 4–10 per cardiac cycle. The differences for MDCT relate to the numbers of cardiac cycles used for imaging and the actual tomographic imaging "speed" – ranging from roughly 80 to 300 milliseconds.

EBCT using the e-Speed scanner is capable of up to eight frames per second acquired simultaneously with 1.5 mm contrast-enhanced slices designed to facilitate imaging of the major epicardial coronary arteries (EBA – electron beam angiography, see Chapters 4, 9). MDCT essentially performs the same methods, albeit with a much thinner slice thickness capability than with EBCT. The number of frames taken per cardiac cycle can be predetermined in each method as the scanning sequences are set up.

In order to employ CT to define the cardiac chambers fully and separate them from the ventricular myocardium, it is necessary to use intravenous contrast. In general this can be accomplished with <100 mL of non-ionic contrast and it is possible, with the latest CT scanners, to accomplish complete imaging of the heart chambers, the coronary arteries, and the proximal great vessels (aorta and pulmonary artery) in a single setting with a single injection of contrast.

First it is necessary to determine what is called the "circulation time" to optimize imaging at and during peak systemic circulation contrast enhancement (opacification). That is, the time for contrast, injected into a peripheral (usually cephalic arm vein) vein, to reach the systemic circulation. This is actually a very old concept, developed in the 1950s. Originally this was done using intravenous indocyanine ("green") dye coupled with a densitometer attached to an arterial line. Later magnesium sulfate was administered and the patient asked to state when a bitter taste developed under the tongue (the "arm–tongue time").

In general this crude measure of the circulation time was helpful in defining contrast timing using early applications of EBCT in the 1980s. Later it was determined that, using the flow mode of the EBCT scanner, a limited (as little as 10 mL) contrast injection could be given and the charac-

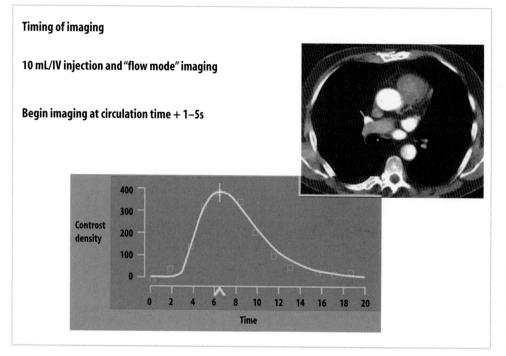

Figure 5.4. Schematic overview of determination of "circulation time" (see text for details). Far right, single image at aortic outflow tract. Region of interest is placed over the aorta. Lower panel shows aortic contrast clearance ("time–density" curve) after bolus intravenous contrast injection.

teristics of the contrast clearance curve in the ascending aorta analyzed to define systemic flow characteristics. This method is still used widely for EBCT imaging (Figure 5.4). "Circulation time" in the normal patient is approximately 12 seconds, but it can be as long as 20–25 seconds in a conditioned athlete with resting bradycardia. Circulation times can also be as long as 45–60 seconds in patients with congestive heart failure. Thus defining circulation time is important so that contrast doses can be kept to a minimum

while maintaining systemic contrast opacification at an adequate level. Current MDCT scanners have "bolus tracking" software installed that basically takes the guesswork out of this calculation. Furthermore, with the more modern 32- and 64-slice scanners, with complete cardiac imaging scanning times on the order of 4–10 seconds, contrast enhancement needs to be at peak for only a short amount of time and under most circumstances optimized imaging is almost assured.

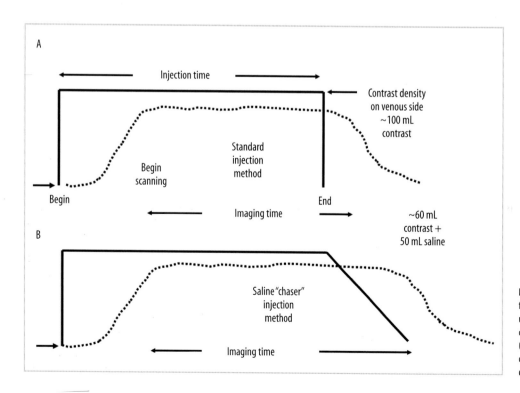

Figure 5.5. Schematic illustration of two different contrast injection methods for CT evaluation of cardiac function. Top: standard contrast injection method at rate of 3–5 mL/s (see text for details). Bottom: "saline chaser" contrast injection method (see text for details).

Contrast injection methods vary largely due to the objective of the imaging. For cardiac size and function by CT, intravenous contrast can be delivered from a standard power-injection, identical to that used in the cardiac catheterization laboratory. Following intravenous contrast injection (nominally at 3–5 mL/s), imaging of the left ventricle can commence at or slightly past the "circulation time." Contrast opacification in the left sided cardiac structures continues as long as contrast is coming into the vein and is still optimized until it then falls off at a time roughly equal to half the circulation time following completion of the intravenous injection. The total time in which the systemic circulation is maximally opacified is called the "imaging time" (Figure 5.5).

Another method that is valuable is to use a dual barreled injection with one barrel filled with iodinated contrast and the other filled with normal saline. At the end of the contrast injection, the saline begins to flow, thus "shoving" the residual contrast in the intravenous line (the "saline chaser") and assisting in moving the residual contrast towards the systemic circulation. The method actually allows for a longer "imaging time" and also can be used to actually reduce the total contrast administered to the patient (Figure 5.5).

Another method that also helps reduce the amount of contrast administered is to take advantage of the inevitable contrast "recirculation." Contrast can be injected at a nominal rate of 3–5 mL/s for a preset time and then reduced to a slower rate (e.g. 1–2 mL/s), taking advantage of venous to systemic recirculation of the earlier injected contrast.

Tumors, Thrombi, Acquired and Congenital Abnormalities

Orthogonal (short and various long axis) CT images with intravenous contrast allow for identification of non-opacified intracardiac thrombi and tumors with, in particular, excellent resolution (especially with the newer MDCT systems) of the left atrium and the left atrial appendage, allowing identification of structures smaller than 1 mm [9, 9a]. CT can also be used to detect tumor neovascularity. CT can additionally be of assistance in defining thrombi or occult occlusion of the venae cavae and other right-sided structures. Cardiac CT can also be a primary method of defining intracardiac shunts such as those caused by inter-atrial and interventricular defects [10].

Ventricular Anatomy and Function

Computed tomography (EBCT and MDCT) can be used to quantitate left and right ventricular volumes [4,11,12], left and right atrial volumes, left and right ventricular muscle mass [6,11,13,14], regional left ventricular function and wall thickening and contractility [15–21], rates of diastolic filling of the right and left ventricles [22–25], post-infarction left and right ventricular remodeling [26–29], cardiac remodeling following cardiac [30] and lung transplantation [31], and ejection fraction [32–34] in patients with no contraindication to the use of iodinated contrast medium. Additional applications include quantitation of uni-valvular regurgitation [35] and assessment of infarct size [36,37]. The majority of these validation studies were performed in the 1980s and 1990s using EBCT and have been adapted and validated in many instances using MDCT at the turn of the century. In most instances, these quantitative aspects can be performed or at least well approximated in patients with generally normal sinus rhythm. Since the number of cardiac cycles imaged per scan is generally single or limited to <5, quantitation may be limited in those patients with significant dysrhythmias, such as atrial fibrillation.

Normal adult values had been established by EBCT in the mid 1980s [38] for left ventricular mass ($98 \pm 18\,g/m^2$), end-diastolic volume ($73 \pm 19\,mL/m^2$), end-systolic volume ($24 \pm 8\,mL/m^2$), and stroke volume ($48 \pm 11\,mL/m^2$). Comparisons of left ventricular ejection fraction with the standard of radionuclide angiography were also established at this time with correlations of $r = 0.94$ across a broad variety of values from 20% to 80%. Reproducibility of CT in performing right and left ventricular volume and function measurements was also firmly established [39] (Figure 5.6).

CT imaging using thin sections allows post-processing of images into end-diastolic and end-systolic short and "long" axis images to facilitate identification of structures and salient features of the ventricular anatomy (Figure 5.7). Using short and long axis imaging also allows for identification of infarct locations and, as noted above, infarct size (Figure 5.8). Demonstrated in this latter example is a common CT finding in contrast-enhanced images from patients with remote myocardial infarction. The "negative" contrast noted in Figure 5.8 is actually due to lack of contrast opacification in the infarcted region causing "contrast rarefaction." Long axis (both vertical and horizontal) imaging of the left ventricle also allows for definition of apical thrombi (Figure 5.9) and apical infarcts and pseudo- and true apical aneurysms (Figure 5.10). Two-dimensional and three-dimensional reconstruction methods, possible in nearly an infinite number of imaging planes, also allows for postoperative assessment of successful left ventricular aneurysectomy (Figure 5.11). The right ventricle can also be imaged. Figure 5.12 shows a dilated right ventricle in a patient with arrhythmogenic right ventricular dysplasia; CT can often be an alternative or a confirmatory method to MRI in the evaluation of such patients.

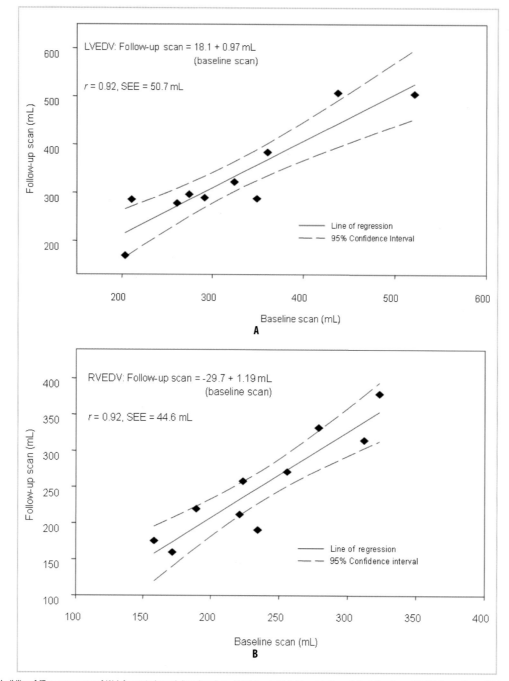

Figure 5.6. Reproducibility of CT measurements of (**A**) left ventricular end-diastolic volume (LVEDV) and (**B**) right ventricular end-diastolic volume (RVEDV). Ten patients with known dilated cardiomy-opathy studied at baseline with repeat studies at 2-week follow-up. (Data adapted from Schmermund et al. [39].)

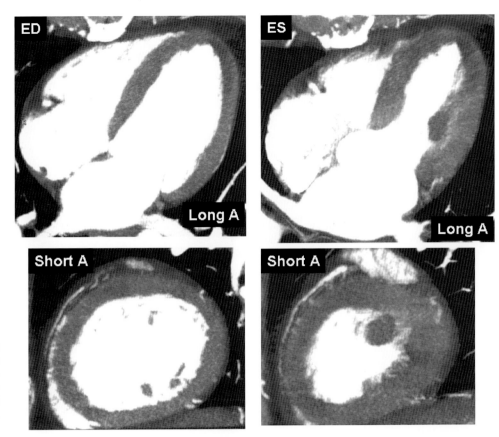

Figure 5.7. Top panels: Vertical long axis (Long A) end-diastolic (ED) and end-systolic (ES) images in a patient with normal left ventricular ejection fraction, but apical hypokinesis. Bottom panels: Short axis end-diastolic and end-systolic images in the same patient. Images are from a 32-slice MDCT scan.

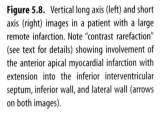

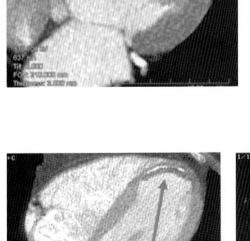

Figure 5.8. Vertical long axis (left) and short axis (right) images in a patient with a large remote infarction. Note "contrast rarefaction" (see text for details) showing involvement of the anterior apical myocardial infarction with extension into the inferior interventricular septum, inferior wall, and lateral wall (arrows on both images).

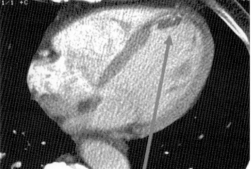

Figure 5.9. Vertical long axis tomograms at two different left ventricular tomographic levels. This patient had a two-dimensional echocardiogram that resulted in incomplete imaging of the ventricular apex and a question of a thrombus. The image on the left shows calcification from a remote mural hemorrhage and the image on the right shows the clearly delineated ventricular thrombus (see arrows).

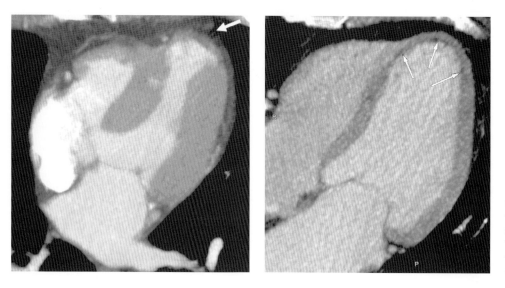

Figure 5.10. Vertical long axis images from two different patients. The image on the left shows an apical aneurysm without thrombus. The image on the right shows a completed transmural infarction with apical thinning (arrows). P = posterior, R = right.

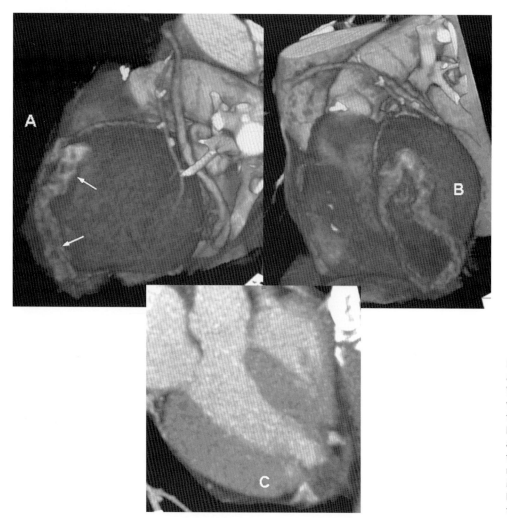

Figure 5.11. Images from a patient who had a left ventricular aneurysectomy and repair. **A** Volume-rendered 3-D image from a lateral view. The repair is indicated by arrows. Incidentally noted is a patent left internal mammary bypass graft to the first obtuse marginal artery and a patent saphenous vein bypass graft to the second obtuse marginal artery. **B** Volume-rendered 3-D image from an anterior view. **C** Maximum intensity projection of the vertical long axis showing the partially opacified ventricular apex and the repair soffits.

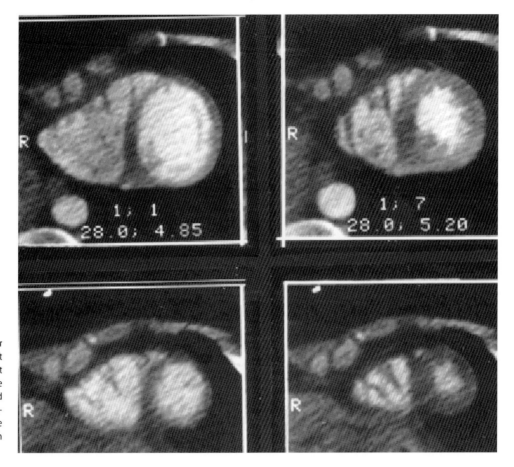

Figure 5.12. Four short axis images at four different ventricular levels showing the left ventricle (right side of images) and the right ventricle (left side of the images). Note that the right ventricle is significantly dilated compared to the left ventricle. Furthermore, the right ventricle has deep trabeculations. Both of these characteristics are common in patients with right ventricular dysplasia.

Chamber Measurements

Three-dimensional calipers available on virtually all CT workstations allow for quantitative measures of ventricular dimensions in any axis (Figure 5.13). Additionally, measures of ventricular muscle thicknesses can be done on all myocardial walls (Figure 5.14). Measures of the aorta and other chambers such as the left atrium (Figure 5.15) can also be helpful and augment data on ventricular volumes, muscle mass, and function by CT.

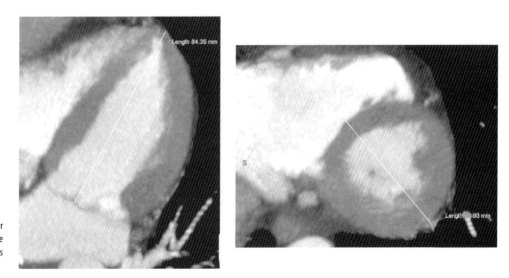

Figure 5.13. Three-dimensional caliber measurements of the left ventricle from the vertical long axis (left) and the short axis (right).

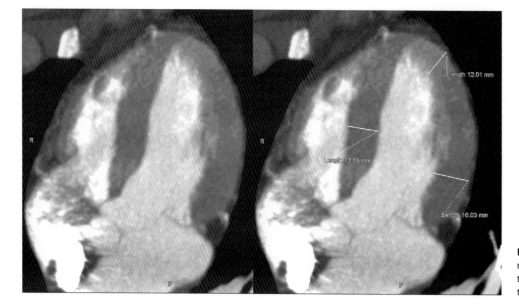

Figure 5.14. Three-dimensional caliber measurements of the myocardial walls in a vertical long axis image. This patient has concentric left ventricular hypertrophy.

Diseases of the Pericardium

Normal layers of fat on the epicardial surface of the heart and the outer surface of the pericardial sac provide natural contrast and permit the examiner to reliably identify the pericardium. Contrast-enhanced CT often allows separating chronic effusive pericarditis from gross pericardial thickening since the parietal and epicardial layers of the pericardium have their own blood supply. CT can be used to define the entire anatomy of the pericardium and may be of greatest value in localization of loculated effusions such as those confined to the posterior areas of the heart (which are difficult to define using surface two-dimensional echocardiography). Tamponade can be identified with CT by right atrial or ventricular collapse or by indirect signs such as an inappropriately enlarged inferior vena cava or enlarged hepatic veins. High-resolution images can define the anatomic localization and extent of pericardial thickening. In the evaluation of a patient for constrictive pericarditis, CT can add considerably to the diagnosis (Figure 5.16). CT has an advantage over traditional echocardiography in that the entire cardiac volume is imaged very quickly and then images of both two-dimensional and three-dimensional views can be rapidly generated (Figure 5.17). Contrast is usually not required to image the pericardium, as the natural delineation of the pericardial surface (usually 100 HU) and adjacent air (minus 1000 HU) is dramatic. Calcified pericardial tissue is even easier to image, as the calcification is usually in the 300–400 HU range.

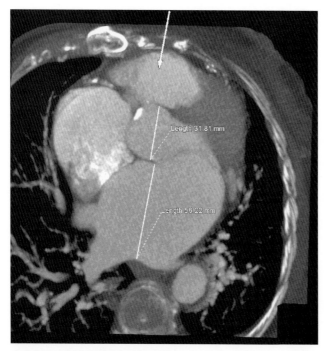

Figure 5.15. Neutral axis CT image of the aorta and a significantly dilated left atrium. The anterior structure (arrow) is the right ventricular outflow tract.

Conclusions

There have been extensive validations using EBCT for virtually all cardiac size, shape, and functional measures and these were established long before such measures were attempted by MRI. Recent improvements in spiral/helical

CT have also accorded this validity to MDCT. CT then becomes a very robust method to define the heart and its detailed anatomy in health and in disease. Furthermore, these types of measures can be accomplished during post-processing of images intended to define coronary artery anatomy, generally without the need for additional imaging. The disadvantage is that additional sets of cardiac data are required at various portions of the cardiac cycle (nominally at end-diastole and end-systole) and this then obligates concomitant increases in radiation exposure to the patient. That said, CT is a very robust method that can function as both a primary method and a complementary method (such as to echocardiography, contrast ventriculography, radionuclide angiography, and MRI) to quantitate details of cardiac anatomy and function.

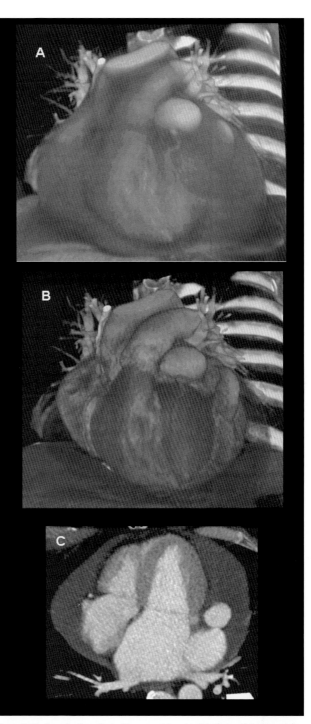

Figure 5.17. Example of a patient with a concentric pericardial effusion. **A** Anterior volume-rendered 3-D image rendered to demonstrate the external cardiac silhouette. **B** Anterior volume-rendered 3-D image as in **A**, but rendered to demonstrate the epicardial surface of the heart. Note the differences in the perceived heart size. **C** Maximum intensity (2-D) horizontal long axis image of the heart showing the four cardiac chambers (opacified) and the circumferential pericardial effusion (lowered attenuation).

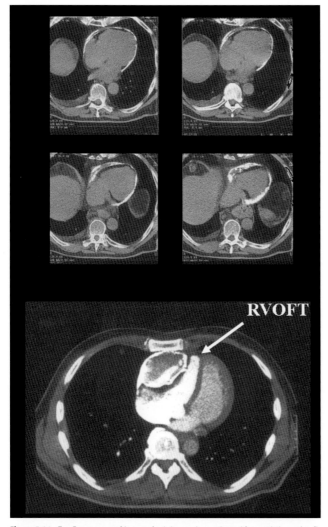

Figure 5.16. Top: Four tomographic neutral axis images in a patient with constrictive pericarditis. Note the concentric, thick calcification. This patient had a remote history of tuberculosis. Bottom: Calcified pericardial cyst causing right ventricular outflow tract (RVOFT) obstruction and mimicking symptoms that initially suggested constrictive pericarditis.

References

1. Hammermeister KE, DeRouen TA, Dodge HT. Variables predictive of survival with coronary disease: selection by univariate and multivariate analyses from the clinical, electrocardiographic, exercise, arteriographic and quantitative angiographic evaluation. Circulation 1979;59:421–450.

2. Norris RW, Barnaby PF, Brandt PWT. Prognosis after recovery from first acute myocardial infarction: determinant of reinfarction and sudden death. Am J Cardiol 1984;53:408–413.

3. White HD, Norris RM, Brown MA, Brandt PWJ, Whitlock RML, Weld CJ. Left ventricular end-systolic volume as the major determinant of survival after recovery from myocardial infarction. Circulation 1987;76:44–51.

4. Reiter SJ, Rumberger JA, Feiring AJ, Stanford W, Marcus ML. Precision of right and left ventricular stroke volume measurements by rapid acquisition cine computed tomography. Circulation 1986;74:890–900.

5. Feiring AJ, Rumberger JA, Reiter SJ, et al. Sectional and segmental variability of left ventricular function: experimental and clinical studies using ultrafast computed tomography. J Am Coll Cardiol 1988;12:415–425.

6. Feiring AJ, Rumberger JA, Skorton DJ, et al. Determination of left ventricular mass in the dog with rapid acquisition cardiac CT scanning. Circulation 1985;72:1355–1362.

7. Rees MJ, Feiring AJ, Rumberger JA, MacMillan RM, Clark DL. Heart evaluation by cine CT: use of two new oblique views. Radiology 1986;159:804.

8. Cerqueira MD, Weissman NJ, Dilsizian V, et al. Standardized myocardial segmentation and nomenclature for tomographic imaging of the heart – a statement for healthcare professions from the Cardiac Imaging Committee of the Council on Clinical Cardiology of the American Heart Association. Circulation 2002;105:539–542.

9. Achenbach S, Sacher D, Ropers D, Pohle K, Nixdorff U, Hoffman U, Muschiol G, Flachskampf PA, Daniel WW. Electron beam computed tomograph for the detection of left atrial thrombi in patients with atrial fibrillation. Heart 2004;90(12):1477–1478.

9a. Meinel JF, Wang G, Jiang M, et al. Spatial variation of resolution and noise in multi-detector row spiral CT. Acad Radiol 2003;10:607–610.

10. Paul JF, Mace L, Caussin C, et al. Multirow detector computed tomography assessment of intraseptal dissection and ventricular pseudoaneurysm in postinfarction ventricular septal defect. Circulation 2001;104:497–498.

11. Yamamuro M, Tadamura E, Kubo S, et al. Cardiac functional analysis with multi-detector row CT and segmental reconstruction algorithm: comparison with echocardiography, SPECT, and MR imaging. Radiology 2005;234:381–390.

12. Halliburton SS, Petersilka M, Schvartzman PR, Obuchowski N, White RD. Evaluation of left ventricular dysfunction using multiphasic reconstructions of coronary multi-slice computed tomography data in patients with chronic ischemic heart disease: validation against cine magnetic resonance imaging. Int J Cardiovasc Imaging 2003;19:73–83.

13. Hajduczok Z, Weiss RM, Marcus ML, Stanford W. Determination of right ventricular mass in humans and dogs with ultrafast computed tomography. Circulation 1990;82:202.

14. Kuroda T, Seward JB, Rumberger JA, Yanagi H, Tajik AJ. Left ventricular volume and mass: comparative study of 2-dimensional echocardiography and ultrafast computed tomography. Echocardiography 1994;11:1–9.

15. Feiring AJ, Rumberger JA, Reiter SJ, et al. Sectional and segmental variability of left ventricular function: Experimental and clinical studies using ultrafast computed tomography. J Am Coll Cardiol 1988;12:415.

16. Lanzer P, Garrett J, Lipton MJ, et al. Quantitation of regional myocardial function by cine computed tomography: pharmacologic changes in wall thickness. J Am Coll Cardiol 1986;8:682.

17. Rumberger JA. Quantifying left ventricular regional and global systolic function using ultrafast computed tomography. Am J Card Imaging 1991;5:29.

18. Rumberger JA. Quantifying left ventricular regional and global systolic function using ultrafast computed tomography. Am J Card Imaging 1991;5(1):29–37.

19. Feiring AJ, Rumberger JA: Ultrafast computed tomography analysis of regional radius-to-wall thickness ratios in normal and volume-overloaded human left ventricle. Circulation 1992;85:1423–1432.

20. Lanzer P, Garrett J, Lipton MJ, et al. Quantitation of regional myocardial function by cine computed tomography: pharmacologic changes in wall thickness. J Am Coll Cardiol 1986;8:682–692.

21. Sehgal M, Hirose K, Reed JE, Rumberger JA. Regional left ventricular systolic thickening and thicknesses during the first year after initial Q-wave myocardial infarction: serial effects of ventricular remodeling. Int J Cardiol 1996;53:45–54.

22. Rumberger, JA, Weiss, RM, Feiring, AJ, et al. Patterns of regional diastolic function in the normal human left ventricle: An ultrafast-CT study. J Am Coll Cardiol 1989;13:119.

23. Lipton MJ, Rumberger JA. The assessment of left ventricular systolic and diastolic function by ultrafast computed tomography. Am J Card Imaging 1991;5:318–327.

24. Rumberger JA, Reed JE. Quantitative dynamics of left ventricular emptying and filling as a function of heart size and stroke volume in pure aortic regurgitation and in normal subjects. Am J Cardiol 1992;70:1045–1050.

25. Hirose K, Reed JE, Rumberger JA. Serial changes in left and right ventricular systolic and diastolic mechanics during the first year after an initial left ventricular Q-wave myocardial infarction. J Am Coll Cardiol 1995;25:1097–1104.

26. Rumberger JA, Behrenbeck T, Breen JR, Reed JE, Gersh BJ. Nonparallel changes in global chamber volume and muscle mass during the first year following transmural myocardial infarction in man. J Am Coll Cardiol 1993;21:673–682.

27. Hirose K, Reed JE, Rumberger JA. Serial changes in left and right ventricular systolic and diastolic mechanics during the first year after an initial left ventricular Q-wave myocardial infarction. J Am Coll Cardiol 1995;25:1097.

28. Hirose K, Shu NH, Reed JE, Rumberger JA. Right ventricular dilatation and remodeling the first year after an initial transmural wall myocardial infarction. Am J Cardiol 1993;72:1126.

29. Chareonthaitawee P, Christian TF, Hirose K, Gibbons, Rumberger JA. Relation of initial infarct size with the extent of left ventricular remodeling in the year after acute myocardial infarction. J Am Coll Cardiol 1995;25:567–573.

30. Vigneswaran WT, Rumberger JA, Rodeheffer RJ, Breen JF, McGregor CGA. Ventricular remodeling following orthotopic cardiac transplantation. Mayo Clin Proc 1996;71:735–742.

31. Rensing BJ, McDougall JC, Breen JR, Vigneswaran WT, McGregor CGA, Rumberger JA. Right and left ventricular remodeling after orthotopic single lung transplantation for end-stage emphysema. J Heart Lung Transplant 1997;16:926–933.

32. Gerber T, Rumberger JA, Gibbons R, Behrenbeck T. Measurement of left ventricular ejection fraction by TC-99M sestamibi first-pass angiography in patients with myocardial infarction: comparison with electron beam computed tomography. Am J Cardiol 1999;83:1022–1026.

32. Schuijf JD, Bax JJ, Jukema JW, et al. Noninvasive angiography and assessment of left ventricular function using multislice computed tomography in patients with type 2 diabetes. Diabetes Care 2004;27:2905–2910.

34. Dirksen JS, Bax JJ, de Roos A, et al. Usefulness of dynamic multislice computed tomography of left ventricular function in unstable angina pectoris and comparison with echocardiography. Am J Cardiol 2002;90;1157–1160.

35. Reiter SJ, Rumberger JA, Stanford W, Marcus ML. Quantitative determination of aortic regurgitant volume by cine computed tomography. Circulation 1986;76:728.

36. Weiss RM, Stark CA, Rumberger JA, Marcus ML. Identification and quantitation of myocardial infarction or risk area size with cine-computed tomography. Am J Card Imaging 1990;4:33–37.

37. Schmermund A, Gerber T, Behrenbeck T, et al. Measurement of myocardial infarct size by electron beam computed tomography: a comparison with ^{99m}Tc sestamibi. Invest Radiol 1998;33:313–321.

38. Rumberger JA, Sheedy PF, Breen JF. Use of ultrafast (cine) x-ray computed tomography in cardiac and cardiovascular imaging. In: Giuliani ER, Gersh BJ, McGoon MD, Hayes DL, Schaff HF (eds) Mayo Clinic practice of cardiology, 3rd edn. St Louis: Mosby, 1996: 303–324.

39. Schmermund A, Breen JF, Sheedy PF, Rumberger JA. Reproducibility of right and left ventricular volume measurements by electron-beam CT in patients with congestive heart failure. Int J Card Imaging 1998;14(3):201–209.

6

Assessment of Cardiovascular Calcium: Interpretation and Relevance of Calcium Scoring Relationship to Lipids and Other Cardiovascular Risk Factors

Harvey S. Hecht

Cardiac risk assessment has traditionally been based on conventional risk factors; the shortcomings of this approach are all too often highlighted by major cardiac events occurring in presumably low-risk people. The annual presentation of 650,000 previously asymptomatic patients with an acute coronary event as the initial manifestation of coronary artery disease (CAD) [1] is a testimony to the failure of our current risk assessment model. Consequently, there has been a focus on markers of subclinical atherosclerosis that may be utilized for risk assessment of individuals, rather than extrapolating from risk factors that reflect trends in large groups of patients in epidemiologic studies. The most powerful of these subclinical markers is coronary artery calcium (CAC).

Background

CAC is pathognomonic for atherosclerosis [2–4]. Mönckeberg's calcific medial sclerosis does not occur in the coronary arteries [5]; atherosclerosis is the only vascular disease known to be associated with coronary calcification. Calcium phosphate (in the hydroxyapatite form) and cholesterol accumulate in atherosclerotic lesions. Circulating proteins that are normally associated with bone remodeling play an important role in coronary calcification, and arterial calcium in atherosclerosis is a regulated active process similar to bone formation, rather than a passive precipitation of calcium phosphate crystals [6–9].

Rumberger et al. [10] demonstrated that the total area of coronary artery calcification is highly correlated ($r = 0.9$) in a linear fashion with the total area of coronary artery plaque on a segmental, individual, and whole coronary artery system basis (Figure 6.1), and the areas of coronary calcification comprise approximately one fifth that of the

associated coronary plaque. Additionally, there were plaque areas without associated coronary calcium, suggesting that there may be a coronary plaque size most commonly associated with coronary calcium but, in the smaller plaques, the calcium is either not present or is undetectable. Intravascular ultrasound [11,12] measures of combined calcified and non-calcified plaque confirm the strong relationship (Figure 6.2).

Methodology

Technical

Until recently the data substantiating the importance of coronary artery calcium has been derived almost exclusively through the use of electron beam tomography (EBT), utilizing a rotating electron beam to acquire prospectively triggered, tomographic 100-millisecond X-ray images at 3 mm intervals in the space of a 30- to 40-second breathhold. The multidetector computed tomography (MDCT) technology is a more recent development and employs a rotating gantry with a special X-ray tube and variable number of detectors (from 4 to 64), with 165–375-millisecond images at 0.5, 1.5, 2.0, or 3.0 mm intervals depending on the protocol and manufacturer.

Scoring

The presence of coronary calcium is sequentially quantified through the entire epicardial coronary system. Coronary calcium is defined as a lesion above a threshold of 130 Hounsfield units (which range from −1000 (air), through 0 (water), and up to +1000 (dense cortical bone)), with an area of three or more adjacent pixels (at least

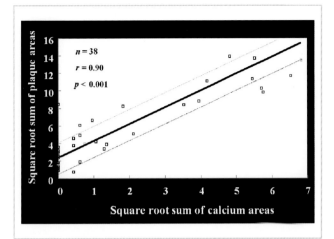

Figure 6.1. Correlation between calcified and total plaque burden in histopathologic coronary artery specimens. (Rumberger JA, Simons DB, Fitzpatrick LA, et al. Coronary artery calcium area by electron-beam computed tomography and coronary atherosclerotic plaque area: A histopathologic correlative study. circulation 1995;92:2157–2162. With permission from Lippincott Williams & Wilkins.)

1 mm^2). The original calcium score developed by Agatston et al. [13] is determined by the product of the calcified plaque area and maximum calcium lesion density (from 1 to 4 based upon Hounsfield units). Standardized categories for the calcium score have been developed with scores of 1–10 considered minimal, 11–100 mild, 101–400 moderate, and >400 severe. Examples are shown in Figure 6.1. The calcium volume score [14] is a more reproducible parameter that is independent of calcium density and is considered to be the parameter of choice for serial studies to track

progression or regression of atherosclerosis. Phantom-based calcium mass scores are being developed that will be applicable to any CT scanner [15], but have yet to be validated. Examples of CAC scans are shown in Figure 6.3.

Epidemiology

By comparing a person's calcium score to others of the same age and gender through the use of large databases of asymptomatic subjects, a *calcium percentile* is generated [16]. This is an index of the prematurity of atherosclerosis; for example, a 50-year-old man in the 76th percentile has more plaque than 75% but less plaque than 24% of asymptomatic 50-year-old men. Although there is an increasing incidence of coronary calcification with increasing age (Figure 6.4), this simply parallels the development of coronary atherosclerosis. Table 6.1 shows coronary calcification incidence by EBT in an unselected patient population of men and women [17]. The amount of coronary artery calcium in women is similar to that in men a decade younger, paralleling the 10-year lag in women of the development of clinical atherosclerosis. Useful though these current nomograms are, variations according to ethnicity have been described and data regarding these variations are still being collected and separated. Blacks have been noted to have either lower [18,19] or similar [20,21] amounts of CAC as Caucasians of the same age; Hispanics may have less CAC than Caucasians [18]. Thus, the application of predictive indices from these tables in non-

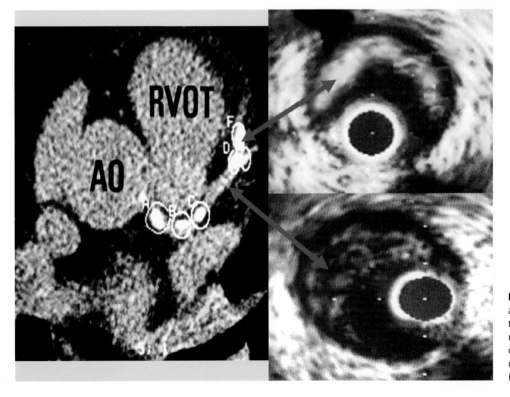

Figure 6.2. EBT scan (left) demonstrating areas of extensive calcification corresponding to heavily calcified plaque on intravascular ultrasound (upper right), and less extensive calcification corresponding to less heavily calcified plaque on intravascular ultrasound (lower right).

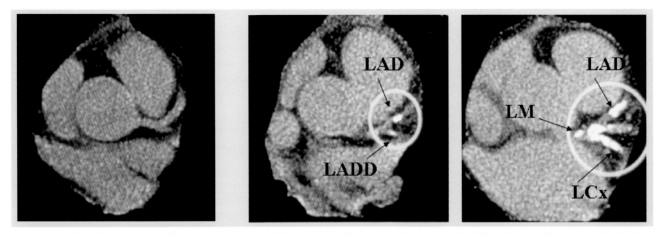

Figure 6.3. Examples of EBT coronary artery calcium scans. Left: normal without CAC. Center: moderate CAC involving the left anterior descending (LAD) and circumflex (LCx) coronary arteries. Right: Extensive CAC involving the left main (LM), anterior descending and circumflex coronary arteries.

Caucasians should be used with caution. Younger patients with a family history of premature CAD have significantly higher CAC scores than similar aged individuals without this risk factor, particularly if there is a sibling history of premature CAD [22].

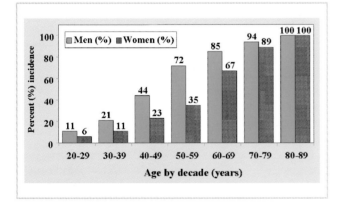

Figure 6.4. Prevalence of CAC in men and women by decades. (Reprinted from Janowitz WR, Agatston AS, Kaplan G, et al. Differences in prevalence and extent of coronary artery oalcium detected by ultrafast computed tomography in asymptomatic men and women. Am J Cardiol 1993;72:251. With permission from Excerpta Medica, Inc.)

Coronary Artery Calcium and Obstructive Disease

Key Correlative Studies

The relationship of CAC to obstructive disease has been extensively investigated, and was misunderstood by the 2000 ACC/AHA Consensus Document on EBT [23], which focused on the low specificity as a critical flaw. While the presence of CAC is nearly 100% specific for atherosclerosis, it is not specific for obstructive disease since both obstructive and non-obstructive lesions have calcification present in the intima. Comparisons with pathology specimens have shown that the degree of luminal narrowing is weakly correlated with the amount of calcification on a site-by-site basis [24–26], whereas the likelihood of significant obstruction increases with the total CAC score [27–29].

Shavelle et al. [30] reported a 96% sensitivity and 47% specificity for a calcium score >0, with a relative risk for obstructive disease of 4.5, compared to a 76% sensitivity

Table 6.1. Calcium percentile database for asymptomatic men and women: EBT coronary calcium scores as a function of patient age at the time of examination

Percentiles	40–45 years	46–50 years	51–55 years	56–60 years	61–65 years	66–70 years	71–75 years
Men (n = 28,250)							
10	0	0	0	1	1	3	3
25	0	1	2	5	12	30	69
50	2	3	15	54	117	166	350
75	11	36	110	229	386	538	844
90	69	151	346	588	933	1151	1650
Women (n = 14,540)							
10	0	0	0	0	0	0	0
25	0	0	0	0	0	1	4
50	0	0	1	1	3	25	51
75	1	2	6	22	68	148	231
90	4	21	61	127	208	327	698

and 60% specificity for treadmill testing, with a relative risk of 1.7. Bielak et al. [31] noted a sensitivity and specificity of 99.1% and 38.6% for a calcium score >0. However, when corrected for verification bias, the specificity improved to 72.4%, without loss of sensitivity (97%). The likelihood ratio for obstruction ranged from 0.03–0.07 in men and women ≥50 years of age for 0 scores to 12.85 for scores >200. In the <50 years cohort, the likelihood ratios ranged from 0.1–0.29 for 0 scores to 54–189 for scores >100. Rumberger et al. [32] demonstrated that higher calcium scores are associated with a greater specificity for obstructive disease at the expense of sensitivity; for example, a threshold score of 368 was 95% specific for the presence of obstructive CAD. In 1764 persons undergoing angiography the sensitivity and negative predictive value in men and women were >99% [33]; a score of 0 virtually excluded patients with obstructive CAD. In a separate study of 1851 patients undergoing CAC scanning and angiography [34], CAC scanning by EBT in conjunction with pretest probability of disease derived by a combination of age, gender, and risk factors, facilitated prediction of the severity and extent of angiographically significant CAD in symptomatic patients.

Prognostic Studies in Symptomatic Patients

The prognostic value of extensive coronary calcium (>1000) in symptomatic males with established advanced CAD was demonstrated in a 5-year follow-up study of 150 patients [35], but does not justify its use in this setting, since maximal therapy is indicated irrespective of the CAC score. CAC scanning is not routinely recommended in patients with classical angina symptoms. However, in those with atypical chest pain, a 0 or very low CAC score would render obstructive disease very unlikely.

Clarification

Despite the apparently reasonable specificities, which are similar to those of stress testing, it must be understood that

the purpose of CAC scanning is not to detect obstructive disease and, therefore, it is inappropriate to even use "specificity" in the context of obstruction. Rather, its purpose is to detect subclinical atherosclerosis in its early stages, for which it is virtually 100% specific.

Key Prognostic Studies in Primary Prevention

The utility of CAC for risk evaluation in the asymptomatic primary prevention population is dependent on prognostic studies documenting the relative risk conferred by calcified plaque quantitation compared to conventional risk factors (Table 6.2). Raggi et al. [36] demonstrated, in 632 asymptomatic patients followed for 32 months, an annualized event rate of 0.1%/year in patients with 0 scores, compared to 2.1%/year with scores of 1–99, 4.1%/year with scores of 100–400, and 4.8%/year with scores >400. Thus, the annualized event rates associated with coronary calcium were in the range considered to warrant secondary prevention classification by the Framingham Risk Score (Figure 6.5). The odds ratio conferred by a calcium percentile >75 % was 21.5 times greater than for the lowest 25%, compared to an odds ratio of 7 for the highest versus lowest quartiles of National Cholesterol Education Program (NCEP) risk factors (Figure 6.6).

Wong et al. [37], in 926 asymptomatic patients followed for 3.3 years, noted a relative risk of 8 for scores >270, after adjusting for age, gender, hypertension, high cholesterol, smoking, and diabetes. Arad et al. [38], in 1132 subjects followed for 3.6 years, reported odds ratios of 14.3–20.2 for scores ranging from >80 to >600; these were 3–7 times greater than for the NCEP risk factors.

In a retrospective analysis of 5635 asymptomatic, predominantly low to moderate risk, largely middle-aged patients followed for 37 ± 12 months, Kondos et al. [39] found that the presence of any CAC by EBT was associated with a relative risk for events of 10.5, compared to 1.98 and 1.4 for diabetes and smoking, respectively. In women, only CAC was linked to events, with a relative risk of 2.6; risk

Table 6.2. Prognostic studies using electron beam computed tomography in asymptomatic patients

Author	Number	Mean age (years)	Follow-up duration (years)	Calcium score cutoff	Comparator group for RR calculation	Risk ratio
Raggi et al. [36]	632	52	2.7	Top quartile	Lowest quartile	13
Wong et al. [37]	926	54	3.3	Top quartile (>270)	First score quartile	8.8
Arad et al. [38]	1,173	53	3.6	CAC >160	CAC <160	20.2
Kondos et al. [39]	5,635	51	3.1	CAC	No CAC	10.5
Shaw et al. [40]	10,377	53	5	CAC 401–1000	CAC <10	2.54[a]
Arad et al. [42]	5,585	59	4.3	CAC ≥100	CAC <100	10.7
Greenland et al. [41]	1,312	66	7.0	CAC >300	No CAC	3.9

CAC = coronary artery calcium score, RR = relative risk.
[a] Patients with scores >1000 had higher risk and were not included in this RR.

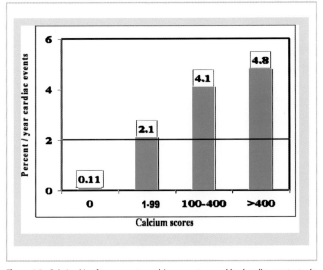

Figure 6.5. Relationship of coronary artery calcium score to annual hard cardiac event rates in 632 asymptomatic patients undergoing EBT calcified plaque imaging. The solid line indicates the 2%/year event rate consistent with secondary prevention risk.

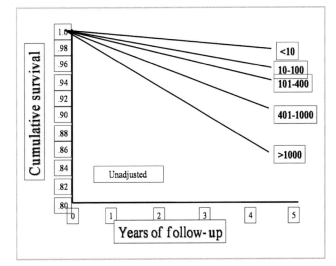

Figure 6.7. Cumulative survival of 10,377 patients from the National Death Registry according to coronary artery calcium categories. (Shaw LJ, Raggi P, Schisterman E, et al. Prognostic value of cardiac risk factors and coronary artery calcium screening for all-cause mortality. Radiology 2003;28:831.)

factors were not related. The presence of CAC provided prognostic information incremental to age and other risk factors.

Shaw et al. [40] retrospectively analyzed 10,377 asymptomatic patients with a 5-year follow-up after an initial EBT evaluation. All-cause mortality increased proportional to CAC (Figure 6.7), which was an independent predictor of risk after adjusting for all of the Framingham risk factors ($p < 0.001$). Superiority of CAC to conventional Framingham risk factor assessment was demonstrated by a significantly greater area under the ROC curves (0.73 versus 0.67, $p < 0.001$). Incremental value of CAC to Framingham risk was also established by a significant increase of the area under the ROC curves, from 0.72 for Framing-

ham risk to 0.78 with the addition of CAC ($p < 0.001$). Risk stratification was present in each risk group, and was particularly strong in the 10–20-year Framingham risk group. Stratification of mortality risk by CAC score was as effective in women as in men.

Greenland et al. [41] analyzed a population-based study of 1461 prospectively followed, asymptomatic subjects who were predominantly moderate to high risk, and found that CAC scores >300 significantly added prognostic information to Framingham risk analysis in the 10–20% Framingham risk category.

The results of the St Francis Heart Study by Arad et al. [42] in a prospective, population-based study of 5585 asymptomatic, predominantly moderate- to moderately high-risk men and women, mirrored previous retrospective studies [7,18–20], and confirmed the higher event rates associated with increasing CAC scores. CAC scores >100 were associated with relative risks of from 12 to 32, and were secondary prevention equivalent, with event rates >2%/year (Figure 6.8). Incremental information over Framingham scores was documented, with areas under the ROC curves of 0.81 for CAC and 0.71 for Framingham ($p < 0.01$). Importantly, classification by CAC tertiles changed the risk group of approximately 67% of patients classified in the Framingham 10–20% 10-year event rate group to either lower or higher risk. The appropriateness of this change was confirmed by outcome measures of cardiac events. Furthermore, in the Framingham high-risk category (>20% 10-year event rate), 45% were correctly moved to lower-risk categories by CAC tertile reclassification. Finally, in the Framingham <10% 10-year risk group, 29% had scores >100 with an associated 1.7%/year event rate (Figure 6.9).

The prognostic significance of very high calcium scores was provided in a study of 98 asymptomatic patients with

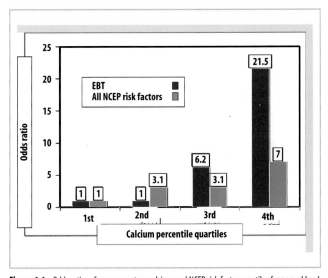

Figure 6.6. Odds ratios of coronary artery calcium and NCEP risk factor quartiles for annual hard cardiac event rates in asymptomatic patients undergoing EBT calcified plaque imaging.

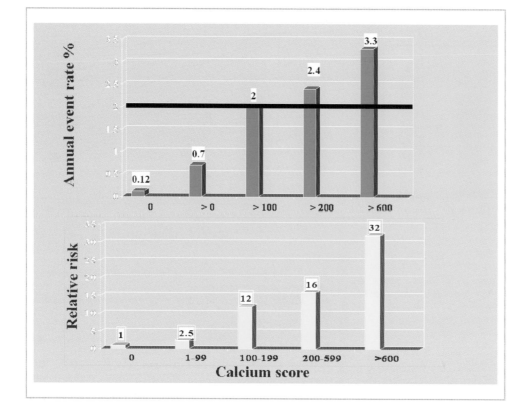

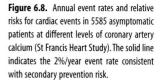

Figure 6.8. Annual event rates and relative risks for cardiac events in 5585 asymptomatic patients at different levels of coronary artery calcium (St Francis Heart Study). The solid line indicates the 2%/year event rate consistent with secondary prevention risk.

a CAC score >1000 who were followed for 17 months [43] during which 35 patients (36%) suffered a hard cardiac event (myocardial infarction or cardiac death). The annualized event rate of 25% refuted the erroneous concept that extensive calcified plaque may confer protection against plaque rupture and events.

Coronary Artery Calcium and Guidelines

Guidelines have been increasingly positive regarding the value of CAC scanning. The American College of Cardiology/American Heart Association expert consensus document (2000) concluded that:

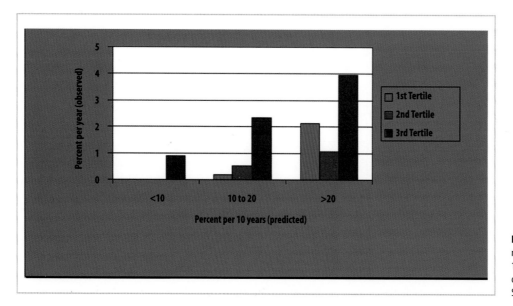

Figure 6.9. Annual event rates in asymptomatic patients in the different Framingham 10-year risk groups according to the tertile of coronary artery calcium score (St Francis Heart Study).

1. A negative EBCT test makes the presence of atherosclerotic plaque, including unstable plaque, very unlikely. 2. A negative test is highly unlikely in the presence of significant luminal obstructive disease. 3. Negative tests occur in the majority of patients who have angiographically normal coronary arteries. 4. A negative test may be consistent with a low risk of a cardiovascular event in the next 2 to 5 years. 5. A positive EBCT confirms the presence of a coronary atherosclerotic plaque. 6. The greater the amount of calcium, the greater the likelihood of occlusive CAD, but there is not a 1-to-1 relationship, and findings may not be site specific. 7. The total amount of calcium correlates best with the total amount of atherosclerotic plaque, although the true "plaque burden" is underestimated. 8. A high calcium score may be consistent with moderate to high risk of a cardiovascular event within the next 2 to 5 years. [23]

The American Heart Association Prevention V Update (2000) suggested that CAC be considered for risk assessment in the 6–20% Framingham 10-year risk category [44]. The final report of the NCEP guidelines [45] made the following recommendation on the basis of existing data at the time of publication (2002): "Therefore, measurement of coronary calcium is an option for advanced risk assessment in appropriately selected persons. In persons with multiple risk factors, high coronary calcium scores (e.g. >75th percentile for age and sex) denotes advanced coronary atherosclerosis and provides a rationale for intensified LDL-lowering therapy." The European Guidelines on Cardiovascular Disease Prevention in Clinical Practice (2003) state "Coronary calcium scanning is thus especially suited for patients at medium risk," and use CAC to qualify conventional risk analysis [46]. The American Heart Association Guidelines for Cardiovascular Disease Prevention in Women (2004) listed coronary calcification as an example of subclinical cardiovascular disease placing patients in the 10–20% Framingham 10-year risk category and acknowledged that "some patients with subclinical CVD will have >20% 10-year CHD risk and should be elevated to the high-risk category" [47].

Zero Coronary Artery Calcium Scores and the Vulnerable Plaque

Individuals with zero CAC scores have not yet developed detectable, calcified coronary plaque but they may have fatty streaking and early stages of plaque. Non-calcified plaques are present in many young adults [48]. Nonetheless, the event rate in patients with CAC score 0 is very low [36,41,42]. Raggi et al. [36] have demonstrated an annual event rate of 0.11% in asymptomatic subjects with 0 scores, and in the St Francis Heart Study [42], scores of 0 were associated with a 0.12% annual event rate over the ensuing 4.3 years. Greenland et al. [41], in a higher-risk asymptomatic cohort, noted a higher annual event rate (0.62%) with 0 CAC scores; a less sensitive CAC detection technique and

marked ethnic heterogeneity may have contributed to their findings [49].

While non-calcified, potentially "vulnerable" plaque is by definition not detected by CAC testing, CAC can identify the pool of higher-risk patients out of which will emerge approximately 95% of the patients presenting each year with sudden death or an acute myocardial infarction (MI). While the culprit lesion contains calcified plaque in only 80% of the acute events [50], of greater importance is the observation that exclusively soft, non-calcified plaque has been seen in only 5% of acute ischemic syndromes in both younger and older populations [12,51]. CAC identifies the vulnerable patient, which is more important than identifying the vulnerable plaque for which there is no specific therapy in asymptomatic patients. While it is uncommon that a patient with an imminent acute ischemic syndrome would have a 0 CAC score, it is clear that patients with typical anginal or anginal equivalent symptoms and/or stress test results documenting ischemia in the setting of a 0 calcium score warrant aggressive therapy and coronary angiography.

Correlation with Risk Factors

Correlation in Individual Patients

Conventional risk factors do correlate with CAC [52–54], even though CAC is superior to conventional risk factors in predicting outcomes. There is a clear association of CAC with a premature family history of CAD, diabetes, and lipid values in large groups of patients. However, the difficulty of equating risk factors with CAC in individual patients has been highlighted by the work of Hecht et al. in 930 consecutive primary prevention subjects undergoing EBT [53]. They found increasing likelihoods of CAC with increasing levels of low-density lipoprotein cholesterol (LDL-C) and decreasing levels of high-density lipoprotein cholesterol (HDL-C) in the population as a whole, but found no differences in the amount of plaque between groups and demonstrated a total lack of correlation in *individual* patients between the EBT calcium percentile and the levels of total, LDL- and HDL-cholesterol, total/HDL-cholesterol, triglycerides, lipoprotein(a) (Lp(a)), homocysteine and LDL particle size (Figure 6.10). This discrepancy underscores the difficulties inherent in applying population-based guidelines derived from statistical analyses to decision-making in the real world of individual patient care. Postmenopausal women presented a striking example of the inability of conventional risk analysis to predict the presence or absence of subclinical atherosclerosis [55]. There were no differences in any lipid parameters or in the Framingham Risk Scores between postmenopausal women with and without calcified plaque, rendering therapeutic decisions that are not plaque imaging based extremely problematic.

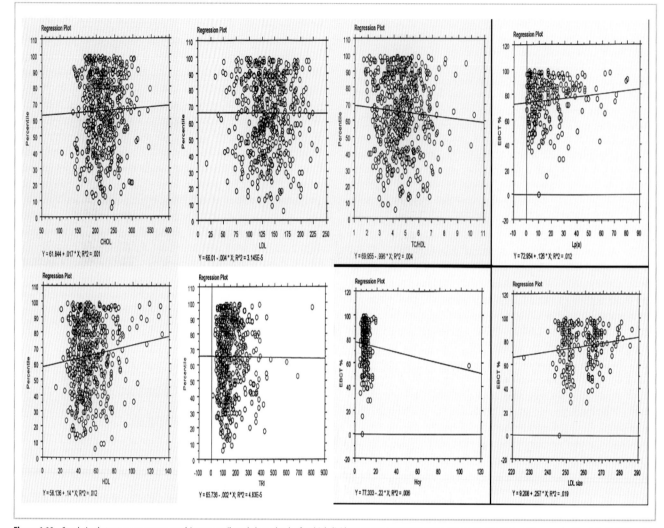

Figure 6.10. Correlation between coronary artery calcium percentile and plasma levels of multiple lipid parameters in 930 asymptomatic patients. Not all correlations are significant. Hecht HS. Translating tomographic plaque imaging into treatment: interventional lipidology. Progress in Cardiovascular Diseases. Am J Cardiol 2001;87:406–412.

Further support for the poor correlation of conventional risk factors with subclinical atherosclerosis was provided by Taylor et al. in 630 active duty US Army personnel aged 39–45 years, undergoing EBT [56]. The area under the ROC curve was only 0.62 for the Framingham Risk Score and 0.61 for LDL-C alone. The authors conclude: "In this age-homogeneous, low-risk screening cohort, conventional coronary risk factors significantly under-estimated the presence of premature, subclinical calcified coronary atherosclerosis."

hs-CRP and Coronary Artery Calcium

Although not acknowledged as a risk factor, high-sensitivity C-reactive protein (hs-CRP) has been clearly linked to the inflammatory process inherent in CAD. Extensive investigations have led to the suggestion that it be used to screen large segments of the asymptomatic population [57] despite the absence of data demonstrating that

hs-CRP is additive to standard risk factors in predicting events. There is, however, evidence that it is significantly inferior to CAC in this capacity. Park et al., in 967 asymptomatic patients, demonstrated that the relative risk of an MI or cardiac death, after adjustment for conventional risk factors, increased 4–5-fold from low to high calcium scores at any hs-CRP level, and only 0.25–0.7-fold from low to high hs-CRP at any calcified plaque level (Figure 6.11). In multivariate analysis after adjustment for risk factors, CAC was significantly predictive of events ($p < 0.005$); hs-CRP was not significantly predictive ($p = 0.09$,) before or after adjustment for CAC [58]. In 1005 asymptomatic patients randomized to treatment with atorvastatin or placebo in the St Francis Heart Study [59], only the calcium score was significantly associated with disease events ($p < 0.0001$) in a multivariate analysis including standard coronary disease risk factors, hs-CRP, and baseline coronary calcium score. Hs-CRP did not predict events independently of the calcium score ($p = 0.47$). There were no correlations between CAC and hs-CRP in either study. In addition, in a

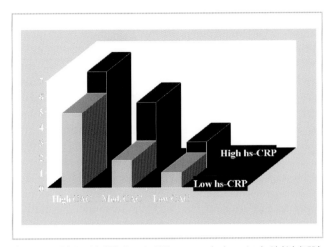

Figure 6.11. Relative risks (RR) of non-fatal MI or coronary death associated with high (≥75th percentile = 4.05 mg/L) and low (<4.05 mg/L) levels of CRP and high (>142.1), medium (3.7 to 142.1), and low (<3.7) tertiles of calcium scores. (Park R, Robert Detrano R, Xiang M, et al. Combined use of computed tomography coronary calcium scores and c-reactive protein levels in predicting cardiovascular events in nondiabetic individuals. Circulation 2002;106:2076. With permission from Lippincott Williams & Wilkins.)

separate study of 914 asymptomatic patients, there was no significant relation between hs-CRP and CAC [60]. The absence of additional predictive value of hs-CRP and its lack of correlation with CAC do not challenge the inflammatory aspects of the disease process. Rather, it emphasizes the greater value of evidence of the disease itself, namely CAC, compared to a risk marker, such as hs-CRP.

Unknown Factors

The lack of clear relationship between lipid levels and subclinical plaque in individual patients does not negate the atherogenic effect of these metabolic disorders. Rather, it highlights the variations in individual susceptibility to the atherogenic effects at a given plasma level, very likely mediated by as yet undetermined genetic factors. O'Donnell et al. [61], in an analysis of abdominal aortic calcium in 2151 patients in 1159 families in the Framingham Study, noted a heritability component accounting for up to 49% of the variability in calcified plaque, and concluded that "AAC deposits are heritable atherosclerotic traits. A substantial portion of the variation is due to the additive effects of genes, which have yet to be characterized." Peyser et al. [62], analyzing coronary calcium in 698 patients in 302 families, found a variance of up to 48% associated with additive polygenes after adjustment for covariates. They concluded that there is a "substantial genetic component for subclinical CAD variation . . . even after accounting for effects of genes acting through measured risk factors. These genes may act through other measurable risk factors or through novel pathways that have not or cannot be measured in vivo. Identification of such genes will provide a better basis for prevention and treatment of subclinical CAD."

Advanced Metabolic Testing

The discovery of significant CAC in patients with ostensibly unremarkable lipid values has led to more extensive metabolic analysis in these patients in the search for treatable disorders. In 296 asymptomatic patients with CAC, Superko and Hecht [63] reported a 66% incidence of small, dense LDL; 27% had elevated Lp(a) and 7% had elevated homocysteine. While there is no clear-cut evidence for event reduction by treatment of these abnormalities, consideration should be given to the administration of niacin for small, dense LDL and Lp(a) and folic acid for homocysteine elevations. The combination of tomographic plaque imaging with metabolic testing and aggressive treatment of identifiable abnormalities has been termed "interventional lipidology" [64].

Clinical Applications

Patient Selection

Moderately High Risk

Hecht et al. [65] have proposed recommendations for the application of CAC scanning. The Framingham Risk Score [66], incorporating both age and gender, is recommended as the initial step in selecting the appropriate test populations. Asymptomatic patients in the National Cholesterol Education Adult Treatment Program III [67] classified 10–20% Framingham 10-year risk category (moderately high risk) comprise the group that presents the greatest challenge to the treating physician, and are those in whom the application of CAC scoring is most appropriate; the CAC score can assist the physician in decisions regarding recommendations for the use of medications and the degree of emphasis to be placed on lifestyle modifications.

Lower Risk

Selected patients with less than moderately high Framingham risk may also benefit from CAC scoring to guide management decisions. For instance, most young patients with a family history of premature CAD will not have sufficient risk factors to even warrant Framingham scoring (lower NCEP risk) or will be in the moderate (1–10% 10-year Framingham risk group), since family history, while an NCEP risk factor, does not contribute points to the Framingham score. In 222 young patients presenting with an MI as the first sign of CAD (mean age 50 years), Akosah et al. [68] demonstrated that 70% were in these lesser risk categories and would not have been started on a statin using NCEP guidelines. Data from Schmermund at al. [12] and Pohle et al. [51] indicate that 95% of acute MI patients would have been identified by EBT plaque imaging irrespective of age. On the basis of these observations, the use of CAC scoring should be considered in patients with a family history of premature CAD, even when their Framingham risk is moderate or even low.

Higher Risk

Selective application of CAC scanning to patients with Framingham high risk may also be warranted. For instance, some Framingham high-risk patients may be intolerant of statins or may strongly prefer alternative medicine approaches. In these patients, CAC evidence of high risk may be used to reinforce the necessity for finding a statin that can be tolerated and for persuading the refractory patient of the need for aggressive treatment. Conversely, the absence of significant CAC may permit relaxation of the treatment goals.

Initiation and Goals of Drug Therapy

New Paradigm

The presence or absence and the amount of CAC can be useful for clinical decision-making, as previously recommended in the AHA Prevention V Update [44]. As an extension of this report, based on recent data, Table 6.3 [65] provides simple, easily implemented treatment paradigms for combining the risks of varying CAC scores with the most recent NCEP recommendations [67].

Conversion to Higher or Lower Risk

Patients in the moderately high (10–20% 10-year risk) category who are then identified to be at higher risk by CAC become candidates for secondary prevention lipid goals [67] irrespective of their baseline lipid level. This would apply even for patients with LDL-C <100 mg/dL, as implied by the Heart Protection Study [69] and stated in the most recent NCEP report [67].

Based on prognostic data, CAC >100 or >75th percentile defines a CAD equivalent. In the St Francis Heart Study [42], the CAC cutpoint for initiating secondary prevention therapy was a score >100, and the >75th percentile was suggested by the NCEP guidelines [45]. Since it has become accepted therapy to administer beta blockers to patients with established CAD, it is also reasonable to consider their use in primary prevention patients in the highest CAC risk categories. In this regard, CAC scores >400 [36] or >90th percentile [70] are associated with a very high annual risk (4.8% and 6.5% respectively) and are candidates for this more aggressive approach. These recommendations also apply to initiation of the NCEP guided therapeutic life changes [71] that are an essential component of aggressive prevention. The transformation of a moderately high-risk to a high-risk patient is shown in Figure 6.12. A 57-year-old man with hypertension, total cholesterol 235 mg/dL, LDL-C 150 mg/dL, HDL-C 75 mg/dL, and a 10-year Framingham risk of 12%, was referred for CAC scanning. The CAC score was 1872, in the >99th % for his age, placing him in the highest risk category with LDL-C treatment goal of <70 mg/dL.

In the Framingham 10–20% 10-year risk population, patients with CAC scores ≤100 and ≤75th percentile remain in the same risk group or are transformed to lower-risk categories depending on the score, and are treated accordingly. CAC scores from 10 to 100 and <75th percentile maintain the patient in the moderately high-risk group (10–20% 10-year risk). Patients with CAC scores from 1 to 10 and <75th percentile are reclassified as moderate risk (<10% 10-year risk), and CAC scores of 0 reclassify the patient to the lower-risk category.

As noted above, some patients in the lower-risk groups based on Framingham scores, such as younger patients (35–45 years of age) with a strong family history of premature coronary heart disease, are appropriate candidates for CAC scanning. In such patients, the recommendations in Table 6.3 would also apply. Figure 6.13a displays the CAC scan of a 41-year-old woman whose mother experienced a myocardial infarction at age 55. The total cholesterol was 188 mg/dL, LDL-C 112 mg/dL, HDL-C 50 mg/dL and triglycerides 132 mg/dL. She was in the 0–1 risk factor

Table 6.3. Guidelines for treatment in asymptomatic, NCEP classified moderately high-risk patients based upon CAC score

CAC score/percentile	Framingham risk group equivalent	LDL goal (mg/dL)	Drug therapy (mg/dL)
0	Lower risk; 0–1 risk factors; Framingham risk assessment not required	<160	≥190 160–189: drug optional
1–10 and ≤75th %	Moderate risk; 2+ risk factors (<10% Framingham 10-year risk)	<130	≥160
11–100 and ≤75th %	Moderately high; 2+ risk factors (10–20% Framingham 10-year risk)	<130	≥130 100–129: consider drug
101–400 or >75th %	High risk; CAD risk equivalent (>20% Framingham 10-year risk)	<100 Optional goal <70	≥100 <100: consider drug
>400 or >90th %	Highest risk[a]	<100 Optional goal <70	Any LDL level

[a] Based on CAC score; consider beta blockers.

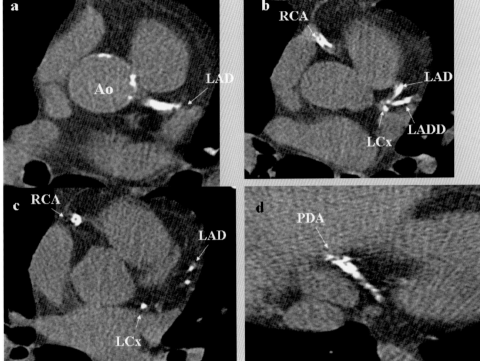

Figure 6.12. A 57-year-old man with hypertension, total cholesterol 235 mg/dL, LDL-C 150 mg/dL, HDL-C 75 mg/dL, and a 10-year Framingham risk of 12% referred for CAC scanning; CAC score was 1872, in the >99th percentile. Slices from base (**a**) through apex (**d**) reveal significant CAC in all coronary arteries and the ascending aorta. Ao = aorta, LAD = left anterior descending coronary artery, LADD = diagonal branch of left anterior descending coronary artery, LCx = left circumflex coronary artery, PDA = posterior descending branch of right coronary artery, RCA = right coronary artery.

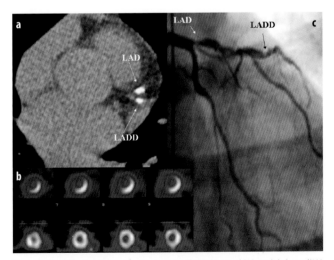

Figure 6.13. A 41-year-old woman with a premature family history of CAD, total cholesterol 188 mg/dL, LDL-C 112 mg/dL, HDL-C 50 mg/dL, and triglycerides 132 mg/dL, in the lowest Framingham risk group. **a** CAC score of 110, in the left anterior descending and diagonal branch, in the >99th percentile. **b** Dual isotope nuclear stress testing revealing severe anteroseptal ischemia. **c** Angiography demonstrating 95% ostial LAD stenosis and severe LADD disease. LAD = left anterior descending coronary artery, LADD = diagonal branch of left anterior descending coronary artery.

group in which a Framingham Risk Score need not be calculated. The CAC score was 110, in the left anterior descending (LAD) and diagonal branch, in the >99th percentile for her age, placing her in a high-risk category. She underwent dual isotope nuclear stress testing (Figure 6.13b), which revealed severe anteroseptal ischemia, followed by angiography and placement of a stent to treat a 95% ostial LAD stenosis (Figure 6.13c). Statin therapy was implemented to reduce the LDL-C to <70 mg/dL.

Patients in the high-risk category (10-year Framingham risk >20%) may be downgraded if the CAC scores do not warrant the highest risk category. CAC scores ≤100, and, in particular, ≤10, imply a lower than expected risk and should reduce the intensity of therapy. For instance, a 65-year-old male hypertensive smoker, with an LDL-C of 140 mg/dL and a 10-year Framingham risk of 25%, was very reluctant to take a statin prescribed for his LDL-C. A CAC scan was performed (Figure 6.14), which demonstrated total absence of calcified plaque, despite the presumed high risk. Therapeutic life changes, rather than statins, were recommended.

Diabetes

Diabetic patients deserve special consideration. The NCEP ATP-III guidelines characterize diabetes as a CAD risk equivalent. Raggi et al. [72] (Figure 6.15), however, have demonstrated that diabetic patients with 0 CAC scores have the same excellent prognosis as patients without diabetes; it is reasonable to treat those with 0 CAC scores less aggressively than would be dictated as a CAD risk equivalent. At the same time, diabetic patients have CAC scores corresponding to older people [73,74] and have a worse prognosis than those without diabetes and similar CAC scores [72], and should be treated more aggressively.

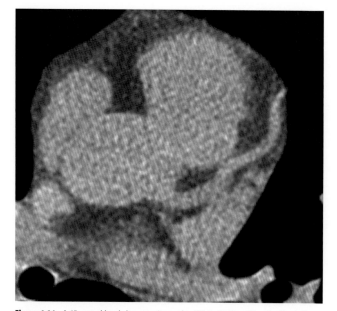

Figure 6.14. A 65-year-old male hypertensive smoker, LDL-C of 140 mg/dL and a 10-year Framingham risk of 25%. CAC scan demonstrated total absence of calcified plaque.

Evaluation of Therapy

The use of serial CAC scanning to evaluate the progression of disease and the effects of therapy will be covered in great detail in Chapter 7. For this purpose, patients with established CAD who would not ordinarily be candidates for CAC scanning may undergo evaluation as a baseline for future examinations. This may include patients who have had stent placement; the stented area must be excluded

from the scoring. In Figure 6.16, the patient underwent stent placement in the right coronary artery. Calcified plaque was noted in the left main and left anterior descending coronary arteries. The non-stented areas are suitable for tracking plaque progression. Patients with coronary artery bypass grafting are not good candidates for CAC scanning; the profusion of surgical clips makes scoring difficult, and the importance of plaque progression in bypassed areas is unknown.

Stress Testing

The important relationship of stress testing to CAC scanning will be discussed in great detail in Chapter 17 and will be mentioned here only in the context of the utility of CAC in clarifying the results of stress testing in symptomatic and asymptomatic patients. While CAC scanning is almost always reserved for patients without symptoms, it may be employed following stress tests in equivocal situations to determine the need for invasive evaluation, irrespective of the symptomatic status. In a series of 118 patients, the absence of coronary calcium accurately identified those with a false-positive treadmill test with a negative predictive value of 90% [75], suggesting that CAC may be useful to enhance the accuracy of abnormal stress tests in patients with a low clinical suspicion of obstructive disease, prior to recommending angiography. In 323 primary prevention patients referred for angiography who underwent electrocardiographic stress testing and calcified plaque imaging, Schmermund et al. reported that CAC significantly improved angiographic classification of patients with an equivocal or normal stress evaluation, but not of those with abnormal tests [76]. Figure 6.17 displays the CAC scan of a

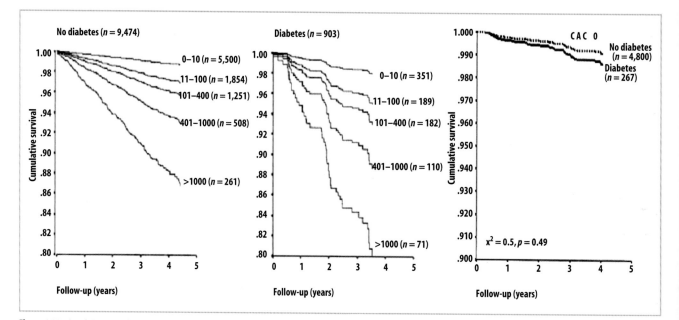

Figure 6.15. Cumulative survival in non-diabetics (left) and diabetics (center) in relation to CAC score, and in diabetics and non-diabetics with 0 CAC scores (right). (Raggi P, Shaw LJ, Berman DS, et al. Prognostic value of coronary artery calcium screening in subjects with and without diabetes. J Am Coll Cardiol 2004;43:1666.)

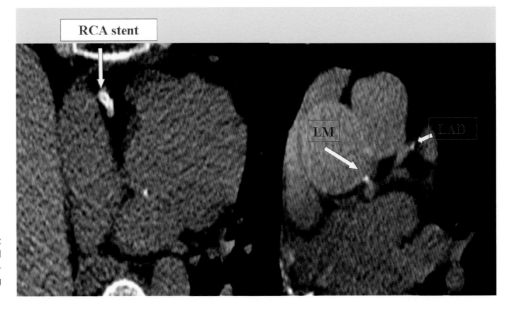

Figure 6.16. CAC scan demonstrating a stent in the right coronary artery (RCA) and calcified plaque in the LM and LAD. LM = left main coronary artery, LAD = left anterior descending coronary artery.

51-year-old male smoker with atypical chest pain, obtained after an equivocal nuclear stress test. Extensive plaque and aneurysmal dilatation were demonstrated in both the left anterior descending (LAD) and right coronary arteries. Subsequent coronary arteriography confirmed the coronary aneurysms and revealed critical LAD stenosis and thrombus.

Cardiomyopathy

CAC may be used to differentiate ischemic from non-ischemic cardiomyopathies. Budoff et al. [77] demonstrated in 120 patients with heart failure of unknown etiology that the presence of CAC was associated with a 99% sensitivity for ischemic cardiomyopathy.

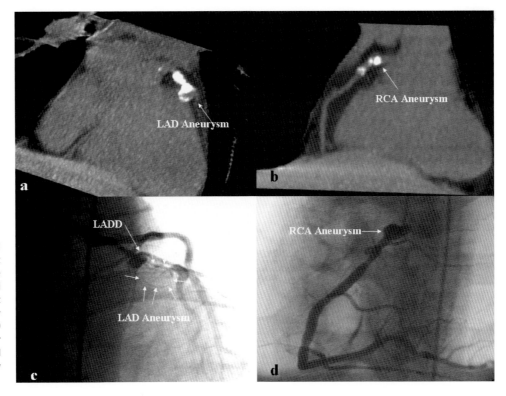

Figure 6.17. CAC imaging in a 51-year-old male smoker with atypical chest pain, post equivocal nuclear stress test. Extensive plaque and aneurysmal dilatation were demonstrated in both the LAD (**a**) and RCA (**b**). Subsequent coronary arteriography confirmed the coronary aneurysms (**c** and **d**) and revealed critical LAD stenosis and thrombus. LAD = left anterior descending coronary artery, LADD = diagonal branch of left anterior descending coronary artery, RCA = right coronary artery.

Emergency Department Chest Pain Evaluation

Emergency department triage of chest pain patients may be accomplished effectively by CAC. Laudon et al. [78] reported on 105 patients. Of the 46 with positive scores (>0), 14 had abnormal follow-up inpatient testing. Of the 59 with 0 calcium scores, stress evaluation and/or coronary arteriography were normal in the 54 who underwent further testing and all were free of cardiac events 4 months later (100% negative predictive value). Georgiou et al. [79] noted 41 cardiac events in 192 emergency room patients followed for 37 months; all but 4 were associated with calcium scores ≥ 4.

A CAC score of 0 in a chest pain patient with normal electrocardiogram and cardiac enzymes warrants discharge without stress testing.

Conclusions

The validation of CAC scanning as a risk assessment tool may well represent one of the most significant advances in the history of preventive medicine. It offers the possibility of accurately identifying the vast majority of patients destined to suffer acute cardiac events, and in so doing, will allow for substantial reduction of cardiovascular mortality and morbidity by increasingly effective pharmacologic therapy of the underlying disease process.

References

1. Heart and Stoke Statistical Update. Dallas, TX: American Heart Association, 2001.
2. Blankenhorn DH, Stern D. Calcification of the coronary arteries. Am J Roentgenol 1959;81:772–777.
3. Frink RJ, Achor RWP, Brown AL, et al. Significance of calcification of the coronary arteries. Am J Cardiol 1970;26:241–247.
4. Wexler L, Brundage B, Crouse J, et al. Coronary artery calcification: pathophysiology, epidemiology, image methods and clinical implications. A scientific statement from the American Heart Association. Circulation 1996;94:1175–1192.
5. Faber A. Die Arteriosklerose, from Pathologische Anatomie, from Pathogenese Und Actiologie. G. Fischer, 1912.
6. Bostrom K, Watson KE, Horn S, et al. Bone morphogenetic protein expression in human atherosclerotic lesions. J Clin Invest 1993;91:1800–1809.
7. Ideda T, Shirasawa T, Esaki Y, et al. Osteopontin mRNA is expressed by smooth muscle-derived foam cells in human atherosclerotic lesions of the aorta. J Clin Invest 1993;92:2814–2820.
8. Hirota S, Imakita M, Kohri K, et al. Expression of osteopontin messenger RNA by macrophages in atherosclerotic plaques. A possible association with calcification. Am J Pathol 1993;143:1003–1008.
9. Shanahan CM, Cary NR, Metcalfe JC, Weissberg PL. High expression of genes for calcification-regulating proteins in human atherosclerotic plaque. J Clin Invest 1994;93:2393–2402.
10. Rumberger JA, Simons DB, Fitzpatrick LA, et al. Coronary artery calcium areas by electron beam computed tomography and coronary atherosclerotic plaque area: A histopathologic correlative study. Circulation 1995;92:2157–2162.
11. Baumgart D, Schmermund A, Goerge G, et al. Comparison of electron beam computed tomography with intracoronary ultrasound and coronary angiography for detection of coronary atherosclerosis. J Am Coll Cardiol 1997;30:57–64.
12. Schmermund A, Baumgart D, Gorge G, et al. Coronary artery calcium in acute coronary syndromes: a comparative study of electron beam CT, coronary angiography, and intracoronary ultrasound in survivors of acute myocardial infarction and unstable angina. Circulation 1997;96:1461–1469.
13. Agatston AS, Janowitz WR, Hildner FJ, et al. Quantification of coronary artery calcium using ultrafast computed tomography. J Am Coll Cardiol 1990;15:827–832.
14. Callister TQ, Cooil B, Raya SP, et al. Coronary artery disease: improved reproducibility of calcium scoring with an electron-beam CT volumetric method. Radiology 1998;208:807–814.
15. Becker CR, Kleffel T, Crispin A, et al. Coronary artery calcium measurement. Agreement of multirow detector and electron beam CT. AJR Am J Roentgenol 2001;176:1295–1298.
16. Janowitz WR, Agatston AS, Kaplan G, Viamonte M. Differences in prevalence and extent of coronary artery calcium detected by ultrafast computed tomography in asymptomatic men and women. Am J Cardiol 1993;72:247–254.
17. Hoff JA, Chomka EV, Krainik AJ, et al. Age and gender distributions of coronary artery calcium detected by electron beam tomography in 35,246 adults. Am J Cardiol 2001;87:1335–1339.
18. Budoff MJ, Yang TP, Shavelle RM. Ethnic differences in coronary atherosclerosis. J Am Coll Cardiol 2002;39:408–412.
19. Newman AB, Naydeck BL, Whittle J, et al. Racial differences in coronary artery calcification in adults. Arterioscler Thromb Vasc Biol 2002;22:424–430.
20. Khuran C, Rosenbaum CG, Howard BV, et al. Coronary artery calcification in black women and white women. Am Heart J 2003;145:724–729.
21. Jain T, Peshock R, Darren K. McGuire DK, et al. African Americans and Caucasians have a similar prevalence of coronary calcium in the Dallas Heart Study. J Am Coll Cardiol 2004;44:1011–1017.
22. Nasir K, Michos ED, Rumberger JA, et al. Coronary artery calcification and family history of premature coronary heart disease: sibling history is more strongly associated than parental history. Circulation 2004;110:2150–2156.
23. O'Rourke RA, Brundage BH, Froelicher VF, et al.: American College of Cardiology/American Heart Association expert consensus document on electron beam computed tomography for the diagnosis and prognosis of coronary artery disease. Circulation 2000;102:126–140.
24. Simons DB, Schwartz RS, Edwards WD, et al: Noninvasive definition of anatomic coronary disease by ultrafast computed tomographic scanning: a quantitative pathologic comparison study. J Am Coll Cardiol 1992;20:1118–1126.
25. Detrano R, Tang W, Kang X, et al. Accurate coronary calcium phosphate mass measurements from electron beam computed tomograms. Am J Card Imaging 1995;9:167–173.
26. Mautner GC, Mautner SL, Froelich J, et al. Coronary artery calcification: assessment with electron beam CT and histomorphometric correlation. Radiology 1994;192:619–623.
27. Budoff MJ, Georgiou D, Brody A, et al. Ultrafast computed tomography as a diagnostic modality in the detection of coronary artery disease-a multicenter study. Circulation 1996;93:898–904.
28. Wexler L, Brundage B, Crouse J et al. Coronary artery calcification: pathophysiology, epidemiology, imaging methods, and clinical implications: a statement for health professionals from the American Heart Association. Circulation 1996;94:1175–1192.
29. Guerci AD, Spadaro LA, Popma JJ, et al. Electron Beam tomography of the coronary arteries: relationship of coronary calcium score to arteriographic findings in asymptomatic and symptomatic adults. Am J Cardiol 1997;79:128–133.
30. Shavelle DM, Budoff MJ, LaMont DH, Shavelle RM, Kennedy JM, Brundage BH. Exercise testing and electron beam computed tomography in the evaluation of coronary artery disease. J Am Coll Cardiol 2000;36:32–38.

31. Bielak LF, Rumberger JA, Sheedy PF, Schwartz RS, Peyser PA. Probabilistic model for prediction of angiographically defined obstructive coronary artery disease using electron beam computed tomography calcium score strata. Circulation 2000;102:380–385.

32. Rumberger JA, Sheedy PF, Breen FJ, et al: Electron beam CT coronary calcium score cutpoints and severity of associated angiography luminal stenosis. J Am Coll Cardiol 1997;29:1542–1548.

33. Haberl R, Becker A, Leber A, et al. Correlation of coronary calcification and angiographically documented stenoses in patients with suspected coronary artery disease: results of 1,764 patients. J Am Coll Cardiol 2001;37:451–457.

34. Budoff MJ, Raggi P, Berman D, et al. Continuous probabilistic prediction of angiographically significant coronary artery disease using electron beam tomography. Circulation 2002;105(15):1791–1796.

35. Mohlenkamp S, Lehmann N, Schmermund A, et al. Prognostic value of extensive coronary calcium quantities in symptomatic males – a 5-year follow-up study. Eur Heart J 24:2003;24, 845–854.

36. Raggi P, Callister TQ, Cooil B, et al. Identification of patients at increased risk of first unheralded acute myocardial infarction by electron beam computed tomography. Circulation 2000;101:850–855.

37. Wong ND, Hsu JC, Detrano RC, Diamond G, Eisenberg H, Gardin JM. Coronary artery calcium evaluation by electron beam computed tomography and its relation to new cardiovascular events. Am J Cardiol 2000;86:495–498.

38. Arad Y, Spadaro LA, Goodman K, Newstein D, Guerci AD. Prediction of coronary events with electron beam computed tomography. J Am Coll Cardiol 2000;36:1253–1260.

39. Kondos GT, Hoff JA, Sevrukov A, et al. Electron-beam tomography coronary artery calcium and cardiac events: a 37-month follow-up of 5,635 initially asymptomatic low to intermediate risk adults. Circulation 2003;107:2571–2576.

40. Shaw LJ, Raggi P, Schisterman E, et al. Prognostic value of cardiac risk factors and coronary artery calcium screening for all-cause mortality. Radiology 2003;28:826–833.

41. Greenland P, LaBree L, Azen SP, et al. Coronary artery calcium score combined with Framingham score for risk prediction in asymptomatic individuals. JAMA 2004;291:210–215.

42. Arad Y, Goodman KJ, Roth M, Newstein D, Guerci AD. Coronary calcification, coronary risk factors, and atherosclerotic cardiovascular disease events. The St Francis Heart Study. J Am Coll Cardiol 2005;46(1):158–165.

43. Wayhs R, Zelinger A, Raggi P. High coronary artery calcium scores pose an extremely elevated risk for hard events. J Am Coll Cardiol 2002;39:225–230.

44. Smith SC, Greenland P, Grundy SM. Prevention Conference V: beyond secondary prevention: identifying the high-risk patient for primary prevention. Executive summary. Circulation 2000;101:111–116.

45. Third Report of the National Cholesterol Education Program (NCEP) Expert Panel on Detection, Evaluation, and Treatment of High Blood Cholesterol in Adults (Adult Treatment Panel III). Final Report. NIH Publication No. 02–5215. September 2002.

46. De Backer G, Ambrosioni E, Borch-Johnson K, et al. European guidelines on cardiovascular disease prevention in clinical practice. Third joint task force of European and other societies in cardiovascular disease prevention in clinical practice. Eur J Cardiovasc Prev Rehab 2003;10(Suppl 1):S1–S10.

47. Mosca L, Appel LJ, Benjamin EJ, et al. Evidence-based guidelines for cardiovascular disease prevention in women. Expert Panel/Writing Group. Circulation 2004;109:672–693.

48. Tuzcu EM, Kapadia SR, Tutar E, et al. High prevalence of coronary atherosclerosis in asymptomatic teenagers and young adults: evidence from intravascular ultrasound. Circulation 2001;103:2705–2710.

49. Budoff MJ, Ehrlich J, Hecht HS, Rumberger JR. Letter to the Editor. JAMA 2004;291:1822.

50. Mascola A, Ko J, Bakhsheshi H, et al. Electron beam tomography comparison of culprit and non-culprit coronary arteries in patients with acute myocardial infarction. Am J Cardiol 2000;85:1357–1359.

51. Pohle K, Ropers D, Mäffert R, et al. Coronary calcifications in young patients with first, unheralded myocardial infarction: a risk factor matched analysis by electron beam tomography. Heart 2003;89:625–628.

52. Kuller LH, Matthews KA, Sutton-Tyrrell K, et al. Coronary and aortic calcification among women 8 years after menopause and their premenopausal risk factors: The Healthy Women Study. Arterioscler Thromb Vasc Biol 1999;19:2189–2198.

53. Hecht HS, Superko HR, Smith LK, et al. Relation of coronary artery calcium identified by electron beam tomography to serum lipoprotein levels and implications for treatment. Am J Cardiol 2001;87:406–412.

54. Daviglus ML, Pirzada A, Liu K, et al. Comparison of low risk and higher risk profiles in middle age to frequency and quantity of coronary artery calcium years later. Am J Cardiol 2004;94:367–369.

55. Hecht HS, Superko HR. Electron beam tomography and national cholesterol education program guidelines in asymptomatic women. J Am Coll Cardiol 2001;37:1506–1511.

56. Taylor AJ, Feuerstein I, Wong H, et al. Do conventional risk factors predict subclinical coronary artery disease? Results from the Prospective Army Coronary Calcium Project. Am Heart J 2001;141:463–468.

57. Ridker PM, Wilson PW, Grundy SM. Should C-reactive protein be added to metabolic syndrome and to assessment of global cardiovascular risk? Circulation 2004;109:2818–2825.

58. Park R, Robert Detrano R, Xiang M, et al. Combined use of computed tomography coronary calcium scores and C-reactive protein levels in predicting cardiovascular events in nondiabetic individuals. Circulation 2002;106:2073–2077.

59. Arad Y, Spadaro LA, Roth M, Newstein D, Guerci AD. Treatment of asymptomatic adults with elevated coronary calcium scores with atorvastatin, vitamin C, and vitamin E: The St Francis Heart Study randomized clinical trial. J Am Coll Cardiol 2005;46(1):166–172.

60. Reilly MP, Wolfe ML, Localio AR, Rader DJ. C-reactive protein and coronary artery calcification: The Study of Inherited Risk of Coronary Atherosclerosis (SIRCA). Arterioscler Thromb Vasc Biol 2003;23:1851–1856.

61. O'Donnell CJ, Chazaro I, Wilson PWF, et al. Evidence for heritability of abdominal aortic calcific deposits in the Framingham Heart Study. Circulation 2002;106:337–341.

62. Peyser PA, Bielak LF, Chu J, et al. Heritability of coronary artery calcium quantity measured by electron beam computed tomography in asymptomatic adults. Circulation 2002;106:304–308.

63. Superko HR, Hecht HS. Metabolic disorders contribute to subclinical atherosclerosis in patients with coronary calcification. Am J Cardiol 2001;88:260–264.

64. Hecht HS. "Interventional lipidology": Tomographic plaque imaging and aggressive treatment of metabolic disorders. Am J Cardiol 2002;90:268–270.

65. Hecht HS, Budoff M, Ehrlich J, Rumberger J. Coronary artery calcium scanning: clinical recommendations for cardiac risk assessment and treatment. J Am Coll Cardiol 2005: In press.

66. Wilson PWF, D'Agostino B, Levy D, et al. Prediction of coronary heart disease using risk factor categories. Circulation 1998;97:1837–1847.

67. Grundy SM, Cleeman JI, Merz CNB, et al. Implications of recent clinical trials for the National Cholesterol Education Program Adult Treatment Panel III guidelines. Circulation 2004;110:227–239.

68. Akosah K, Schaper A, Cogbill C, Schoenfeld P. Preventing myocardial infarction in the young adult in the first place: How do the National Cholesterol Education Panel III guidelines perform? J Am Coll Cardiol 2003;41:1475–1479.

69. Heart Protection Study Collaborative Group. MRC/BHF Heart Protection Study of cholesterol lowering with simvastatin in 20 536

high-risk individuals: a randomised placebo-controlled trial. Lancet 2002;360:7–22.

70. Raggi P, Cooil B, Callister TQ. Use of electron beam tomography data to develop models for prediction of hard coronary events. Am Heart J 2001;141:375–382.

71. Expert Panel on Detection, Evaluation, and Treatment of High Blood Cholesterol in Adults. Executive Summary of The Third Report of The National Cholesterol Education Program (NCEP) (Adult Treatment Panel III). JAMA 2001;285:2486–2497.

72. Raggi P, Shaw LJ, Berman DS, Callister TQ. Prognostic value of coronary artery calcium screening in subjects with and without diabetes. J Am Coll Cardiol 2004;43:1663–1669.

73. Kuller LH, Velentgas P, Barzilay J, et al. Diabetes mellitus, subclinical cardiovascular disease and risk of incident cardiovascular disease and all-cause mortality. Arterioscler Thromb Vasc Biol 2000;20: 823–829.

74. Hoff JA, Quinn L, Sevrukov A, et al. The prevalence of coronary artery calcium among diabetic individuals without known coronary artery disease. J Am Coll Cardiol 2003;41:1008–1012.

75. LaMont DH, Budoff MJ, Shavelle DM, et al. Coronary calcium screening identifies patients with false positive stress tests (abstract). Circulation 1997;96:306-I.

76. Schmermund A, Baumgart D, Sack S, et al. Assessment of coronary calcification by electron-beam computed tomography in symptomatic patients with normal, abnormal or equivocal exercise stress test. Eur Heart J 2000;21:1674–1682.

77. Budoff MJ, Shavelle DM, Lamont DH, et al. Usefulness of electron beam computed tomography scanning for distinguishing ischemic from non-ischemic cardiomyopathy. J Am Coll Cardiol 1998;32: 1173–1178.

78. Laudon DA, Vukov LF, Breen JF, et al. Use of electron-beam computed tomography in the evaluation of chest pain patients in the emergency department. Ann Emerg Med 1999;33:15–21.

79. Georgiou D, Budoff MJ, Kaufer E, et al. Screening patients with chest pain in the emergency department using electron beam tomography: a follow-up study. J Am Coll Cardiol 2001;38:105–110.

7

Natural History and Impact of Interventions on Coronary Calcium

Paolo Raggi

Preface

Coronary artery calcification has long been known to be associated with atherosclerosis and is intimately associated with atherosclerotic plaque development. Similarly, aortic valve degeneration and calcification appear to follow a pathophysiologic process very similar to atherosclerosis. Non-invasive imaging technologies such as electron beam tomography (EBT) and multidetector computer tomography (MDCT) scanners allow the accurate detection and quantification of cardiovascular calcification, offering an opportunity to monitor the effectiveness of therapy initiated to retard the progression of disease. It has recently become apparent that continued progression of coronary calcification represents a marker of risk of myocardial infarction and cardiac death both in patients on treatment and those untreated. Furthermore, aortic valve sclerosis and calcification have been associated with a high risk of cardiovascular events. Therefore, there is currently a considerable interest in utilizing non-invasive CT imaging modalities to follow the progression of cardiovascular calcification in a variety of patient settings. In this chapter, we present a review of the studies published to date on the use of CT technology to gauge the effects of medical therapy on coronary and valvular calcification.

Development of Vascular Calcifications and Animal Studies of Plaque Regression

In Western society changes in the arterial walls begin very early in life. Necropsy data from 2876 subjects between the ages of 15 and 34 revealed intimal lesions in the aortas of all patients and more than half of the right coronary arteries of the youngest age group (15–19 years old) with increasing prevalence and extent of disease with advancing age [1]. Though coronary artery calcification (CAC) has long been known to be associated with atherosclerosis, it was only recently suggested that plaque calcification may

be dependent upon an active process of mineralization resembling bone formation [2–5]. Several enzymes necessary for the assembly of normal bone have been found in the context of human atherosclerotic plaques [2–4] and cells normally found in the vessel wall, such as smooth muscle cells and macrophages, can transform into osteoblast-like cells with bone generating potential [5]. As a result, in advanced stages of atherosclerotic disease true ossification can be observed in pathologic specimens.

It is currently unknown if arterial calcification is a part of the ongoing inflammatory phenomena at the level of the plaque or an attempt at repairing the damage brought to the vascular wall by various stimuli. Indeed, some investigators have suggested that calcium deposition simply results from recurrent intra-lesional hemorrhage and thrombosis [6]. Nonetheless, as the process of calcification of a plaque appears to be dependent upon active phenomena of mineralization, it is plausible that formation and degradation of calcium deposits may be an ongoing dynamic phenomenon in the atherosclerotic plaque as in bone tissue and that these processes may be activated or inhibited by external interventions.

Several investigators have conducted animal studies of atherosclerosis regression to analyze the morphologic plaque changes induced by various treatments. In one such experiment, 59 rhesus monkeys were fed a high-cholesterol diet for several years and then exposed to a severely cholesterol restricted diet [7]. Animals were killed at different times during the experimental period and findings revealed typical accumulation of plaques with a lipid-rich core and scattered calcific granules. As plaques expanded, more extensive calcific deposits became visible. However, after exposing the animals to about 3 years of a severely restricted diet, the plaques became more fibrotic, with a lower cholesterol content and, although the calcium did not disappear, its burden did not increase either [7].

In a more recent experiment Williams et al. [8] used a monkey model of atherosclerosis to study the effect of medical therapy in addition to diet on atherosclerosis progression and regression. Thirty-two adult (7 to 10 years of age) male cynomolgus monkeys were fed an atherogenic diet containing 0.61 mg of cholesterol per kilocalorie of diet for 2 years (progression phase). The monkeys were divided into two well-balanced groups as far as iliac artery size and baseline lipid levels were concerned. In each animal, one iliac artery was surgically removed at the beginning of the treatment phase to serve as a baseline measure of plaque regression. During the treatment phase both animal groups consumed a lipid-lowering diet containing 0.11 mg of cholesterol per kilocalorie of diet for an additional 2 years. Since some monkeys also received ($n = 14$) and others did not receive ($n = 18$) pravastatin (20 mg/kg body weight per day), the diets were adjusted throughout the treatment phase to maintain equal changes in plasma lipoproteins. At the end of the treatment phase the animals' total low-density (LDL) and high-density lipoprotein (HDL) cholesterol levels were similar in both groups. However, histologic analysis of the coronary, carotid, and iliac arteries revealed important differences between treatment groups. While the lumen area was not different, pravastatin-treated animals showed a reduction in intimal neovascularization and plaque macrophage infiltration and a decrease in calcification of early as well as advanced plaques. These findings suggested that pravachol (and potentially other statins) might benefit the arterial wall in more ways than just lowering serum lipoprotein levels. Furthermore, the deposition of calcium in the atherosclerotic plaque appears to be a dynamic process of deposition and removal.

Unlike the investigators mentioned above, Daoud et al. [9] and Clarkson et al. [10] did not find any reduction in atherosclerotic plaque calcium deposition in experiments conducted in swine and monkeys, respectively. It should be remembered, however, that all animal experiments were cross-sectional since no true pathologic longitudinal study on living beings can be conducted. Hence, although attractive, the histologic proof that cardiovascular calcification may regress remains a matter of debate at this time.

Technical Considerations

CAC can be accurately detected by EBT and MDCT but it usually becomes visible in the intermediate to late stages of development of an atherosclerotic plaque. The degree of calcification is assessed by means of quantitative calcium-scores. Agatston et al. [11] developed a scoring system that correlates well with the underlying atherosclerotic plaque burden [12] and has been widely used in research and clinical trials. This score is a unitless number derived from the multiplication of the area of calcification by an arbitrarily chosen density coefficient rated 1 through 4. This scoring method has been known to have a limited interscan reproducibility, especially when used with the older CT technologies, and has been replaced by a new scoring method for the performance of sequential studies [13]. The new method, known as calcium volume score, is derived using

an isotropic interpolation principle and it represents a direct measurement of the volume of calcium in an atherosclerotic plaque (measured in picoliters). This score, found to be substantially more reproducible than the Agatston method [13], takes into consideration the likely pathophysiologic changes that occur in a plaque undergoing aggressive medical management. In fact, it is conceivable that volumetric contraction and increase in density due to the loss of soft-core contents in the plaque would cause an increase in the Agatston score (dependent on density) rather than a decrease. More recently, a third type of score has been introduced, the mass score [14]. Though reportedly more reliable and reproducible than the other scores, to date this measurement has not yet been employed in sequential studies of atherosclerosis.

Effect of Lipid-Lowering Therapy with Statins on Progression of Coronary Artery Calcium

Human studies of atherosclerosis progression and regression have mainly been conducted by means of quantitative coronary angiography [15,16] and only recently with sequential measurements of coronary artery calcification and carotid artery intimal medial thickness [17–21]. The cardiovascular event reduction associated with luminal stenosis improvements seen on quantitative angiography far outweighed the magnitude of often minimal regression [22]. This observation became germane to the concept that induction of plaque regression is an important surrogate marker worth achieving since it may translate into substantial cardiovascular risk reduction.

Nonetheless, the invasive nature of coronary angiography greatly limits the utility of this tool for sequential studies, especially in asymptomatic people. In this vein, several human studies have addressed the utility of CT technology, as well as that of several other technologies not discussed in this chapter, to assess the effect of various medical interventions on cardiovascular disease. This notion suffers from an inherent limitation, however, since it assumes that limiting the progression or inducing the regression of atherosclerosis in asymptomatic individuals will provide the same benefit observed in symptomatic patients studied with invasive modalities. Indeed, symptomatic patients may have a very different substrate for their ongoing atherosclerotic disease compared to asymptomatic subjects harboring subclinical disease.

Callister et al. [17] published the first report of sequential EBT scanning in asymptomatic patients. They conducted an observational study on 149 patients referred by primary care physicians for CAC screening. Since the reproducibility of the calcium volume score is very high for scores above 30 [13], a minimum score of 30 was required for patients' inclusion in the study. Treatment with HMG-CoA reductase inhibitors was advised for all patients, but

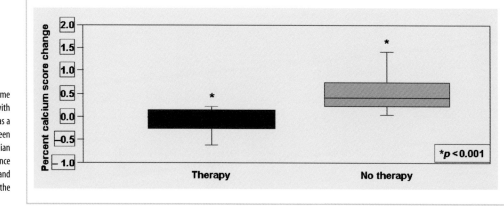

Figure 7.1. Progression of calcium volume score in 105 patients treated for a year with statins and 44 untreated patients. There was a significant difference in progression between the two groups. The box plots indicate median (line in the middle of the box), confidence intervals (vertical lines) as well as 25th and 75th percentiles (lower and top borders of the box). (Created from Callister et al. [17].)

the initiation of such therapy was left to the discretion of the referring physician. Patients underwent a baseline and follow-up EBT scan at a minimum of 12-month interval (range 12–15 months) and serial LDL-cholesterol measurements were obtained. Of the 149 patients, 105 received treatment with HMG-CoA reductase inhibitors and 44 did not. Progression of calcium volume score was seen in all untreated patients (mean LDL ± SD: 147 ± 22 mg/dL) and averaged 52 ± 36% per year (Figure 7.1). In contrast, the mean yearly calcium volume score change for all treated patients (mean LDL: 114 ± 23 mg/dL) was 5 ± 28% ($p <$ 0.001 versus untreated patients). Among the treated patients, 65 individuals attained an LDL level <120 mg/dL (mean LDL: 100 ± 17 mg/dL) and showed a net regression of their calcium volume score (–7 ± 22%, Figure 7.2). For the patients who received HMG-CoA reductase inhibitors but maintained an average LDL >120 mg/dL (mean LDL: 139 ± 18 mg/dL) the mean yearly calcium volume score progression was 25 ± 22% (Figure 7.2). All intergroup comparisons were highly statistically significant ($p <$ 0.0001). The study provided the first indication that there might be a direct correlation between the aggressiveness of LDL treatment and effectiveness with which the atherosclerotic process is halted as demonstrated by EBT imaging.

An example of progression of coronary calcification in a patient who remained symptom free through time is shown in Figure 7.3. Other emerging lipid or non-lipid factors, such as lipoprotein(a) (Lp(a)), low HDL levels, homocysteine, high C-reactive protein (CRP) etc., that could have affected the outcome of the analysis were not taken into consideration. This might help explain the apparent failure to treat a portion of the study cohort.

In the next published report, Budoff at al. [18] followed a total of 299 asymptomatic patients with various risk factors for atherosclerosis for 1 to 6.5 years. All patients underwent sequential EBT scans at a minimum of 12-month interval. The follow-up scan indicated a significant increase in calcium score in all untreated patients, regardless of the underlying risk factor/s. However, treatment with statins resulted in a statistically significant slowing of calcium score progression (15 ± 8% per year on treatment versus 39 ± 12% per year without treatment).

Achenbach et al. [19] conducted a small prospective cohort study and compared the rate of change in the amount of coronary calcium prior to and during lipid-lowering therapy with cerivastatin. A total of 66 patients with known coronary calcium and LDL levels >130 mg/dL were evaluated. An EBT scan was performed at baseline and repeated after a period of 14 months without therapy. Cerivastatin therapy was then initiated at a dose of 0.3 mg/day and a final EBT scan was performed after 12 months of treatment. Therapy with cerivastatin lowered

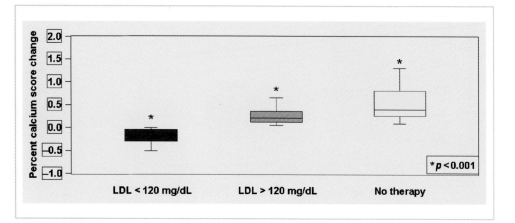

Figure 7.2. Progression of calcium volume score in 65 patients exposed to intensive treatment with statins for one year (mean LDL <120 mg/dL), 40 patients treated with a moderate statin regimen for a year (mean LDL >120 mg/dL on treatment), and 44 untreated patients. There was a significant difference in progression between the three groups. The box plots indicate median (line in the middle of the box), confidence intervals (vertical lines) as well as 25th and 75th percentiles (lower and top borders of the box). (Created from Callister et al. [17].)

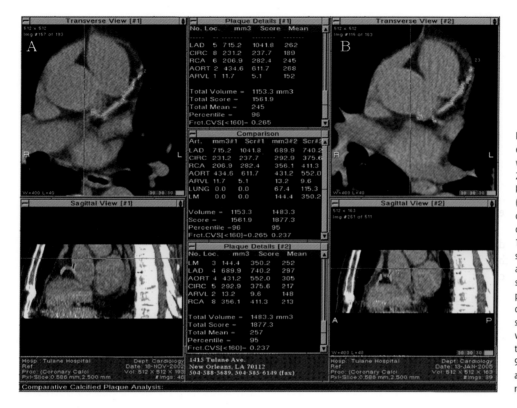

Figure 7.3. Asymptomatic patient with extensive coronary calcification (calcium volume score = 1153.3) at baseline (**A**). After 26 months of intensive treatment with lipid-lowering drugs and antihypertensive drugs (**B**) there was a mild progression of calcification (follow-up score = 1483.3). This corresponds to an annualized score increase of 12%, which is smaller than the 15% annual score increase necessary for the test to indicate actual progression. **A** and **B** show transverse sections of the heart with calcification in the proximal and mid portion of the left anterior descending coronary artery. The central inset shows a comparison of baseline and follow-up volume scores and Agatston scores. Note that the calcium score percentile diminished from 96th at baseline to 95th at follow-up despite an increase in absolute score. This suggests a relative slowing of the progression of disease.

the cholesterol level from an average of 164 ± 30 to 107 ± 21 mg/dL. The median calcium volume score increase during the drug-free period was 25% (Figure 7.4). However, the median score progression was only 8.8% at the end of one year's treatment with cerivastatin ($p < 0.0001$). In 32 patients who attained an average LDL <100 mg/dL with treatment, the median annual calcium volume score change was −3.4% while the same patients had progressed 27% during the untreated period ($p = 0.0001$). Though small, this prospective study confirmed and expanded the findings of the earlier observational studies that suggested

that a decline in the rate of progression in coronary calcification can be attained with aggressive medical treatment of hypercholesterolemia.

More recently, a trial of LDL apheresis and sequential coronary artery calcium scoring was conducted in 8 patients with familial hypercholesterolemia in whom diet and optimum pharmacotherapy had not resulted in desired levels of LDL [20]. The mean patient age was 46 ± 8 years. All patients had been on treatment with simvastatin 40 mg/day prior to initiation of LDL apheresis, but were switched to atorvastatin 80 mg/day during apheresis

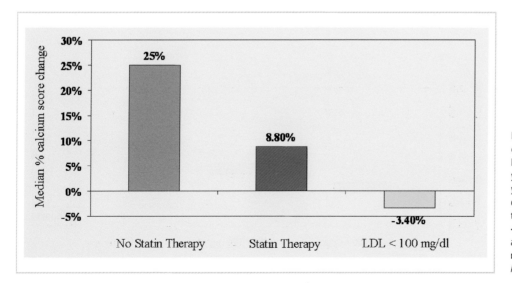

Figure 7.4. Median yearly progression of coronary calcium volume score in 66 hypercholesterolemic patients left untreated for one year (score increase = 25%), followed by one year of treatment with 0.3 mg of cerivastatin daily (score increase = 8.8%). Thirty-two patients attained a mean level of LDL <100 mg/dL with treatment, and their median annual calcium score change was slightly negative (change: −3.4%). (Created from Achenbach et al. [19].)

and continued treatment for an average period of 29 months. Total cholesterol, LDL, triglycerides, and HDL levels were obtained at baseline and at several time points during the study period. Baseline imaging of the coronary arteries was performed by EBT and follow-up scans were done by means of multidetector spiral CT scanning. CT measurements included calcium volume scores, mean plaque density and Agatston scores. At the end of the study the calcium volume score decreased in all patients by an average of $23 \pm 15\%$ ($p < 0.01$). The Agatston scores also decreased by an average of $26 \pm 14\%$ ($p < 0.01$). In contrast the mean plaque density increased by $17 \pm 11\%$ ($p < 0.01$), suggesting that healing of the plaque may be associated with reduction in plaque size and – potentially – collapse of the plaque into a denser and smaller volume. This study constituted further proof of the fact that aggressive lipid-lowering therapy slows the progression of coronary artery calcification and it can be measured effectively with sequential CT imaging.

Two studies addressed the issue of slowing of progression of CAC with statins in women. In a subanalysis of the Women's Health Initiative Observational Study, Hsia et al. [23] evaluated prospectively the rate and determinants of progression of CAC in healthy postmenopausal women. Of 914 postmenopausal women enrolled in the main study, 305 women with a baseline calcium score ≥10 were invited for a repeat scan. The progression analysis included the 94 women who agreed to undergo a second scan. The mean age of the study participants was 65 ± 9 years and the mean interval between scans was 3.3 ± 0.7 years. A wide range of changes in coronary calcium score was observed, with variations from -53 to $+452$ Agatston score units per year. Women with lower scores at baseline had smaller annual increases in absolute calcium score. Coronary calcium scores increased 11, 31, and 79 units per year among women with baseline calcium score in the lowest, middle, and highest tertiles of score. In multivariate analysis, age was not an independent predictor of change in coronary calcium score. Statin use at baseline was a negative predictor ($p = 0.015$), whereas baseline calcium score was a strong positive predictor ($p < 0.0001$) of progression of coronary calcification.

The BELLES trial (Beyond Endorsed Lipid Lowering with EBT Scanning) was a prospective randomized study of postmenopausal and dyslipidemic women with a minimal calcium volume score of 30 at baseline [24]. After the initial EBT scan, the 615 women enrolled were randomized to treatment with atorvastatin 80 mg/day or pravastatin 40 mg/day and a second scan was repeated after 12 months (Figure 7.5). The mean age of the 475 women who completed the study was 64 years. The attained mean LDL-cholesterol level was significantly lower with atorvastatin (94 mg/dL) than with pravastatin (129 mg/dL). Nonetheless, the median relative change in the calcium volume score was not different between the two treatment arms (15.1% and 14.3% for atorvastatin and pravastatin respectively, $p = $ NS). This study failed to demonstrate the superiority of an aggressive lipid-lowering treatment over a more moderate treatment in slowing progression of coronary artery calcification, therefore partly disputing the findings of the observational study previously published by Callister et al. [17]. Furthermore, the findings were not consonant with other trial results that demonstrated the superiority of aggressive lipid-lowering therapy with atorvastatin as far as both reduction of cardiovascular events [25] and slowing of plaque growth assessed by transcutaneous and intravascular ultrasound were concerned [21,26,27].

The reasons for such discrepancies are likely multifaceted. The spatial resolution of transcutaneous, and especially intravascular, ultrasound is several-fold greater than that of the EBT technology employed for the BELLES study. Furthermore, prior research efforts were focused on higher-risk individuals (patients with familial hypercholesterolemia, and patients suffering from angina with an indication for coronary angiography) than the patients

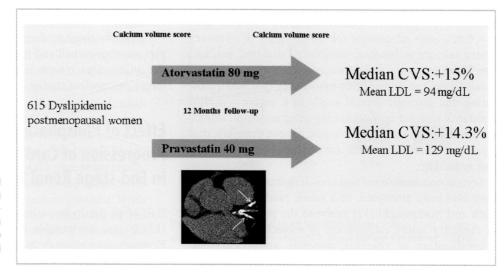

Figure 7.5. Design of the BELLES trial and main study results. Aggressive lipid-lowering therapy with atorvastatin did not slow progression of coronary artery calcium more than moderate treatment with pravastatin. CVS = calcium volume score. (Created from Raggi et al. [24].)

0.02 for all intergroup comparisons). Of note, the mean LDL-cholesterol was significantly lower in the sevelamer group, though patients in the calcium groups were more likely to be receiving a statin during the treatment period. This is a known additional effect of sevelamer that appears to effectively reduce intestinal absorption of cholesterol [46] with potential additional anti-inflammatory effects [47]. However, the changes in calcification severity seen at 52 weeks were independent of the levels of LDL-cholesterol, HDL-cholesterol and CRP attained and the use of statins. This study provided evidence, therefore, that the lack of calcification progression with sevelamer was attributable to the absence of calcium overload induced by calcium-based phosphate binders. Finally, while serum phosphorus and calcium levels were controlled similarly in the calcium-salts and sevelamer groups, over-suppression of PTH was more frequent in patients receiving calcium phosphate binders than sevelamer, and this was accompanied by a simultaneous loss in bone mineral density [48]. Interestingly, an inverse relationship between coronary calcification and bone density has also been observed in non-uremic individuals [49,50] and suggests an intriguing interaction between bone and vascular health.

The Treat-to-Goal study along with other clinical and laboratory data [51,52] provided evidence that absorption of elemental calcium from calcium-based phosphate binders is linked to rapid and severe progression of cardiovascular calcification and should be carefully monitored in ESRD.

Clinical Implications

It is obvious that the main question related to the measurement of coronary calcification progression is its clinical relevance. Indeed, the clinical significance of slowing of the calcification process has been addressed in two observational studies to date. Raggi et al. [53] followed 817 asymptomatic individuals referred by primary care physicians for sequential EBT imaging at an average interval of 2.2 ± 1.3 years. Patients were treated with statins at the discretion of the treating physician. After several years from the initial EBT scan, telephone interviews were conducted to determine the occurrence of myocardial infarction in all individuals. A myocardial infarction had to have occurred after the second EBT scan for the event to be related to an actual change in calcium score. The mean yearly calcium volume score change for the individuals who suffered a myocardial infarction was 47 ± 50% while it averaged 26 ± 32% in those free of an event at follow-up ($p < 0.001$). Treatment of hyperlipidemia (a probable marker of greater baseline risk) and calcium score change were independent predictors of myocardial infarction.

In a second publication, Raggi et al. [54] estimated the occurrence of myocardial infarction in a cohort of 495 asymptomatic individuals submitted to sequential EBT scanning while undergoing treatment with statins. The

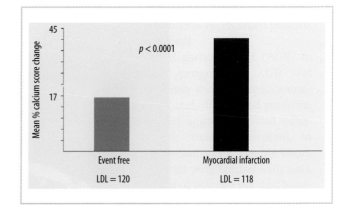

Figure 7.8. Mean coronary calcium volume score in patients treated with statins who suffered a myocardial infarction during follow-up and event-free subjects. Despite attaining a similar mean LDL level with treatment, the calcium score progression was significantly different between groups. (Created from Raggi et al. [54].)

mean follow-up was 3 years, men and women were enrolled in equal proportions, and the mean age of the enrolled subject was 57 ± 8 years. Unlike the previous study, in this case the investigators were able to assess the progression of coronary artery calcium in event-free and myocardial infarction patients in relation to the attained LDL level while on treatment. In spite of an identical average LDL level (~120 mg/dL in each group), the 41 patients who suffered a myocardial infarction showed a much greater yearly calcium score progression than the 454 event-free survivors (42 ± 23% versus 17 ± 25%, $p < 0.001$, Figure 7.8). The investigators further analyzed the data after dividing the patients according to a relative calcium score change greater than 15% per year. This value had been identified in prior publications as representing a true score change as opposed to a measurement reproducibility error [13]. In a multivariable model the best predictors of a yearly calcium score increase ≥15% were smoking ($p = 0.032$), male gender ($p = 0.014$), and baseline calcium score ($p = 0.002$). Independent of the baseline calcium score, patients demonstrating a score change smaller than 15% per year (essentially representing no progression from baseline) suffered very few events ($n = 5$) and the events occurred late during follow-up. In contrast, the majority of events ($n = 36$) occurred in patients showing score progression greater than 15% per year and the events occurred sooner during the follow-up period as the baseline score increased. Therefore, this study indicated that statins are not effective in every patient to curb the atherosclerotic process and their effectiveness cannot be merely based on a serum lipoprotein test. On the other hand, an objective measurement of the effects of these drugs on the atherosclerotic disease may provide a window on the anatomical correlate of therapy.

Conclusion

The data presented in this chapter provide evidence that non-invasive CT imaging can be used to monitor the effectiveness of medical therapy by following changes in burden of calcified plaque. Nonetheless, there are some limitations inherent with the technology currently available. There is a strong need to standardize the scoring methods and assess the equivalence of the existing CT equipment. Additionally, the rigid application of a density threshold of 130 HU to define the presence of vascular or valvular calcification in all patients limits our ability to identify more recent, less densely calcified and therefore softer plaques. Though further prospective studies will be necessary to confirm the clinical significance of the findings herein summarized, it is quite evident that the effectiveness of anti-atherosclerotic therapy can be gauged with sequential CT imaging. The application of this technology will greatly facilitate primary and secondary prevention studies by allowing a great reduction in the number of patients needed to show effectiveness of therapy. Simultaneously, a physician's effort to implement preventive measures could be gratified by the ability to measure the effectiveness of the applied remedies. Interventions directed at modifying risk factors associated with atherosclerosis besides LDL such as small-density LDL, Lp(a), low HDL, elevated homocysteine levels, and use of anti-viral and anti-bacterial agents will likely be the focus of future research.

With continued improvements in CT technology and expanded clinical experience, it is hoped that the role of coronary calcium in primary and secondary prevention will be further defined and become more readily accepted by a wider circle of physician users.

References

1. Strong JP, Malcom GT, McMahan A, et al. Prevalence and extent of atherosclerosis in adolescents and young adults. The Pathobiological Determinants of Atherosclerosis in Youth Study. JAMA 1999; 281:727–735.
2. Bostrom K, Watson KE, Horn S, Wortham C, Herman IM, Demer LL. Bone morphogenic protein expression in human atherosclerotic lesions. J Clin Invest 1993;91:1800–1809.
3. Fitzpatrick LA, Severson A, Edwards WD, Ingram RT. Diffuse calcification in human coronary arteries: association of osteopontin with atherosclerosis. J Clin Invest 1994;94:1597–1604.
4. Shanahan CM, Cary NR, Metcalfe JC, Weissberg PL. High Expression of genes for calcification-regulating proteins in human atherosclerotic plaques. J Clin Invest 1994;93:2393–2402.
5. Proudfoot D, Davies JD, Skepper JN, Weissberg PL, Shanahan CM. Acetylated low-density lipoprotein stimulates human vascular smooth muscle cell calcification by promoting osteoblastic differentiation and inhibiting phagocytosis. Circulation 2002;106:3044–3050.
6. Bini A, Mann KG, Kudryk BJ, Schen FJ. Noncollagenous bone matrix proteins, calcification and thrombosis in carotid artery atherosclerosis. Arterioscl Thromb Vasc Biol 1999;19:1852–1861.
7. Stary HC. Natural history of calcium deposits in atherosclerosis progression and regression. Z Kardiol 2000;89(suppl 2):28–35.
8. Williams JK, Sukhova GK, Herrington DM, Libby P. Pravastatin has cholesterol-lowering independent effects on the artery wall of atherosclerotic monkeys. J Am Coll Cardiol 1998;31:684–691.
9. Daoud AS, Jarmolych J, Augustyn JM, et al. Sequential morphologic studies of regression of advanced atherosclerosis. Arch Pathol 1981; 105:233–239.
10. Clarkson TB, Bond MG, Bullock BC, et al. A study of atherosclerosis regression in *Macaca mulatta*. IV. Changes in coronary arteries from animals with atherosclerosis induced for 19 months and then regressed for 24 months or 48 months at plasma cholesterol concentrations of 300 or 200 mg/dl. Exp Mol Pathol 1981;34:345–368.
11. Agatston AS, Janowitz WR, Hildner JR, Zusmer NR, Viamonte M Jr, Detrano R. Quantification of coronary artery calcium using ultrafast computed tomography scanning. J Am Coll Cardiol 1990;15:827–832.
12. Sangiorgi G, Rumberger JA, Severson A, et al. Arterial calcification and not lumen stenosis is highly correlated with atherosclerotic plaque burden in humans: a histologic study of 723 coronary artery segments using non-decalcifying methodology. Electron beam computed tomography and coronary artery disease: scanning for coronary artery calcification. J Am Coll Cardiol 1998;31:126–133.
13. Callister TQ, Cooil B, Raya S, Lippolis NJ, Russo DJ, Raggi P. Coronary artery disease: improved reproducibility of calcium scoring with electron-beam CT volumetric method. Radiology 1998;208: 807–814.
14. Rumberger JA, Kaufman L. A rosetta stone for coronary calcium risk stratification: Agatston, volume, and mass scores in 11,490 individuals. AJR Am J Roentgenol 2003;181:743–748.
15. Jukema JW, Bruschke AV, van Boven AJ, et al. Effects of lipid lowering by pravastatin on progression and regression of coronary artery disease in symptomatic men with normal to moderately elevated serum cholesterol levels. The Regression Growth Evaluation Statin Study (REGRESS). Circulation 1995;91:2528–2540.
16. Brown G, Albers JJ, Fisher LD, et al. Regression of coronary artery disease as a result of intensive lipid-lowering therapy in men with high levels of apolipoprotein B. N Engl J Med 1990;323:1289–1298.
17. Callister TQ, Raggi P, Cooil B. Effects of HMG-CoA reductase inhibitors on coronary artery disease. N Engl J Med 1998;339: 1972–1977.
18. Budoff MJ, Lane KL, Bakhsheshi H, et al. Rates of progression of coronary calcium by electron beam tomography. Am J Cardiol 2000; 86:8–11.
19. Achenbach S, Dieter R, Pohle K, et al. Influence of lipid-lowering therapy on the progression of coronary artery calcification. Circulation 2002;106:1077–1082.
20. Hoffmann U, Derfler K, Haas M, Stadler A, Brady TJ, Kostner K. Effects of combined low density lipoprotein apheresis and aggressive statin therapy on coronary calcified plaque as measured by computed tomography. Am J Cardiol 2003;91:461–464.
21. Taylor AJ, Kent SM, Flaherty PJ, Coyle LC, Markwood TT, Vernalis MN. ARBITER: Arterial Biology for the Investigation of the Treatment Effects of Reducing Cholesterol: a randomized trial comparing the effects of atorvastatin and pravastatin on carotid intima medial thickness. Circulation 2002;106:2055–2060.
22. Levine GN, Keaney JF Jr, Vita JA. Cholesterol reduction in cardiovascular disease: clinical benefits and possible mechanisms. N Engl J Med 1995;332:512–521.
23. Hsia J, Klouj A, Prasad A, Burt J, Adams-Campbell LL, Howard BV. Progression of coronary calcification in healthy postmenopausal women. BMC Cardiovasc Disord 2004;4:21.
24. Raggi P, Davidson M, Callister TQ, et al. Aggressive versus moderate lipid-lowering therapy in hypercholesterolemic post-menopausal women: Beyond Endorsed Lipid Lowering With EBT Scanning (BELLES). Circulation 2005;112(4):563–571.
25. Cannon CP, Braunwald E, McCabe CH, et al. Comparison of intensive and moderate lipid lowering with statins after acute coronary syndromes. N Engl J Med 2004;350:1495–1504.
26. Smilde TJ, van Wissen S, Wollersheim H, Trip MD, Kastelein JJ, Stalenhoef AF. Effect of aggressive versus conventional lipid lowering on atherosclerosis progression in familial hypercholesterolaemia (ASAP): a prospective, randomised, double-blind trial. Lancet 2001; 357:577–581.

27. Nissen SE, Tuzcu EM, Schoenhagen P, et al. Effect of intensive compared with moderate lipid-lowering therapy on progression of coronary atherosclerosis. A randomized controlled trial. JAMA 2004;291:1071–1080.

28. Hecht HS, Harman SM. Comparison of the effects of atorvastatin versus simvastatin on subclinical atherosclerosis in primary prevention as determined by electron beam tomography. Am J Cardiol 2003;91:42–45.

29. Hecht HS, Harman SM. Relation of aggressiveness of lipid-lowering treatment to changes in calcified plaque burden by electron beam tomography. Am J Cardiol 2003;92:334–336.

30. Wong ND, Kawakubo M, LaBree L, Azen SP, Xiang M, Detrano R. Relation of coronary calcium progression and control of lipids according to the National Cholesterol Education Program guidelines. Am J Cardiol 2004;94:431–436.

31. Snell-Bergeon JK, Hokanson JE, Jensen L, et al. Progression of coronary artery calcification in type 1 diabetes: the importance of glycemic control. Diabetes Care 2003;26:2923–2928.

32. Rath M, Niedzwiecki A. Nutritional supplement program halts progression of early coronary atherosclerosis documented by ultrafast computed tomography. J Appl Nutr 1996;48:67–78.

33. Budoff MJ, Takasu J, Flores FR, et al. Inhibiting progression of coronary calcification using Aged Garlic Extract in patients receiving statin therapy: a preliminary study. Prev Med 2004;39:985–991.

34. Maniscalco BS, Taylor KA. Calcification in coronary artery disease can be reversed by EDTA-tetracycline long-term chemotherapy. Pathophysiology 2004;11:95–101.

35. US Renal Data System. USRDS 2004 Annual Data Report: Atlas of End-Stage Renal Disease in the United States. National Institutes of Health, National Institute of Diabetes and Digestive and Kidney Diseases, Bethesda, MD, 2004.

36. Longenecker JC, Coresh J, Powe NR, et al. Traditional cardiovascular disease risk factors in dialysis patients compared with the general population: the CHOICE Study. J Am Soc Nephrol 2002;13: 1918–1927.

37. Block G, Hulbert-Shearon T, Levin N, et al. Association of serum phosphorus and calcium × phosphate product with mortality risk in chronic hemodialysis patients: a national study. Am J Kidney Dis 1998;31:607–617.

38. Guerin AP, London GM, Marchais SJ, et al. Arterial stiffening and vascular calcifications in end-stage renal disease. Nephrol Dial Transplant 2000;15:1014–1021.

39. Blacher J, Guerin AP, Pannier B, et al. Arterial calcifications, arterial stiffness, and cardiovascular risk in end-stage renal disease. Hypertension 2001;38:938–942.

40. Raggi P, Boulay A, Chasan-Taber S, et al. Cardiac calcification in adult hemodialysis patients. A link between end-stage renal disease and cardiovascular disease? J Am Coll Cardiol 2002;39:695–701.

41. London GM, Guerin AP, Marchais SJ, et al. Arterial media calcification in end-stage renal disease: impact on all-cause and cardiovascular mortality. Nephrol Dial Transplant 2003;18:1731–1740.

42. London GM. Cardiovascular calcifications in uremic patients: clinical impact on cardiovascular function. J Am Soc Nephrol 2003; 14:S305–309.

43. Block GA, Klassen PS, Lazarus JM, et al. Mineral metabolism, mortality, and morbidity in maintenance hemodialysis. J Am Soc Nephrol 2004;15:2208–2218.

44. Goodman WG, Goldin J, Kuizon BD, et al. Coronary-artery calcification in young adults with end-stage renal disease who are undergoing dialysis. N Engl J Med 2000;342:1478–1483.

45. Chertow GM, Burke SK, Raggi P. Sevelamer attenuates the progression of coronary and aortic calcification in hemodialysis patients. Kidney Int 2002;62:245–252.

46. Chertow GM, Burke SK, Dillon MA, Slatopolsky E. Long-term effects of sevelamer hydrochloride on the calcium × phosphate product and lipid profile of haemodialysis patients. Nephrol Dial Transplant 1999,14:2907–2914.

47. Ferramosca E, Burke S, Chasan-Taber S, Ratti C, Chertow GM, Raggi P. Potential antiatherogenic and anti-inflammatory properties of sevelamer in maintenance hemodialysis patients. Am Heart J 2005; 149(5):820–825.

48. Raggi P, James G, Burke S, et al. Decrease in thoracic vertebral bone attenuation with calcium-based phosphate binders in hemodialysis. J Bone Min Res 2005;20(5):764–772.

49. Barengolts EI, Berman M, Kukreja SC, Kouznetsova T, Lin C, Chomka EV. Osteoporosis and coronary atherosclerosis in asymptomatic postmenopausal women. Calcif Tissue Int 1998;62:209–213.

50. Sirola J, Sirola J, Honkanen R, et al. Relation of statin use and bone loss: a prospective population-based cohort study in early postmenopausal women. Osteoporos Int 2002;13:537–541.

51. Yang H, Curinga G, Giachelli CM. Elevated extracellular calcium levels induce smooth muscle cell matrix mineralization in vitro. Kidney Int 2004;66:2293–2299.

52. Reynolds JL, Joannides AJ, Skepper JN, et al. Human vascular smooth muscle cells undergo vesicle-mediated calcification in response to changes in extracellular calcium and phosphate concentrations: a potential mechanism for accelerated vascular calcification in ESRD. J Am Soc Nephrol 2004;15:2857–2867.

53. Raggi P, Cooil B, Shaw LJ, et al. Progression of coronary calcification on serial electron beam tomography scanning is greater in patients with future myocardial infarction. Am J Cardiol 2003;92:827–829.

54. Raggi P, Callister T, Budoff M, Shaw L. Progression of coronary artery calcium and risk of first myocardial infarction in patients receiving cholesterol-lowering therapy. Arterioscler Thromb Vasc Biol 2004; 24:1272–1277.

8

Extra-Coronary Calcium

David M. Shavelle and Junichiro Takasu

Introduction

Calcification can occur in a several extra-coronary structures including the aorta, the aortic and mitral valve and both the carotid and peripheral arteries. Recent studies have found that the process by which calcium accumulates within these geographically distant locations is similar and represents various manifestations of atherosclerosis [1–4]. This chapter will focus on extra-coronary calcification as it relates to imaging by computed tomography (CT).

Aortic Calcium

Background

The aorta begins at the aortic annulus and extends to the bifurcation of the iliac arteries. Calcification can be present at various sites along this course and can be classified as involving the ascending aorta and arch, the descending aorta, and the abdominal aorta. The aortic arch and the infrarenal segments of the abdominal aorta have a higher prevalence of calcified plaques than the other segments (Figure 8.1) [5]. The presence of calcification within the aorta predicts cardiovascular mortality, independent of major cardiovascular risk factors [2,6,7].

Prevalence and Association with Cardiovascular Risk Factors

The prevalence of calcification of the aorta varies according to the population studied and the imaging modality used for detection. The majority of available data is based upon population studies of healthy adults using imaging by chest radiography [2,6,7]. More recently electron beam computed tomography (EBT) has been used to detect and quantify aortic calcification (Figure 8.2) [8–10].

The Kaiser Permanente Medical Care Program of Northern California found the prevalence of calcification of the aortic arch as detected by chest radiograph to be 10.6% for elderly men and 15.6% for elderly women [2]. This study included 139,849 individuals and therefore would appear to be a good approximation of a random sample from the United States population. In a relatively large, population-based study from the Netherlands, the prevalence of abdominal aortic calcification by radiograph was 34.8% for men and 58.3% of women [6]. The Framingham Study reported similar findings, with a prevalence of 57% for men and 47% for women in the ages of 60 to 69 years [7].

The ability to detect calcification by radiography (fluoroscopy) is lower than that for CT. Therefore, the prevalence of CT-measured calcification would be expected to be higher than that by radiography (Table 8.1). Allison et al. performed whole-body EBT scanning of 650 asymptomatic individuals [8]. The mean age of the study group was 57 years with 53% male. For men and women aged 50 to 60 years, the prevalence of calcification of the descending aorta was 29% and 29%, respectively. This prevalence increased to 98% for men and 96% for women above the age of 70 years. For men and women aged 50 to 60 years, the prevalence of calcification of the abdominal aorta was 55% and 50%, respectively. As with the descending aorta, calcification of the abdominal aorta also increased in prevalence with age, occurring in 98% for men and 93% for women above the age of 70 years. Kuller et al. evaluated 169 women with a mean age of 58 years participating in the Healthy Women Study [9]. The aorta was imaged from the aortic root to the iliac bifurcation; however, the investigators did not characterize the exact location of calcification but referred to any calcium within the ascending, descending, or abdominal aorta as "aortic" calcification. By this general definition, aortic calcification was present in 71% of the study group. Reaven and Sacks evaluated 309 patients with type 2 diabetes mellitus and suboptimal glycemic control, defined as a $HgA_1C > 7.5\%$ [11]. Calcification within the descending aorta was present in 14%. Raggi et al. evaluated 245 patients self-referred for EBT coronary scanning and found a prevalence of 37% for "aortic" (ascending, descending, and abdominal aorta) calcification [10]. Cury et al. studied 416 asymptomatic patients undergoing routine EBT coronary and aortic scanning, and found the prevalence of descending aortic calcium to be 51% [12].

Given that calcium within the aorta is related to the systemic process of atherosclerosis, it is not surprising that its presence is associated with traditional coronary risk factors [8–10]. Age, hypertension, cigarette smoking, LDL and HDL levels, systolic blood pressure, and glucose levels are all predictors of aortic calcification [8,9,12]. Although lipoprotein (a) (Lp(a)) is associated with coronary artery calcium, it does not appear to be associated with aortic calcium [10]. In a small study of 28 patients, elevated levels

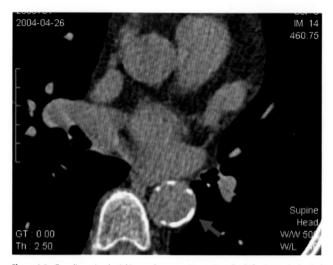

Figure 8.2. Two-dimensional axial image demonstrating aortic wall calcification at the level of the thoracic descending aorta (red arrow). The calcification is easy to visualize and quantitate.

of homocysteine were associated with a higher degree of aortic calcification by CT [13].

The presence of aortic calcification is also associated with more extensive angiographic coronary artery disease [14] and higher coronary artery calcium scores [9,12,15,16]. In a series of 97 patients, the presence of aortic calcification had a specificity of 72% for diagnosing obstructive coronary artery disease [16]. These findings suggest that evaluating the presence and extent of aortic calcification may provide additional prognostic information to that obtained from coronary calcium scoring alone. Studies evaluating the prognostic significance of aortic calcium on future cardiovascular events are ongoing [17].

Aortic Calcium Scoring and Natural History

The natural history of aortic calcification has not been adequately studied by CT imaging and the majority of studies to date have used radiography [18,19]. In a report from the Framingham Heart Study, Kauppila and colleagues developed a semi-quantitative scoring system in 617 patients undergoing a baseline and follow-up lumbar radiograph at 25 years [20]. The scoring system appeared to be reproducible, leading the authors to suggest that it could be used as a simple, low-cost assessment of subclinical vascular disease. However, given the ability to accurately, noninvasively and rapidly quantify calcium throughout the entire aorta by CT imaging, it would seem that plain radiography would be less than ideal. Despite the potential benefits of CT imaging of the aorta, there have been no studies to date that have specifically addressed the issue of reproducibility with serial scanning using the Agatston or volumetric scoring methods.

Several scoring methods have been proposed to quantify the amount of aortic calcification [5,21–26]. These include

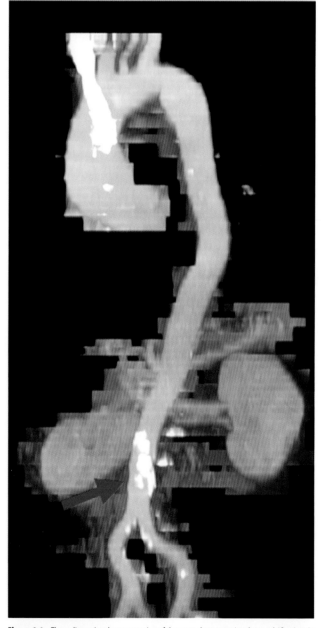

Figure 8.1. Three-dimensional reconstruction of the aorta, demonstrating dense calcifications in the infrarenal region (red arrow).

Table 8.1. Prevalence of calcium in the aorta by CT imaging

Author/Year	No of subjects	Study inclusion criteria	Mean Age (years)	Prevalence of Calcification
Kuller et al. 1999 [9]	169	Asymptomatic, premenopausal women participating in Healthy Women Study	58	Aortic: 71%
Allison et al. 2004 [8]	650	Asymptomatic, referred for preventive medicine evaluation at University Hospital	57	Men 50–60 years: ASC Ao: 29% DESC Ao: 55% Woman 50–60 years: ASC Ao: 29% DESC Ao: 50%
Reaven and Sacks 2005 [11]	309	Veterans with type 2 diabetes mellitus, over the age of 40 with HgA₁C >7.5%	61	DESC Ao: 14%
Raggi et al. 2003 [10]	245	Asymptomatic, self-referred for electron beam tomography coronary calcium scanning	55	Aortic: 37%
Cury et al. 2004 [12]	416	Asymptomatic, participating in age-related bone loss and vascular calcification study	68	DESC Ao: 51%

Aortic = ascending aorta, aortic arch, descending aorta and abdominal aorta.
Asc Ao = ascending aorta; DESC Ao = descending aorta.

the: (1) Agatston method with total score and total number of calcifications, (2) percentage of calcified aortic volume against whole vascular volume (%ACV), (3) arterial calcification volume (ACV), (4) aortic calcification index (ACI), (5) aortic calcification area (ACA), and (6) aortic wall and calcification volume (AWCV). In a small series of 11 patients, the interobserver variability for AWCV and ACV was 5.5 and 4.7%, respectively; the intraobserver and interscan variabilities were not evaluated [22].

The natural history of aortic calcification by CT imaging largely remains unknown. There have been no studies to date that have evaluated sufficient numbers of patients to make conclusions regarding the natural history. However, there have been three small series of patients that applied different scoring systems and determined factors associated with more rapid progression of aortic calcium (see below). These studies are limited by small patient numbers and lack of standardization of scoring methods. As such, the true natural history of aortic calcification remains unclear. The ongoing Multi-Ethnic Study of Atherosclerosis (MESA) trial will hopefully provide this information [17].

Aortic Calcium Progression

Only three studies to date have evaluated progression of aortic calcium on serial CT scans [27–29]. The methods used to quantify aortic calcium in each of these studies were different. In 80 middle-aged women, Sutton-Tyrrell et al. performed EBT of the coronary arteries and aorta at baseline and at 18 months [27]. The mean change in aortic score by the Agatston method was an increase of 112, and 71% of patients had an increase in score at follow-up scan compared to baseline. An increase in aortic calcium score over time (i.e. progression) was associated with higher baseline aortic scores, higher pulse pressure, and higher total cholesterol and LDL levels.

Miwa et al. evaluated 116 patients undergoing serial CT scanning and used %ACV to quantify aortic calcium [29]. This aortic calcification score was determined using an image color analysis program that calculated the percentage of calcified aortic volume against the whole vascular volume. The study population included those with aortic wall calcification on baseline scan and patients achieving optimal control of lipids. Only the abdominal aorta was imaged and the mean follow-up period was 6.3 ± 3.2 years. The rate of progression of %ACV was determined as the absolute change in %ACV divided by the interscan interval in years. %ACV increased (i.e. progression) in 89% of the patients over the study period. The rate of progression of %ACV was related to age, body mass index, systolic blood pressure, and pulse pressure. Pulse pressure was the strongest risk factor for progression. Baseline lipid values and the use of HMG-CoA reductase inhibitors were not related to progression. However, 79% of the patients were receiving HMG-CoA reductase inhibitors and 50% were receiving either fibrates or probucol. Given that all patients in the cohort had "optimal" control of lipids at study entry and the high rate of lipid-lower medications, it would seem difficult to show a treatment effect related to lipid lowering.

Arai et al. used plain and enhanced CT to evaluate the abdominal aorta in 29 patients undergoing treatment with an HMG-CoA reductase inhibitor [28]. ACV was evaluated at baseline and after 2 years of therapy. Progression of ACV was not associated with any of the study variables, including cholesterol levels, blood pressure, measures of coagulation (fibrinogen), or body mass index. Given the small number of patients included and treatment of all study patients with lipid-lowering therapy, conclusions regarding the clinical factors associated with aortic calcium progression in this study remain unclear. To date, no studies have been done using CT imaging to evaluate interventions to decrease aortic calcium progression.

In menopausal women, the natural history of aortic calcification appears to be related to osteoporosis [18,19].

These data are derived from population-based studies using lumbar spine radiographs and there are currently no data with CT imaging. Kiel et al. found that women developing the greatest amount of bone loss throughout the lumbar spine (osteoporosis) also experienced the most severe progression of abdominal aortic calcification [19]. This relationship was not observed in men. Hak et al. extended these observations and studied 236 initially premenopausal women and performed a baseline and follow-up abdominal radiographs at 9 years [18]. The baseline study reflected the premenopausal state and the follow-up study represented the postmenopausal state. There was a significant association between progression of aortic calcification and the degree of osteoporosis. Other investigators have suggested that the link between osteoporosis and vascular calcification is mediated through the estrogen-deficient state of menopause and oxidized lipids [30,31].

A specific subgroup of patients with extensive vascular calcification, including aortic, are those with end-stage renal disease receiving hemodialysis [32–34]. Hashiba et al. evaluated 18 patients with end-stage renal disease on hemodialysis and found that ACA progression was reduced in those receiving etidronate, a bisphosphonate used for the treatment of osteoporosis [23]. In a study of 36 patients on hemodialysis, Bommer et al. found that progression of abdominal aortic calcification was associated with levels of uric acid, cholesterol, and the calcium-phosphorus product [34]. While it is generally accepted that aortic wall calcification is atherosclerosis, the influence of statins, blood pressure agents, and other therapies (e.g. fish oils) have not been reported. Furthermore, the incremental risk associated with this "disease state" has not been measured. The MESA study is evaluating this, both to establish the relationship with atherosclerotic risk factors, as well as the incremental prognostic value of this measure.

Comparison of CT Imaging of the Aorta with Other Imaging Methods

Few studies have compared CT imaging of the aorta with other imaging modalities, such as transesophageal echocardiography (TEE) or magnetic resonance imaging (MRI). Furthermore, there have been no direct comparison studies for the assessment of aortic calcium by different imaging methods. Tenenbaum et al. compared dual helical CT and TEE for the detection of aortic atheromas [35]. CT was found to be accurate for detecting atheromas of the ascending aorta. However, the ability of either EBT or multidetector CT to evaluate plaque has not been determined.

Summary

Calcification of the aorta is a manifestation of systemic atherosclerosis and its presence is associated with increased cardiovascular mortality. The prevalence of aortic calcium increases with age and is associated with coronary risk factors. Progression of aortic calcium in women is associated with osteoporosis, although the underlying mechanisms remain unclear. Additional studies with CT imaging are required to evaluate interventions to reduce aortic calcium progression.

Carotid Artery

Background

Atherosclerosis of the carotid artery accounts for up to 30% of all strokes and cerebrovascular disease is currently the third leading cause of death in the United States [36]. Noninvasive imaging of the carotid artery is typically done with ultrasound and MR angiography. While studies of CT angiography for the assessment of stenosis severity are promising [37], relatively few investigators have specifically focused on imaging of calcium [8,38,39].

Pathologic studies have found that calcium is present within a significant number of carotid artery plaques [40, 41]. Carotid artery calcification typically occurs at the carotid bulb at the region of the bifurcation (Figure 8.3) [40]. The amount of atherosclerosis and calcification appears to be relatively similar between the left and right carotid arteries [42].

Prevalence and Association with Cardiovascular Risk Factors

Two studies have specifically evaluated the prevalence of calcification within the carotid arteries by CT imaging [8,39]. Allison et al. evaluated 650 asymptomatic patients referred for a preventive medicine evaluation at a University Hospital who underwent whole-body CT imaging [8]. For men aged 50 to 60 years, the prevalence of carotid artery calcium within the right and left carotid arteries was the same at 23%. For women aged 50 to 60 years, the prevalence of carotid artery calcium within the right and left carotid arteries was 10% and 11%, respectively. With increasing age, the prevalence of carotid artery calcium increased to approximately 80% for men and 60% for women. Wagenknecht et al. studied 438 asymptomatic individuals with a family history of type 2 diabetes mellitus and quantified carotid calcium using the calcium mass score [39]. For men and women younger than 60 years, the prevalence of carotid artery calcium (calcium mass score >0) was 62% and 52%, respectively. For men and women older than 60 years, the prevalence of carotid artery calcium increased to 90% and 88%, respectively.

In the study by Allison et al, increasing age and hypertension were associated with the presence of carotid artery calcium [8]. No other studies have evaluated the relationship between coronary risk factors and carotid artery calcium by CT imaging.

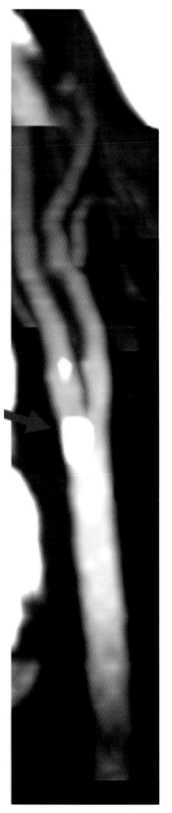

Figure 8.3. A carotid CT angiogram demonstrating dense calcification at the bifurcation of the common carotid (arrow).

The presence of carotid artery and coronary artery calcium are related, but this relationship appears to be complex [8,38]. For patients undergoing elective coronary artery bypass grafting, severe carotid artery stenosis of greater than 80% occurs in up to 12% [43]. Furthermore, patients with established peripheral vascular disease have a high incidence of coexisting coronary artery disease [44]. However, additional studies using CT imaging of both the carotid and coronary arteries are needed to determine true rates of prevalence.

Carotid Calcium Scoring and Natural History

Carotid artery calcium has been quantified by the methods described for coronary artery calcium scoring [8,38,39] (Table 8.2). For asymptomatic patients over the age of 70 years, the median calcium score by the method of Agatston was 73 for men and 79 for women [8]. Using the calcium mass score, Wagenknecht et al. found a median score of 228 for men and 70 for women over the age of 60 years [39]. Arad et al. reported on a smaller cohort of 50 symptomatic patients undergoing CT imaging of the carotid arteries following coronary angiography [38]. The mean age of the study group was 67 years and the median carotid calcium score by the Agatston method was 142 for the entire study group.

To date, no study has addressed the natural history of carotid artery calcification by CT imaging. In addition, there is no information regarding the reproducibility of carotid artery calcium scoring during serial scans, excluding the in vitro study by Adams et al. discussed below [42].

Comparison to Histology and Other Imaging Methods

The accuracy of CT imaging in quantifying the amount of calcium within the carotid arteries was evaluated by Denzel et al. [45]. In this in vitro study of 92 carotid artery plaques, there was good correlation between the CT-derived calcium score and histopathologic grading of plaque composition (correlation coefficient 0.55, $p < 0.001$). Adams et al. evaluated 50 carotid arteries from cadaveric donors and performed both MR and CT imaging [42]. The reproducibility of the Agatston and volumetric scores was excellent with a median variability of 6.2% and 4.8%, respectively. These values are similar to those achieved with coronary and aortic valve calcium scanning [46,47]. In addition, the carotid artery volume measurement by MRI correlated well with both the Agatston and volumetric carotid scores.

Carotid artery intima-media thickness (IMT) is a widely accepted non-invasive measure of atherosclerosis [48]. Further, multiple studies have documented the ability of IMT to predict future cardiovascular events [49,50]. Arad et al. evaluated whether carotid artery calcium by CT correlated with carotid artery IMT [38]. In this study of 50 patients, there was no correlation between IMT and carotid artery calcium. In a larger trial of 438 asymptomatic

Table 8.2. Quantification of carotid artery calcium by CT imaging

Author/Year	No of subjects	Study inclusion criteria	Mean age (years)	Scoring method	Carotid artery calcification score (median)
Allison et al. 2004 [8]	650	Asymptomatic, referred for preventive medicine evaluation at University Hospital	57	Agatston	Men 50–60 years: RCAR: 10 LCAR: 0 Men >70 years: RCAR: 92 LCAR: 54 Women 50–60 years: RCAR: 0 LCAR: 0 Women >70 years: RCAR: 72 LCAR: 86
Wagenknecht et al. 2004 [39]	438	Asymptomatic, family history of type 2 diabetes mellitus	438	Calcium mass score	Men <60 years: Carotid: 16 Men >60 years: Carotid: 228 Women <60 years: Carotid: 1 Women >60 years: Carotid: 70
Arad et al. 1998 [38]	50	Symptomatic, referred following coronary angiography	67	Agatston	142

RCAR = right carotid artery, LCAR = left carotid artery.

patients, Wagenknecht et al. did find a correlation between IMT and carotid artery calcium (correlation coefficient 0.45, $p < 0.0001$) [39]. To date, there have been no studies evaluating the relationship between carotid artery calcium by CT imaging and the severity of stenosis as determined by either ultrasound or angiography.

Although not specifically related to CT assessment of carotid artery calcium, there has been significant progress in the ability of CT angiography to assess the severity of carotid artery stenosis. In a review of 28 studies of CT angiography, Koelemay et al. found an overall sensitivity of 85% and a specificity of 93% for detection of a 70–99% carotid artery stenosis [37].

Summary

Carotid artery disease is a significant cause of morbidity and mortality in the United States. While calcium is present in a large proportion of carotid artery lesions, relatively few studies have specifically described CT imaging of calcium. As such, the natural history and the impact of interventions on disease progression remain unknown. Additional research with CT imaging of calcium within the carotid arteries is needed.

Peripheral Arteries

Background

The peripheral vessels can be classified into three anatomic zones: (1) the inflow zone includes the infrarenal aorta and iliac arteries; (2) the outflow zone includes the femoral and popliteal arteries; and (3) the run-off zone includes the tibial and peroneal arteries. When atherosclerosis involves these sites it is referred to as peripheral vascular disease (PVD). In patients younger than 40 years, the aorta and iliac arteries are more commonly involved with PVD; whereas the femoral and popliteal vessels are the more common site of involvement in patients older than 40 years [51]. The clinical manifestations of PVD include claudication and non-healing wounds or ulcers of the lower extremities. Patients with PVD have a reduced long-term survival compared to the normal population and the most common cause of death is myocardial infarction or stroke [52].

The proximal segments of the peripheral vessels (aortoiliac and femoropopliteal) have significantly more calcification than the distal vessels (infrapopliteal) (Figure 8.4) [53]. The use of CT imaging for calcium in the peripheral vessels has been described by only one study to date [8] and the majority of information available is based upon CT angiography [53,54].

Prevalence and Association with Cardiovascular Risk Factors

The only study to specifically evaluate the prevalence of calcification within the peripheral vessels by CT imaging was done by Allison et al. [8]. As previously discussed in the sections on carotid and aortic calcium, whole-body CT imaging was performed in 650 asymptomatic individuals referred for a preventive medicine evaluation. The left and

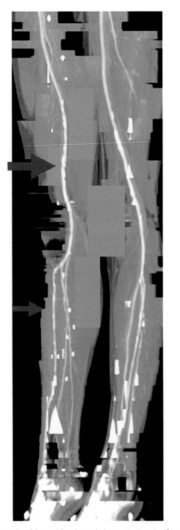

Figure 8.4. CT angiography of the peripheral vessels demonstrating significant calcification of the femoral artery (purple arrow), with virtually no calcification of the tibial vessels (red arrow).

right iliac arteries were imaged and the amount of calcium was quantified using the Agatston score. For men aged 50 to 60 years, the prevalence of calcification of the right and left iliac arteries was 57% and 55%, respectively. These numbers increased to 91% and 89% for the right and left iliac arteries, respectively, for men above the age of 70 years. For women ages 50 to 60 years, the prevalence of calcification of the right and left iliac arteries was 34% and 28%, respectively. For women above the age of 70 years, the prevalence increased to 78% and 73% for the right and left iliac arteries, respectively.

Risk factors associated with iliac artery calcification in both men and women included increasing age and hypertension [8]. In women, cigarette smoking was also associated with the presence of iliac artery calcification.

Calcium Scoring and Natural History

Calcium within the peripheral vessels has been evaluated using a semi-quantitative scale [53] and the method of Agatston [24]. Portugaller et al. found that higher

calcification scores were seen for higher grade stenoses and occlusions, compared to less obstructive lesions (<70% stenosis severity) [53]. In the study by Allison et al, for men ages 50 to 60 years, the median calcium score (Agatston method) of the right and left iliac arteries was 36 and 44, respectively [8]. These values for the right and left iliac arteries increased to 1468 and 1628, respectively, for men above the age of 70 years. For women ages 50 to 60 years, the median calcium score (Agatston method) for both the right and left iliac arteries was 10. For women above the age of 70 years, the median score for the right and left iliac arteries were 1468 and 1628, respectively. To date, no study has used CT imaging to characterize the natural history of calcium within the peripheral vessels.

Comparison to Peripheral Angiography

CT angiography appears to be relatively accurate for the assessment of PVD [53–55]. However, no study has directly compared CT imaging of calcium within the peripheral vessels to the severity of stenosis by CT angiography or conventional angiography. Further, there have been no studies to date evaluating interventions to prevent calcium progression.

Summary

CT imaging for calcium within the peripheral vessels has not been adequately studied. The prevalence of peripheral artery calcium increases with age and is associated with coronary risk factors. The natural history and the impact of interventions on calcium progression remain unknown. Even relatively simple studies such as comparison to ankle-brachial indexes have not been reported. Given the high prevalence of coexisting PVD and coronary artery disease, additional imaging work in this area is needed.

Aortic Valve Calcium

Background

Aortic valve disease is a general term that includes both aortic sclerosis and aortic stenosis (AS). Aortic sclerosis is thought to represent an early stage in the disease process that eventually progresses to result in obstruction to left ventricular outflow or AS. Previously, aortic sclerosis and AS were felt to be "degenerative" diseases that were the result of a "wear and tear" phenomenon and occurred as a consequence of aging. However, newer studies suggest that they are the result of an active disease process within the aortic valve leaflets that has similarities to atherosclerosis including the presence of inflammatory cells [56], the deposition of lipids [57], and involvement of active mediators of calcification [58,59].

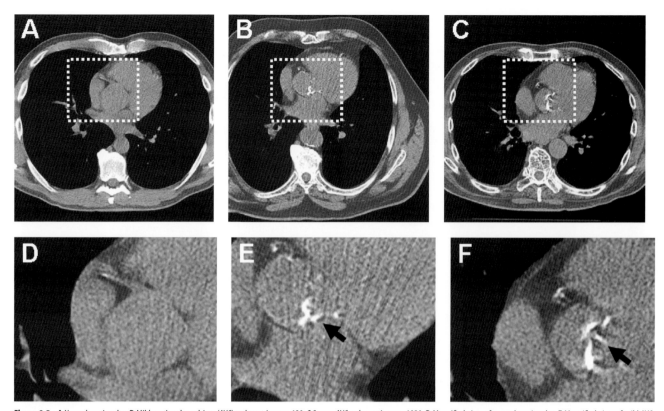

Figure 8.5. **A** Normal aortic valve. **B** Mild aortic valve calcium (AVC); volumetric score 120. **C** Severe AVC; volumetric score 1020. **D** Magnified view of normal aortic valve. **E** Magnified view of mild AVC. **F** Magnified view of severe AVC. Arrows indicate AVC.

Calcification plays a central role in the disease process. Pathologic studies have shown that calcium occurs in areas of lipoprotein deposition and macrophages within the valve leaflets locally produce proteins such as osteopontin that are involved in calcium metabolism [58–60]. Echocardiographic studies have found that the severity of aortic valve calcium (AVC) is associated with more rapid disease progression and predicts clinical outcome [61,62].

In 1988, MacMillan et al. first used EBT to evaluate the aortic valve in 8 patients with AS [63]. EBT assessment of the aortic valve area was similar to that obtained at the time of cardiac catheterization. The initial study to evaluate the reproducibility of EBT scanning of aortic valve calcium was done by Kizer et al. in 2001 [64]. In this study, 19 patients underwent two EBT scans 30 seconds apart. The results showed excellent reproducibility of serial EBT scanning and the authors suggested that EBT would be useful

to quantify AVC during longitudinal studies. Given the ease of scanning, the ability to provide a quantitative measurement of AVC (Figure 8.5), and the excellent reproducibility, EBT assessment of the aortic valve has recently been used in trials evaluating medical therapy for AS [65–67].

Prevalence and Association with Cardiovascular Risk Factors

The development of AVC appears to be a relatively late finding in patients with atherosclerosis and is rarely found in the absence of coronary artery calcium. The prevalence of AVC varies depending upon the population studied (Table 8.3). In asymptomatic patients referred for coronary artery calcium scanning, AVC is present in 7.5–17.7% [66–68]. Additional information regarding the prevalence

Table 8.3. Prevalence of aortic valve calcium by CT imaging

Author/Year	Type of scanner	No of subjects	Study inclusion criteria	Mean age (years)	Prevalence
Pohle et al. 2001 [67]	EBT	2124	Asymptomatic, referred for EBT coronary calcium scanning	65	12.8%
Shavelle et al. 2002 [66]	EBT	640	Asymptomatic, referred for EBT coronary calcium scanning	59	7.5%
Walsh et al. 2004 [68]	EBT	327	Asymptomatic, referred for EBT coronary calcium scanning	60	14%
Pohle et al. 2004 [71]	EBT	1000	Asymptomatic, referred for EBT coronary calcium scanning	57	17.7%
Yamamoto et al. 2002 [14]	EBT	99	Referred for coronary angiography for angina symptoms	56.6	30%
Cowell et al. 2003 [70]	MSCT	157	Aortic stenosis (aortic jet velocity by echocardiography ≥2.5 m/s)	68	98.7%

EBT = electron beam computed tomography; MSCT = multislice computed tomography.

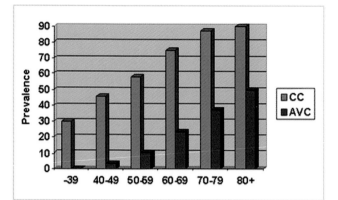

Figure 8.6. Prevalence of coronary artery and aortic valve calcium in a population of 620 persons, based upon age. AVC = aortic valve calcium, CC = coronary calcium. (Reprinted with permission from Takasu et al. [82].)

of AVC in larger numbers of asymptomatic individuals will be obtained from the ongoing MESA trial [17]. For patients with chest pain referred for invasive coronary angiography, AVC is present in approximately 30% [14]. In patients with known AS, the prevalence of AVC ranges from 20% to 99% depending upon the severity of AS [69,70].

Cardiovascular risk factors including hypertension, diabetes mellitus, tobacco use, and hyperlipidemia are commonly present in patients with AVC [71]. Increasing age is strongly associated with increasing prevalence of AVC (Figure 8.6). Patients with AVC usually have associated coronary artery calcium, which appears to predominantly affect the left anterior descending artery (Figure 8.7) [70,71].

Aortic Valve Calcium Scoring

AVC can be measured by the volumetric method, the Agatston method or a modified Agatston method. The volumetric method involves identifying calcium within the aortic valve as areas of at least 2 contiguous pixels with a density of 130 Hounsfield units (HU) or more [72]. The total volume of all the calcifications is then determined. Most studies evaluating AVC have excluded aortic wall calcium from the analysis and have included only calcium that is contained within the actual aortic valve leaflets. The Agatston method was initially described by Agatston et al. in 1990 to evaluate coronary artery calcium [24]. This involves multiplying the lesion area by a density factor derived from the maximal HU. The density factor is 1 for lesions with a maximum density of 130 to 199; 2 for lesions with a maximum density of 200 to 299; 3 for lesions with maximum density of 300 to 399; and 4 for lesion with a maximum density of >400. The total score is determined by adding all the individual lesion scores. The modified Agatston method is being used with multislice CT in the ongoing SALTIRE trial and involves using a threshold of 90 HU to compensate for non-gated imaging [70]. However, non-gated studies can have significant motion artifacts (Figure 8.8), especially if the image is obtained during systole when the aortic valve is actively opening.

Several studies have evaluated the reproducibility of AVC scanning [64,73,74]. Kizer et al. studied 19 patients EBT scans repeated 30 seconds apart and found excellent correlation between scans [64]. Budoff et al. evaluated the Agatston and volumetric method in 44 patients undergoing two EBT scans on the same day [73]. The median interscan variability was 7% and 6.2% for the Agatston and volumetric method, respectively. For the volumetric method, the median interobserver and intraobserver

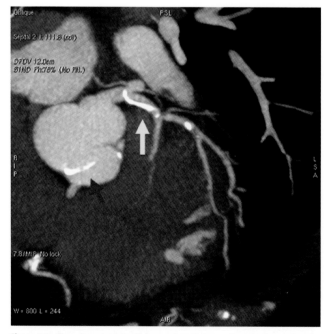

Figure 8.7. Three-dimensional (multiplanar reformat) image demonstrating aortic valve calcification (red arrow) as well as left anterior descending artery calcification (yellow arrow).

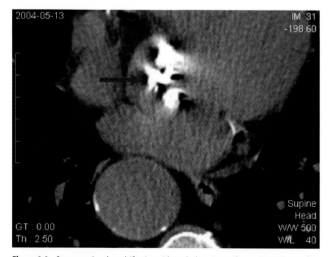

Figure 8.8. Severe aortic valve calcification with marked motion artifacts, taken with a 16-slice multidetector CT (ungated study). The images demonstrate severe motion, making quantification of aortic valve calcification impossible.

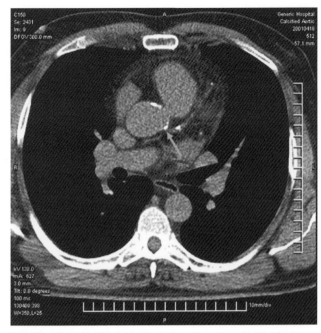

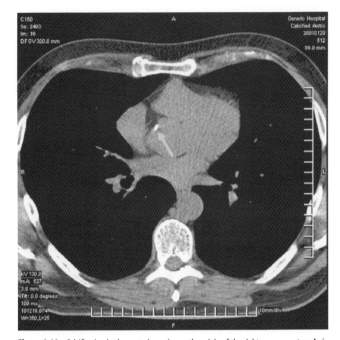

Figure 8.9. The location of the aortic calcification (arrow) is near the origin of the left main coronary artery. Since the calcium is linear and does not extrude toward the coronary artery, it is not considered coronary artery calcification, and would not contribute to the person's coronary calcium score.

Figure 8.10. Calcification in the aorta (arrow) near the origin of the right coronary artery. As in Figure 8.9, the calcium is considered aortic wall and not coronary artery.

variability was 5% and 1%, respectively. Messika-Zeitoun et al. found a mean interobserver variability of 4% and a mean intraobserver variability of 3.7% [74].

The methodology for determining the location of calcification, whether it is considered in the wall of the aorta, the aortic valve or coronary artery has undergone standardization. In the above studies and others, the methodology employed is as follows: if the calcification is linear and in the ring of the aorta, it is considered aortic calcification and not valve or coronary calcification (cc) (Figures 8.9–8.11). This can be appreciated best on the two-dimensional images (Figures 8.9 and 8.10), but also on three-dimensional reconstruction (Figures 8.7 and 8.11). If the calcification is within the center of the aorta, or extending from the wall toward the center, it is considered aortic valve calcification (Figures 8.7, 8.12, and 8.13).

In summary, the interscan, interobserver, and intraobserver variabilities of EBT assessment of the AVC are low, thus allowing for accurate assessment of AVC change over time. The prognostic importance of this measure, as well as factors that may influence change, are being studied in SALTIRE and MESA, among other studies. Given high reproducibility and easy measure on non-contrast study, the potential to non-invasively track therapies with CT imaging is high.

Comparison to Echocardiography

EBT measurement of AVC has been compared to echocardiographic assessment of AS severity [68–70,74,75].

Increasing severity of AS is associated with higher AVC scores [70]. A study of 48 patients found that an AVC volumetric score of >100 had a sensitivity of 100% and a specificity of 77% for identifying patients with an aortic jet velocity of >2.5 m/s, considered hemodynamically

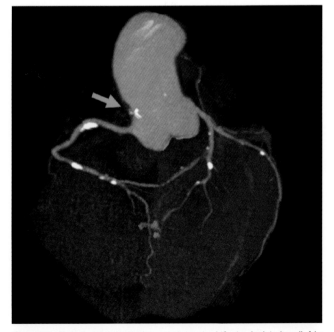

Figure 8.11. Three dimensional image demonstrating aortic calcification clearly in the wall of the aorta (arrow), several centimeters above the aortic valve and ostium of the coronaries. This patient also has calcifications in all three coronary arteries.

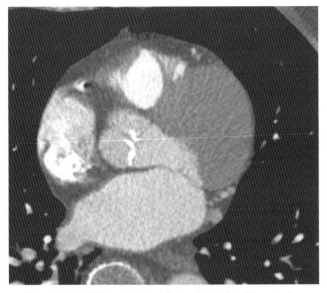

Figure 8.12. Axial CT image showing calcification of two leaflets of the aortic valve.

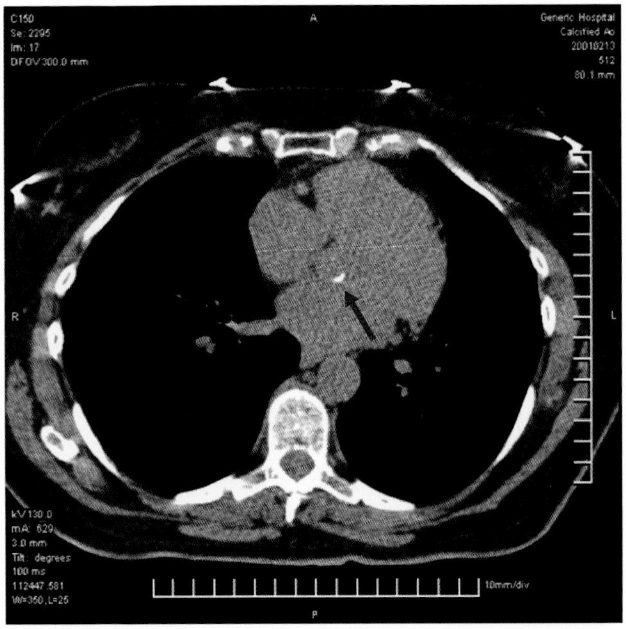

Figure 8.13. Calcified aortic valve in the classic "J" appearance (arrow). The calcification is in the middle of the aortic valve region, so it is unlikely to be in the wall of the aorta or coronary arteries, but rather on the aortic valve leaflet itself.

significant AS [14]. A study of 100 patients found a curvilinear relationship between the AVC score and aortic valve area by echocardiography [74]. In this study, an AVC Agatston score of ≥1100 had a 93% sensitivity and a 82% specificity for detecting severe AS (aortic valve area <1.0 cm²).

Natural History

The initial study to evaluate the natural history of AVC as measured by EBT was done by Pohle et al. in 2001 [67]. Changes in AVC in 104 patients followed for an average of 1.25 years were expressed as the difference between the follow-up score and the initial score, divided by the initial score and the interscan interval in years:

$$\%\Delta AVC/year$$
$$= \frac{\left(Score_{follow\text{-}up\,scan} - Score_{initial\,scan}\right)}{\left(Score_{initial\,scan} \times Interscan\,interval\,in\,years\right)}$$

For the entire group of patients, the mean (± standard deviation) %ΔAVC/year was 25% ± 38%. In a smaller study of 65 patients, the mean (± standard deviation) %ΔAVC/year was 29.8 ± 46% [66] (Table 8.4).

The prognostic role of AVC as detected by EBT with regard to future cardiovascular events largely remains unclear. Data from the South Bay Heart Watch Study suggests that it provides important prognostic information above and beyond that obtained from coronary artery calcium scanning in asymptomatic individuals [76]. A small trial of 100 patients with known AS found that the presence of AVC by EBT was associated with increased future cardiovascular events including death, congestive heart failure, and need for aortic valve replacement [74].

Impact of Interventions on Progression

Given the similarities between aortic valve disease and atherosclerosis and the clinical benefit of lipid lowering therapy in patients with atherosclerosis, two trials retrospectively evaluated whether use of HMG-CoA reductase inhibitors (statins) would reduce AVC progression [66,67] (Table 8.5). Both trials showed a reduction in the rate of AVC progression. In the study by Pohle et al., there was no effect of statins on AVC progression [67]. However, if patients were compared based on LDL status, those with an

Table 8.4. Natural history of aortic valve calcium progression by CT imaging

Author/Year	No of subjects	Mean age (years)	Mean F/U interval (years)	Progression AVC (%Δ/year) Mean ± standard deviation
Pohle et al. 2001 [67]	104	65	1.25	Volumetric score: 25 ± 38%
Shavelle et al. 2002 [66]	65	67	2.5	Volumetric score: 29.8 ± 46%
				Agatston score: 46.8 ± 84%

F/U = Follow-up.

Table 8.5. Effect of medical therapy on aortic valve calcium progression by CT imaging

Author/Year	No of subjects	Mean age (years)	Mean progression AVC (%Δ/year) Study groups	p value	Study findings
Pohle et al. 2001 [67]	104	65	LDL <130: 9% LDL >130: 43%	0.001	↓AVC progression with LDL <130
Shavelle et al. 2002 [66]	65	67	Statin therapy: 12% No statin therapy: 32%	0.006	↓AVC progression with statin therapy

AVC = aortic valve calcium.

LDL <130 had less AVC progression compared to those with an LDL >130. Four retrospective echocardiographic trials showed similar findings with a reduction in the decrease in aortic valve area and a reduction in the increase in aortic jet velocity in patients receiving statin therapy [77–80]. Several prospective trials using statins and either EBT or echocardiography to assess for disease progression are under way [70,81,82].

Summary

AVC plays a central role in the pathogenesis of aortic sclerosis and AS. CT imaging allows AVC to be accurately and non-invasively measured, thus providing insight into the disease process. Given the accuracy of serial CT scanning, measurement of AVC can be used to follow disease progression. The MESA trial will provide additional information regarding the prevalence of AVC in asymptomatic individuals. The ongoing SALTIRE trial is assessing whether statin therapy for patients with AS reduces AVC progression.

Mitral Annular Calcification

Background

Calcification of the mitral valve or mitral valve annulus has similarities to AVC and may also represent a form of atherosclerosis [83]. Mitral annular calcification (MAC) is thought to play a role in a variety of disease processes, including left atrial enlargement, atrial fibrillation, mitral regurgitation and stenosis, and bacterial endocarditis [84–86]. Imaging of the mitral valve by CT has not been extensively studied and the majority of the available data on MAC is related to echocardiography. However, cardiac CT provides an excellent means to image both the mitral valve and mitral annulus (Figures 8.14–8.17).

Prevalence and Association with Coronary Risk Factors

MAC is associated with standard cardiovascular risk factors and also encountered in association with aortic stenosis and chronic renal failure [87,88].

The prevalence of MAC by CT imaging has been evaluated in 3 recent studies [89–91]. Adler et al. evaluated 329 elderly patients (above 60 years age) and found 60 (18%) with MAC [89]. Tenenbaum et al. studied 522 hypertensive patients and found 62 (12%) with advanced MAC (calcium thickness ≥5 mm) and 215 (41%) with trivial MAC (calcium thickness <5 mm) [90]. Yamamoto et al. evaluated 99 patients referred for coronary angiography that also underwent EBT coronary scanning and found 19 (19%) with MAC [91].

Clinical Significance

Echocardiographic studies have found that the presence of MAC predicts subsequent strokes and cardiac related death [92,93]. The presence of MAC is also associated with higher CC scores, more extensive and severe coronary artery

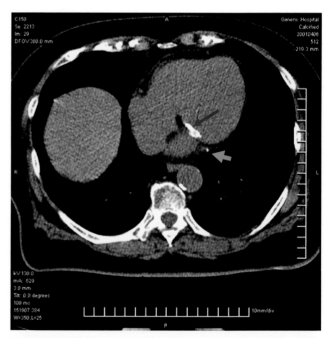

Figure 8.14. Axial CT image showing calcified mitral annulus. The red arrow demonstrates fairly significant calcification of the posterior portion of the leaflet. This is important to distinguish from the circumflex, as this would add hundreds to the "calcium score." The circumflex is seen with a small amount of calcification epicardially (green arrow). The calcified descending aorta is also seen (blue arrow).

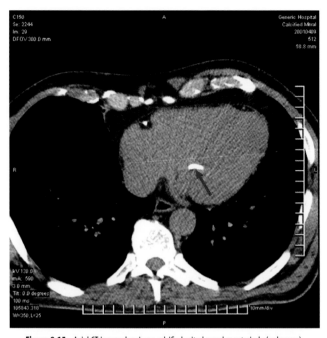

Figure 8.15. Axial CT image showing a calcified mitral annulus anteriorly (red arrow).

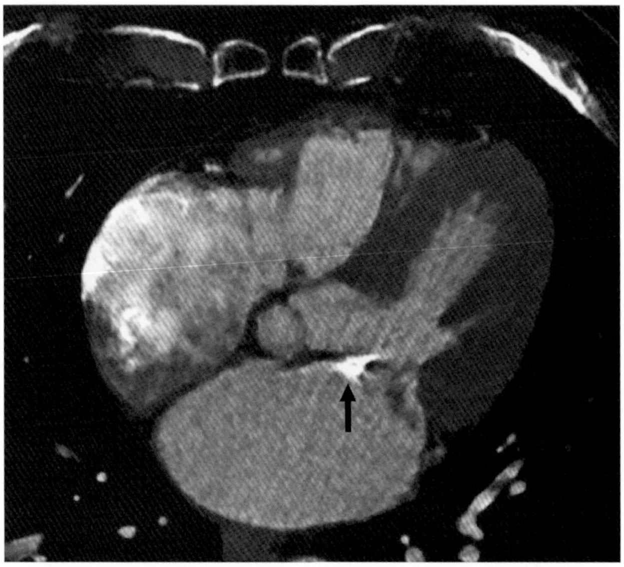

Figure 8.17. Axial CT image showing a densely calcified anterior mitral valve (arrow).

disease and the presence of asymptomatic and symptomatic peripheral vascular disease [93–96].

To date, only 2 studies have been reported that evaluated the significance of MAC by CT imaging to predict coronary artery disease. In the study by Adler et al. of 329 elderly patients, the presence of MAC by helical CT imaging was associated with higher CC scores and the presence of established coronary artery disease [89]. However, Yamamoto et al. reported that the presence of MAC by EBT imaging did not add incremental value above that achieved with AVC and aortic calcium in determining the angiographic extent and severity of coronary artery disease [91]. The prognostic significance of MAC by CT imaging remains unknown as no prospective studies have been reported.

Summary

The exact pathophysiology of MAC is still debated. Whether MAC increases cardiovascular risk, independent of CC or angiographic coronary disease, needs to be evaluated.

Conclusions

Calcium can be present in several extra-coronary locations including the aortic and mitral valves, aortic wall, and the carotid and peripheral arteries. Aortic valve calcium plays a central role in the pathogenesis of aortic valve disease and initial retrospective studies suggest that medical therapy may decrease progression of AVC. Calcium may also be associated with atherosclerosis of the aorta and the carotid and peripheral arteries. CT imaging provides an accurate and non-invasive assessment of calcium in each of these locations. (Figures 8.18 and 8.19).

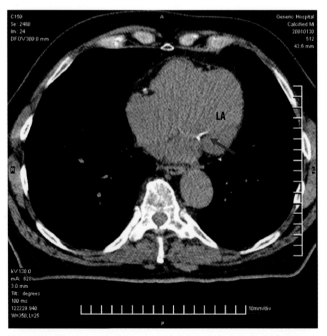

Figure 8.16. This case example demonstrates a calcified mitral valve in the classic "C" appearance (arrow). The valve itself is calcified, with the calcium right in the middle between the left atrium (LA) and ventricle.

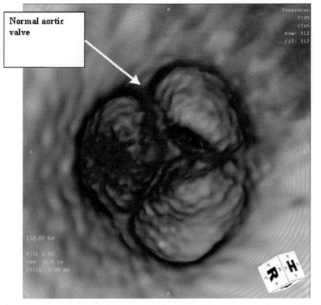

Figure 8.18. A three-dimensional reconstruction using the TerraRecon workstation (San Francisco, CA) showing a normal trileaflet aortic valve and cusps.

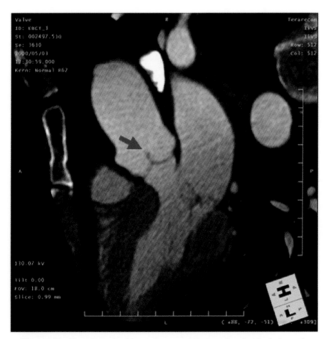

Figure 8.19. Three-dimensional image demonstrating a normal aortic valve (red arrow).

References

1. Simon A, Giral P, Levenson J. Extracoronary atherosclerotic plaque at multiple sites and total coronary calcification deposit in asymptomatic men. Association with coronary risk profile. Circulation 1995;92(6):1414–1421.
2. Iribarren C, Sidney S, Sternfeld B, Browner WS. Calcification of the aortic arch: risk factors and association with coronary heart disease, stroke, and peripheral vascular disease. JAMA 2000;283(21):2810–2815.
3. DeBakey ME, Glaeser DH. Patterns of atherosclerosis: effect of risk factors on recurrence and survival-analysis of 11,890 cases with more than 25-year follow-up. Am J Cardiol 2000;85(9):1045–1053.
4. Khoury Z, Schwartz R, Gottlieb S, Chenzbraun A, Stern S, Keren A. Relation of coronary artery disease to atherosclerotic disease in the aorta, carotid, and femoral arteries evaluated by ultrasound. Am J Cardiol 19971;80(11):1429–1433.
5. Takasu J, Takanashi K, Naito S, et al. Evaluation of morphological changes of the atherosclerotic aorta by enhanced computed tomography. Atherosclerosis 1992;97(2–3):107–121.
6. Witteman JC, Kok FJ, van Saase JL, Valkenburg HA. Aortic calcification as a predictor of cardiovascular mortality. Lancet 1986;ii(8516):1120–1122.
7. Witteman JC, Kannel WB, Wolf PA, et al. Aortic calcified plaques and cardiovascular disease (the Framingham Study). Am J Cardiol 1990;66(15):1060–1064.
8. Allison MA, Criqui MH, Wright CM. Patterns and risk factors for systemic calcified atherosclerosis. Arterioscler Thromb Vasc Biol 2004;24(2):331–336.
9. Kuller LH, Matthews KA, Sutton-Tyrrell K, Edmundowicz D, Bunker CH. Coronary and aortic calcification among women 8 years after menopause and their premenopausal risk factors: the healthy women study. Arterioscler Thromb Vasc Biol 1999;19(9):2189–2198.
10. Raggi P, Cooil B, Hadi A, Friede G. Predictors of aortic and coronary artery calcium on a screening electron beam tomographic scan. Am J Cardiol 2003;91(6):744–746.
11. Reaven PD, Sacks J. Coronary artery and abdominal aortic calcification are associated with cardiovascular disease in type 2 diabetes. Diabetologia 2005;48(2):379–385.
12. Cury RC, Ferencik M, Hoffmann U, et al. Epidemiology and association of vascular and valvular calcium quantified by multidetector computed tomography in elderly asymptomatic subjects. Am J Cardiol 2004;94(3):348–351.
13. Hirose N, Arai Y, Ishii T, Tushima M, Li J. Association of mild hyperhomocysteinemia with aortic calcification in hypercholesterolemic patients. J Atheroscler Thromb 2001;8(3):91–94.
14. Yamamoto H, Shavelle D, Takasu J, et al. Valvular and thoracic aortic calcium as a marker of the extent and severity of angiographic coronary artery disease. Am Heart J 2003;146(1):153–159.
15. Adler Y, Shemesh J, Tenenbaum A, Hovav B, Fisman EZ, Motro M. Aortic valve calcium on spiral computed tomography (dual slice mode) is associated with advanced coronary calcium in hypertensive patients. Coron Artery Dis 2002;13(4):209–213.
16. Takasu J, Mao S, Budoff MJ. Aortic atherosclerosis detected with electron-beam CT as a predictor of obstructive coronary artery disease. Acad Radiol 2003;10(6):631–637.
17. Bild DE, Bluemke DA, Burke GL, et al. Multi-Ethnic Study of Atherosclerosis: objectives and design. Am J Epidemiol 2002;156(9):871–881.
18. Hak AE, Pols HA, van Hemert AM, Hofman A, Witteman JC. Progression of aortic calcificaiton is associated with metacarpal bone loss during menopause: a population-based longitudinal study. Arterioscler Thromb Vasc Biol 2000;20(8):1926–1931.
19. Kiel DP, Kauppila LI, Cupples LA, Hannan MT, O'Donnell CJ, Wilson PW. Bone loss and the progression of abdominal aortic calcification over a 25 year period: the Framingham Heart Study. Calcif Tissue Int 2001;68(5):271–276.
20. Kauppila LI, Polak JF, Cupples LA, Hannan MT, Kiel DP, Wilson PW. New indices to classify location, severity and progression of calcific lesions in the abdominal aorta: a 25-year follow-up study. Atherosclerosis 1997;132(2):245–250.
21. Tsushima M. The clinical classification of arteriosclerosis and noninvasive methods for diagnosis of atherosclerosis (in Japanese). J Jpn Atheroscler Soc 1985;13:783–791.
22. Tsushima M, Koh H, Suzuki M, et al. Noninvasive quantitative evaluation of early atherosclerosis and the effect of monatepil, a new antihypertensive agent. An interim report. Am J Hypertens 1994;7(10 Pt 2):154S–160S.
23. Hashiba H, Aizawa S, Tamura K, Shigematsu T, Kogo H. Inhibitory effects of etidronate on the progression of vascular calcification in hemodialysis patients. Ther Apher Dial 2004;8(3):241–247.

24. Agatston AS, Janowitz WR, Hildner FJ, Zusmer NR, Viamonte M Jr, Detrano R. Quantification of coronary artery calcium using ultrafast computed tomography. J Am Coll Cardiol 1990;15(4):827–832.

25. Mitchell JR, Cranston WI. A simple method for the quantitative assessment of aortic disease. J Atheroscler Res 1965;39:135–144.

26. Williams LR, Flinn WR, Yao JS, et al. Extended use of computed tomography in the management of complex aortic problems: a learning experience. J Vasc Surg 1986;4(3):264–271.

27. Sutton-Tyrrell K, Kuller LH, Edmundowicz D, et al. Usefulness of electron beam tomography to detect progression of coronary and aortic calcium in middle-aged women. Am J Cardiol 2001;87(5):560–564.

28. Arai Y, Hirose N, Yamamura K, et al. Long-term effect of lipid-lowering therapy on atherosclerosis of abdominal aorta in patients with hypercholesterolemia: noninvasive evaluation by a new image analysis program. Angiology 2002;53(1):57–68.

29. Miwa Y, Tsushima M, Arima H, Kawano Y, Sasaguri T. Pulse pressure is an independent predictor for the progression of aortic wall calcification in patients with controlled hyperlipidemia. Hypertension 2004;43(3):536–540.

30. Yamaguchi T, Sugimoto T, Yano S, et al. Plasma lipids and osteoporosis in postmenopausal women. Endocr J 2002;49(2):211–217.

31. Parhami F, Morrow AD, Balucan J, et al. Lipid oxidation products have opposite effects on calcifying vascular cell and bone cell differentiation. A possible explanation for the paradox of arterial calcification in osteoporotic patients. Arterioscler Thromb Vasc Biol 1997;17(4):680–687.

32. Goldsmith D, Ritz E, Covic A. Vascular calcification: a stiff challenge for the nephrologist: does preventing bone disease cause arterial disease? Kidney Int 2004;66(4):1315–1333.

33. Raggi P, Bommer J, Chertow GM. Valvular calcification in hemodialysis patients randomized to calcium-based phosphorus binders or sevelamer. J Heart Valve Dis 2004;13(1):134–141.

34. Bommer J, Strohbeck E, Goerich J, Bahner M, Zuna I. Arteriosclerosis in dialysis patients. Int J Artif Organs 1996;19(11):638–644.

35. Tenenbaum A, Garniek A, Shemesh J, et al. Dual-helical CT for detecting aortic atheromas as a source of stroke: comparison with transesophageal echocardiography. Radiology 1998;208(1):153–158.

36. Kochanek KD, Smith BL. Deaths: preliminary data for 2002. Natl Vital Stat Rep 2004;52(13):1–47.

37. Koelemay MJ, Nederkoorn PJ, Reitsma JB, Majoie CB. Systematic review of computed tomographic angiography for assessment of carotid artery disease. Stroke 2004;35(10):2306–2312.

38. Arad Y, Spadaro LA, Roth M, et al. Correlations between vascular calcification and atherosclerosis: a comparative electron beam CT study of the coronary and carotid arteries. J Comput Assist Tomogr 1998;22(2):207–211.

39. Wagenknecht LE, Langefeld CD, Carr JJ, et al. Race-specific relationships between coronary and carotid artery calcification and carotid intimal medial thickness. Stroke 2004;35(5):e97-e99.

40. Deneke T, Grewe PH, Ruppert S, Balzer K, Muller KM. Atherosclerotic carotid arteries – calcification and radio-morphological findings. Z Kardiol 2000;89(Suppl 2):36–48.

41. Seeger JM, Barratt E, Lawson GA, Klingman N. The relationship between carotid plaque composition, plaque morphology, and neurologic symptoms. J Surg Res 1995;58(3):330–336.

42. Adams GJ, Simoni DM, Bordelon CB Jr, et al. Bilateral symmetry of human carotid artery atherosclerosis. Stroke 2002;33(11):2575–2580.

43. Schwartz LB, Bridgman AH, Kieffer RW, et al. Asymptomatic carotid artery stenosis and stroke in patients undergoing cardiopulmonary bypass. J Vasc Surg 1995;21(1):146–153.

44. Criqui MH, Langer RD, Fronek A, Feigelson HS. Coronary disease and stroke in patients with large-vessel peripheral arterial disease. Drugs 1991;42(Suppl 5):16–21.

45. Denzel C, Lell M, Maak M, et al. Carotid artery calcium: accuracy of a calcium score by computed tomography – an in vitro study with comparison to sonography and histology. Eur J Vasc Endovasc Surg 2004;28(2):214–220.

46. Yamamoto H, Budoff MJ, Lu B, Takasu J, Oudiz RJ, Mao S. Reproducibility of three different scoring systems for measurement of coronary calcium. Int J Cardiovasc Imaging 2002;18(5):391–397.

47. Budoff MJ, Mao S, Takasu J, Shavelle DM, Zhao XQ, O'Brien KD. Reproducibility of electron-beam CT measures of aortic valve calcification. Acad Radiol 2002;9(10):1122–1127.

48. Espeland MA, Craven TE, Riley WA, Corson J, Romont A, Furberg CD. Reliability of longitudinal ultrasonographic measurements of carotid intimal-medial thicknesses. Asymptomatic Carotid Artery Progression Study Research Group. Stroke 1996;27(3):480–485.

49. O'Leary DH, Polak JF, Kronmal RA, Manolio TA, Burke GL, Wolfson SK Jr. Carotid-artery intima and media thickness as a risk factor for myocardial infarction and stroke in older adults. Cardiovascular Health Study Collaborative Research Group. N Engl J Med 1997;340(1):14–22.

50. Hollander M, Hak AE, Koudstaal PJ, et al. Comparison between measures of atherosclerosis and risk of stroke: the Rotterdam Study. Stroke 2003;34(10):2367–2372.

51. Krajewski LP, Olin JW. Peripheral vascular diseases. In: Young JR, Olin JW, Bartholomew JR (eds) St. St Louis, MO: Mosby-Year Book, 1996:208–233.

52. Criqui MH, Langer RD, Fronek A, et al. Mortality over a period of 10 years in patients with peripheral arterial disease. N Engl J Med 1992;326(6):381–386.

53. Portugaller HR, Schoellnast H, Hausegger KA, Tiesenhausen K, Amann W, Berghold A. Multislice spiral CT angiography in peripheral arterial occlusive disease: a valuable tool in detecting significant arterial lumen narrowing? Eur Radiol 2004;14(9):1681–1687.

54. Tins B, Oxtoby J, Patel S. Comparison of CT angiography with conventional arterial angiography in aortoiliac occlusive disease. Br J Radiol 2001;74(879):219–225.

55. Rubin GD, Schmidt AJ, Logan LJ, Sofilos MC. Multi-detector row CT angiography of lower extremity arterial inflow and runoff: initial experience. Radiology 2001;221(1):146–158.

56. Otto CM, Kuusisto J, Reichenbach DD, Gown AM, O'Brien KD. Characterization of the early lesion of "degenerative" valvular aortic stenosis. Histological and immunohistochemical studies. Circulation 1994;90(2):844–853.

57. O'Brien KD, Reichenbach DD, Marcovina SM, Kuusisto J, Alpers CE, Otto CM. Apolipoproteins B, (a), and E accumulate in the morphologically early lesion of "degenerative" valvular aortic stenosis. Arterioscler Thromb Vasc Biol 1996;16(4):523–532.

58. O'Brien KD, Kuusisto J, Reichenbach DD, et al. Osteopontin is expressed in human aortic valvular lesions. Circulation 1995;92(8):2163–2168.

59. Mohler ER, III, Adam LP, McClelland P, Graham L, Hathaway DR. Detection of osteopontin in calcified human aortic valves. Arterioscler Thromb Vasc Biol 1997;17(3):547–552.

60. Mohler ER, III, Gannon F, Reynolds C, Zimmerman R, Keane MG, Kaplan FS. Bone formation and inflammation in cardiac valves. Circulation 2001;103(11):1522–1528.

61. Rosenhek R, Binder T, Porenta G, et al. Predictors of outcome in severe, asymptomatic aortic stenosis. N Engl J Med 2000;343(9):611–617.

62. Bahler RC, Desser DR, Finkelhor RS, Brener SJ, Youssefi M. Factors leading to progression of valvular aortic stenosis. Am J Cardiol 1999;84(9):1044–1048.

63. MacMillan RM, Rees MR, Lumia FJ, Maranhao V. Preliminary experience in the use of ultrafast computed tomography to diagnose aortic valve stenosis. Am Heart J 1988;115(3):665–671.

64. Kizer JR, Gefter WB, deLemos AS, Scoll BJ, Wolfe ML, Mohler ER, III. Electron beam computed tomography for the quantification of aortic valvular calcification. J Heart Valve Dis 2001;10(3):361–366.

65. Morgan-Hughes GJ, Roobottom CA, Marshall AJ. Aortic valve imaging with computed tomography: a review. J Heart Valve Dis 2002;11(5):604–611.

66. Shavelle DM, Takasu J, Budoff MJ, Mao S, Zhao XQ, O'Brien KD. HMG CoA reductase inhibitor (statin) and aortic valve calcium. Lancet 2002;359(9312):1125–1126.

67. Pohle K, Maffert R, Ropers D, et al. Progression of aortic valve calcification: association with coronary atherosclerosis and cardiovascular risk factors. Circulation 2001;104(16):1927–1932.

68. Walsh CR, Larson MG, Kupka MJ, et al. Association of aortic valve calcium detected by electron beam computed tomography with echocardiographic aortic valve disease and with calcium deposits in the coronary arteries and thoracic aorta. Am J Cardiol 2004; 93(4):421–425.

69. Shavelle DM, Budoff MJ, Buljubasic N, et al. Usefulness of aortic valve calcium scores by electron beam computed tomography as a marker for aortic stenosis. Am J Cardiol 2003;92(3):349–353.

70. Cowell SJ, Newby DE, Burton J, et al. Aortic valve calcification on computed tomography predicts the severity of aortic stenosis. Clin Radiol 2003;58(9):712–716.

71. Pohle K, Otte M, Maffert R, et al. Association of cardiovascular risk factors to aortic valve calcification as quantified by electron beam computed tomography. Mayo Clin Proc 2004;79(10):1242–1246.

72. Callister TQ, Cooil B, Raya SP, Lippolis NJ, Russo DJ, Raggi P. Coronary artery disease: improved reproducibility of calcium scoring with an electron-beam CT volumetric method. Radiology 1998; 208(3):807–814.

73. Budoff MJ, Mao S, Takasu J, Shavelle DM, Zhao XQ, O'Brien KD. Reproducibility of electron-beam CT measures of aortic valve calcification. Acad Radiol 2002;9(10):1122–1127.

74. Messika-Zeitoun D, Aubry MC, Detaint D, et al. Evaluation and clinical implications of aortic valve calcification measured by electron-beam computed tomography. Circulation 2004;110(3):356–362.

75. Kaden JJ, Freyer S, Weisser G, et al. Correlation of degree of aortic valve stenosis by Doppler echocardiogram to quantity of calcium in the valve by electron beam tomography. Am J Cardiol 2002;90(5): 554–557.

76. Salami B, Shavelle DM, Xiang M, et al. Aortic valve calcium and c-reactive protein contribute independently to coronary heart disease incidence. J Am Coll Cardiol 2004;43(Suppl A):517A(Abstract).

77. Novaro GM, Tiong IY, Pearce GL, Lauer MS, Sprecher DL, Griffin BP. Effect of hydroxymethylglutaryl coenzyme a reductase inhibitors on the progression of calcific aortic stenosis. Circulation 2001; 104(18):2205–2209.

78. Rosenhek R, Rader F, Loho N, et al. Statins but not angiotensin-converting enzyme inhibitors delay progression of aortic stenosis. Circulation 2004;110(10):1291–1295.

79. Bellamy MF, Pellikka PA, Klarich KW, Tajik AJ, Enriquez-Sarano M. Association of cholesterol levels, hydroxymethylglutaryl coenzyme-A reductase inhibitor treatment, and progression of aortic stenosis in the community. J Am Coll Cardiol 2002;40(10):1723–1730.

80. Aronow WS, Ahn C, Kronzon I, Goldman ME. Association of coronary risk factors and use of statins with progression of mild valvular aortic stenosis in older persons. Am J Cardiol 2001;88(6):693–695.

81. Rossebo AB, Pedersen TR, Skjaerpe T, et al. Design of the simvastatin and ezetimibe in Aortic Stenosis (SEAS) Study. Atherosclerosis 2004;170(Suppl 4):253.

82. Takasu J, Shavelle DM, O'Brien KD, et al. Association between progression of aortic valve calcification and coronary calcification: assessment by electron beam tomography. Acad Radiol 2005;12(3): 298–304.

83. Roberts WC. The senile cardiac calcification syndrome. Am J Cardiol 1986;58(6):572–574.

84. Korn D, Desanctis RW, Sell S. Massive calcification of the mitral annulus. A clinicopathological study of fourteen cases. N Engl J Med 1962;267:900–909.

85. Fulkerson PK, Beaver BM, Auseon JC, Graber HL. Calcification of the mitral annulus: etiology, clinical associations, complications and therapy. Am J Med 1979;66(6):967–977.

86. Aronow WS. Mitral annular calcification: significant and worth acting upon. Geriatrics 1991;46(4):73–80, 85.

87. Boon A, Cheriex E, Lodder J, Kessels F. Cardiac valve calcification: characteristics of patients with calcification of the mitral annulus or aortic valve. Heart 1997;78(5):472–474.

88. Marzo KP, Herling IM. Valvular disease in the elderly. Cardiovasc Clin 1993;23:175–207.

89. Adler Y, Fisman EZ, Shemesh J, Tanne D, Hovav B, Motro M, Schwammenthal E, Tenenbaum A. Usefulness of helical computed tomography in detection of mitral annular calcification as a marker of coronary artery disease. Int J Cardiol 2005;101(3):371–376.

90. Tenenbaum A, Shemesh J, Fisman EZ, Motro M. Advanced mitral annular calcification is associated with severe coronary calcification on fast dual spiral computed tomography. Invest Radiol 2000;35(3):193–198.

91. Yamamoto H, Shavelle D, Takasu J, Lu B, Mao SS, Fischer H, Budoff MJ. Valvular and thoracic aortic calcium as a marker of the extent and severity of angiographic coronary artery disease. Am Heart J 2003;146(1):153–159.

92. Kamensky G, Lisy L, Polak E, Piknova E, Plevova N. Mitral annular calcifications and aortic plaques as predictors of increased cardiovascular mortality. J Cardiol 2001;37 Suppl 1:21–26.

93. Aronow WS, Ahn C, Kronzon I, Gutstein H. Association of mitral annular calcium with new thromboembolic stroke at 44-month follow-up of 2,148 persons, mean age 81 years. Am J Cardiol 1998;81(1):105–106.

94. Adler Y, Koren A, Fink N, Tanne D, Fusman R, Assali A, Yahav J, Zelikovski A, Sagie A. Association between mitral annulus calcification and carotid atherosclerotic disease. Stroke 1998;29(9):1833–1837.

95. Adler Y, Herz I, Vaturi M, Fusman R, Shohat-Zabarski R, Fink N, Porter A, Shapira Y, Assali A, Sagie A. Mitral annular calcium detected by transthoracic echocardiography is a marker for high prevalence and severity of coronary artery disease in patients undergoing coronary angiography. Am J Cardiol 1998;82(10):1183–1186.

96. Park H, Das M, Aronow WS, McClung JA, Belkin RN. Relation of decreased ankle-brachial index to prevalence of atherosclerotic risk factors, coronary artery disease, aortic valve calcium, and mitral annular calcium. Am J Cardiol 2005;95(8):1005–1006.

9

CT Coronary Angiography

Stephan Achenbach

Computed tomography (CT) produces high-resolution cross-sectional imaging. Injection of contrast agent raises the density in the blood pool well above that of the vessel wall and surrounding tissue. Thus, CT "angiography" (CTA) can be performed. CT angiography of the *coronary arteries* poses some unique challenges. Given the small lumen of the coronary vessels (typically 1 to 4 mm) and their constant and rapid motion, CT angiography of the coronary artery lumen requires maximal spatial and temporal resolution. Sufficient temporal resolution was first achieved with electron beam tomography (EBT), with the first successful attempts at angiography of the coronary arteries in the mid 1990s. The recent development of multidetector CT scanners (MDCT) with faster imaging speed has allowed improved coronary artery visualization. This was initially performed with simultaneous acquisition of 4 slices. The technology then advanced to 8, 16, and now up to 64 narrowly collimated slices. This provides high spatial resolution and sufficient temporal resolution to permit adequate and reliable visualization of the coronary artery lumen. Comparison to invasive coronary angiography demonstrates increasing accuracy for stenosis detection. This is expected to bring coronary CTA into the mainstream of cardiology practice.

Imaging Protocol

Preparation

Patient preparation is required to achieve optimal image quality in CT coronary angiography (Table 9.1). Data acquisition protocols have to be tailored to maximize spatial and temporal resolution. The patient must not have contraindications to the administration of iodinated contrast material. Patients must be able to hold their breath in inspiration for 8 to 20 seconds, depending on the CT scanner used (this can be up to 40 seconds for electron beam tomography). Image acquisition and reconstruction

are acquired with electrocardiographic (ECG) gating; therefore, a regular sinus rhythm is necessary. Several studies have shown that a low heart rate during data acquisition – with consequently longer diastolic phases of relatively little coronary motion – substantially improves image quality [1–5]. Furthermore, when using ECG-correlated tube current modulation, full X-ray output is only activated during a fixed time period in diastole, which reduces the radiation dose. A low heart rate with a longer cardiac cycle allows for greater reductions in radiation exposure than faster heart rates with a shorter cardiac cycle [6]. Even though it is possible to obtain high-quality images by MDCT in patients with faster heart rates, slower heart rates will thus improve image quality and reduce radiation exposure. Most experts advocate the use of beta-blocking agents in preparation for the scan in order to achieve heart rates of 60 beats per minute or less during inspiration. At our institution, we use a protocol that combines administration of 100 mg atenolol one hour before the scan to patients with heart rates above 60 beats/min, followed with intravenous injection of up to four doses of 5 mg metoprolol when the patient is on the scanner table until the heart rate is below 60 beats/min. This has proven to be a very safe and effective method in our institution.

For EBT, the overall scan time decreases with *faster* heart rates. Thus, it is favorable to avoid EBT scanning with low heart rates. Many authors suggest the use of intravenous atropine for patients with slow heart rates in order to decrease scan time, thus reducing the necessary amount of contrast agent and breath-hold duration.

Image quality for both EBT and MDCT is further improved through coronary vasodilation. Nitrates are recommended immediately prior to the scan. At our institution, we administer 0.8 mg glyceryl trinitrate sublingually immediately before starting the scan. Other institutions have reported use of 0.4 mg.

Further preparations include placement of ECG leads (making sure contact is not lost during deep inspiration), and instructions to the patient about the importance of breath-holding and the sequence of the examination.

Table 9.1. Preparations for CT imaging of the coronary artery lumen

Contraindications	Non-sinus rhythm
	Inability to follow breath-hold commands
	Contraindications for iodinated contrast
Lower heart rate (MDCT)	Target: heart rate <60 beats/min
	e.g. atenolol 100 mg 1 hour before scan, metoprolol 5 mg, up to 4 doses (20 mg) immediately before scan
Increase heart rate (EBT)	Target: heart rate >70 beats/min
	e.g. atropine
Coronary vasodilation	Sublingual nitrates

Image Acquisition

Image acquisition consists of three steps (Table 9.2). First, a projection image is used for localizing the position of the heart (Figure 9.1). It is important to prescribe a scan volume that is as small as possible, yet covers the entire heart. This assures complete visualization of the coronary vessels with the least possible contrast dose and radiation exposure. To prescribe the scan area, the tracheal bifurcation is frequently used as a reference point. However, we prefer to place the cranial border of the scan volume at the mid left pulmonary artery, which has a less variable relationship with the position of the heart.

The second step of image acquisition is the determination of contrast agent transit time from injection into the peripheral vein to peak enhancement in the ascending aorta, using the smallest amount of contrast possible. Determination of contrast agent transit time can be achieved either through bolus injection and acquisition of repeated low-dose images at the level of the ascending aorta ("test bolus"), or through "bolus tracking" algorithms that automatically start image acquisition when the arrival of contrast agent increases the CT density to a particular value within a predefined region of interest in the ascending aorta [7]. We prefer "test bolus" measurement of the transit time for several reasons: it ensures correct placement of the intravenous line, confirms appropriate starting level of the scan volume, and gives the patient one more opportunity to become familiar with the breath-hold commands.

The scan parameters used for acquisition of data to visualize the coronary arteries vary with scanner specifications.

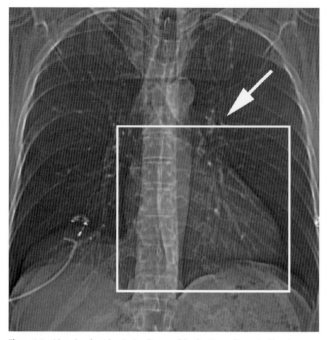

Figure 9.1. A low-dose frontal projectional image of the chest is usually acquired in order to prescribe the scan volume. We typically place the cranial start of the scan volume (white box) at the level of the mid left pulmonary artery (arrow).

Typical image acquisition protocols are listed in Table 9.3. In any case, protocols should be optimized to maximize spatial and temporal resolution, and precautions should be taken to avoid excessive radiation exposure. Contrast agent is typically injected at a rate of 5 mL/s for the duration of the scan (approximately 18 seconds for 16-slice CT, 10 seconds for 64-slice CT). Using a saline bolus to follow the injection of contrast agent is very useful to keep the contrast bolus compact, achieve optimal enhancement in the coronary arteries, and avoid enhancement of right atrium and ventricle (Figure 9.2).

Image Reconstruction

In MDCT, images are reconstructed with retrospective ECG gating. Detailed explanation of reconstruction parameters is beyond the scope of this chapter. In brief, image reconstruction is usually performed in diastole (e.g. around 65% of the cardiac cycle), but may need to be repeated at other periods if motion artifacts are present. A medium soft kernel is used to achieve good balance between sharpness and image noise. The field of view should be chosen as small as possible to completely cover the volume of the heart. Reconstructed slice thickness equals collimation or is a little bit larger (e.g. reconstruction of 0.75 mm slice thickness for data acquired with 0.6 mm collimation). The reconstruction interval is less than the slice thickness. Therefore, overlapping slices are created which again improve the image noise and facilitate image post-processing. The EBT scanner provides axial images with a

Table 9.2. Sequence of scanning for visualization of the coronary artery lumen

1. Localization of heart position	Example: low-dose projectional anteroposterior view of the chest
2. Determination of contrast agent transit time	Example: injection of test bolus followed by repeated acquisition of low-dose images at the level of the ascending aorta
3. High-resolution volume dataset	With intravenous injection of contrast and scan delay according to contrast agent transit time ("Bolus tracking" techniques allow combination of steps 2 and 3 in one acquisition)

Table 9.3. Typical scan parameters for high-resolution imaging of the coronary arteries

Electron beam tomography	Collimation	2 × 1.5 mm
	Image acquisition time	100 ms
	Table increment	Stepwise, 3 mm after each cardiac cycle
	Tube voltage	135 kV
	Tube current	900 mAs
	Scan length	Approximately 120 mm
	Scan duration	Approximately 40 heartbeats (30 seconds)
	Contrast agent	4 mL/s for the duration of the scan (e.g. 120 mL), followed by saline 50 mL at 4 mL/s
16-slice MDCT*[a]*	Collimation	16 × 1.0 mm
	Rotation time	370 ms
	Table increment	Continuous, 3.0 mm/rotation
	Tube voltage	120 kV
	Tube current	500 mAs maximum, reduction in systole
	Scan length	Approximately 120 mm
	Scan duration	Approximately 18 seconds
	Contrast agent	5 mL/s for the duration of the scan (e.g. 90 mL), followed by saline 50 mL at 5 mL/s
64-slice CT*[b]*	Collimation	64 × 0.6 mm
	Rotation time	330 ms
	Table increment	Continuous, 3.8 mm/rotation
	Tube voltage	120 Kv
	Tube current	700 mAs maximum, reduction in systole
	Scan length	Approximately 120 mm
	Scan duration	Approximately 10 seconds
	Contrast agent	5 mL/s for the duration of the scan (e.g. 50 mL), followed by saline 50 mL at 5 mL/s

[a] Suggested scan parameters for Siemens Sensation Cardiac, parameters vary for other scanners.
[b] Suggested scan parameters for Siemens Sensation 64, parameters vary for other scanners.

slice thickness equal to the collimation. A medium sharp reconstruction kernel is usually used.

Data Evaluation

The tortuous course, branching, and small diameters of the coronary arteries can make evaluation challenging and evaluation of the reconstructed axial images usually is not sufficient. For evaluation, coronary CTA datasets are therefore routinely transferred to dedicated workstations. These workstations permit interactive scrolling through the dataset, interactive rendering of oblique multiplanar reconstructions and maximum intensity projections, as well as three-dimensional (3-D) volume rendering. While two-dimensional methods of image post-processing and evaluation will usually be sufficient to evaluate the data, 3-D rendering can provide a useful overview of the anatomy and can effectively convey the findings. Interactive maneuvering through the dataset has been proven to be more effective and accurate than evaluation of pre-rendered reconstructions [8]. Evaluation of the coronary arteries concerning the presence of stenoses will typically be limited to reporting absence of stenosis, presence of non-significant luminal narrowing, presence of a hemodynamically significant luminal narrowing (e.g. more than 50% diameter reduction), or total occlusion. Accurate percent grading of the degree of stenosis is not possible to our current knowledge.

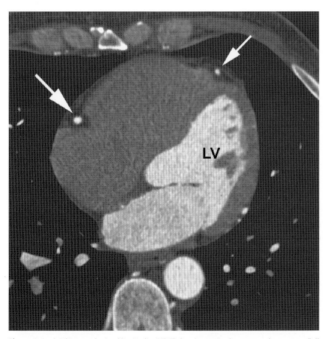

Figure 9.2. Axial image obtained by 64-slice MDCT showing optimal contrast enhancement: Full enhancement within the left ventricular cavity (LV) and coronary arteries (large arrow: right coronary artery, small arrow: left anterior descending coronary artery), but the contrast bolus has already passed the right ventricle, which does not show enhancement.

Clinical Applications

Accuracy for Stenosis Detection

Development of the EBT scanner initially provided the necessary temporal resolution for visualization of the coronary arteries and stenosis detection (Figure 9.3). First comparisons to invasive coronary angiography in the mid 1990s demonstrated the feasibility of stenosis detection [9–20]. However, the limited spatial resolution and long scan time (requiring breath-hold up to 40 seconds) led to image artifacts. Thus, a substantial number of coronary arteries were unevaluable for detection of stenoses [9–20]. Also, the large amount of contrast agent that was necessary to achieve arterial enhancement throughout the long image acquisition interval, and the limited availability of EBT scanners, prevented widespread clinical applications.

The introduction of 4-slice multidetector spiral CT scanners around the year 2000 permitted further advances in coronary artery visualization. Again, comparisons to invasive angiography demonstrated high accuracy for stenosis detection in datasets with high image quality, but artifacts caused mainly by the limited temporal resolution were frequent and the breath-hold time and necessary amount of contrast were similar to electron beam tomography [21–32]. Substantial progress was made with the introduction of scanners with 16 slices starting approximately in the year 2002. These systems provided for data acquisition with collimations of 1.0 mm or less and gantry rotation times of 500 ms or less [33,34]. Sixteen-slice systems are now widely available and are currently regarded as a prerequisite for

CT coronary angiography (Figures 9.4–9.7). However, 16-slice technology has not been able to solve all the problems of the older scanners. Severe calcifications, for example, remain a problem because they can impair image quality and reduce diagnostic accuracy. In a comparison of patients with calcifications of varying degree, Kuettner et al. convincingly showed that both sensitivity and specificity for stenosis detection were 98% in a group of 46 patients with an "Agatston score" equivalent of less than 1000, while only 25 of 35 stenoses were detected correctly in patients with an "Agatston score" equivalent of 1000 or more (sensitivity of 71%) [35].

When comparing studies which evaluate the accuracy of cardiac computed tomography for the detection of coronary stenoses by means of validation against invasive coronary angiography, it has to be considered that the results of different investigations are not immediately comparable. Next to differences in the scanner technology used, the studies differ widely in the selection of included patients and prevalence of significant stenoses. Similarly, studies differ in the number and location of coronary segments that were included in the analysis. For example, some investigators excluded coronary segments with reduced image quality from analysis while others did not. Regardless of these differences, the published studies uniformly reported high sensitivities for the detection of coronary artery stenoses, ranging from 82% to 95% (Table 9.4). Similarly, specificity for stenosis detection ranged from 86% to 98% [33,34,36–41]. Of note, the negative predictive value was uniformly found to be 97% or higher, but it has to be considered that the low prevalence of significant coronary

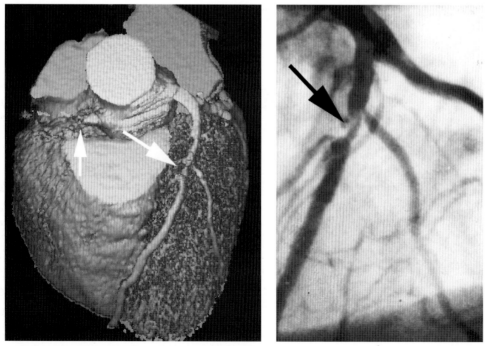

a   b

Figure 9.3. a 3-D reconstruction of the heart and coronary arteries obtained by electron beam tomography in a patient with a stenosis of the left anterior descending coronary artery (large arrow) and occlusion of the right coronary artery (small arrow). **b** Invasive angiogram of the left anterior descending coronary artery. Corresponding high-grade stenosis in mid-vessel (black arrow).

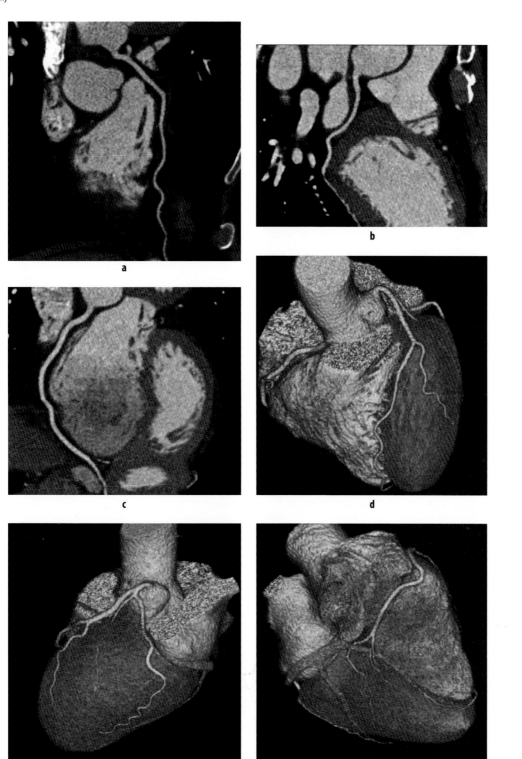

Figure 9.4. Two-dimensional multiplanar reconstructions of the coronary arteries obtained by 16-slice MDCT: left main and left anterior descending coronary artery (**a**), left circumflex coronary artery (**b**), right coronary artery (**c**). Three-dimensional visualization of the coronary arteries (**d**, **e**, **f**).

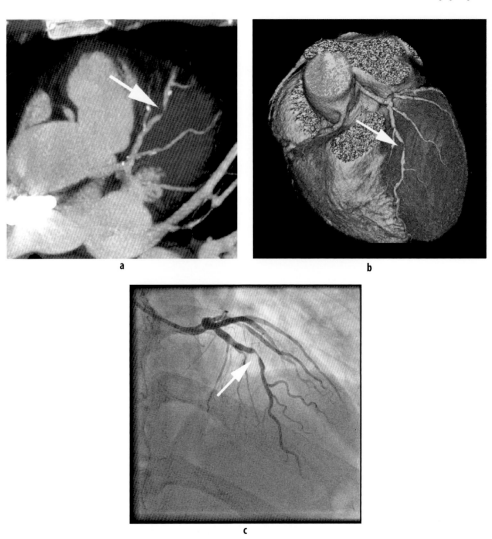

Figure 9.5. An 8 mm thick maximum intensity projection in a slightly oblique para-axial projection (**a**) and 3-D reconstruction (**b**) in a patient with left anterior descending coronary artery stenosis (arrow). Corresponding coronary angiography (**c**).

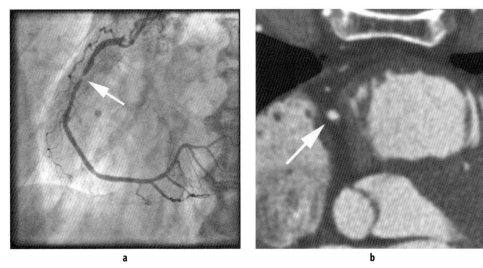

Figure 9.6. Stenosis of the right coronary artery (arrow, **a** – invasive coronary angiogram). Three consecutive axial images (each 1 mm slice thickness) show normal coronary artery lumen proximal to the stenosis (arrow, **b**), absence of a contrast-enhanced lumen at the level of the stenosis (arrow, **c**), and re-establishment of a patent and normal coronary lumen distal to the stenosis (arrow, **d**). Same stenosis in curved multiplanar reconstructions (arrows, **e** and **f**), and in 3-D volume-rendered reconstruction (**g**, **h**).

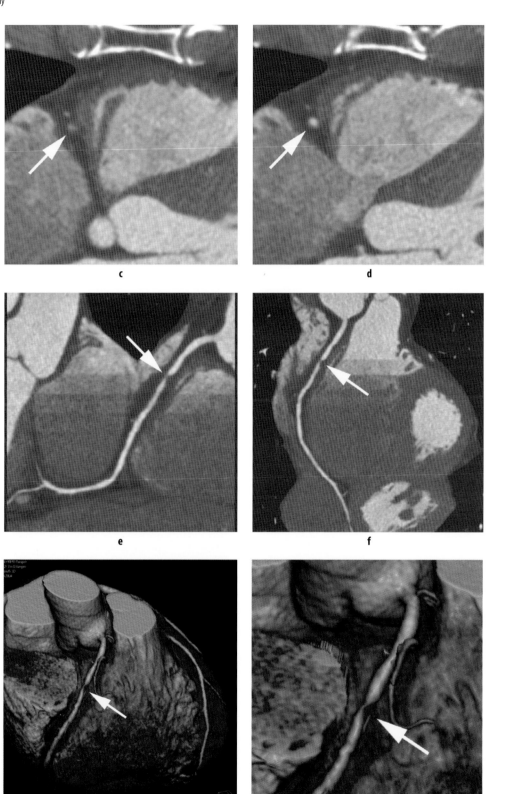

c

d

e

f

g

h

Figure 9.6. (*Continued*)

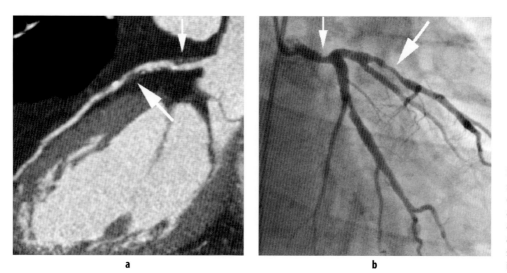

a   b

Figure 9.7. a Multiplanar reconstruction showing an eccentric stenosis of the left main coronary artery (small arrow) and of the left anterior descending coronary artery (large arrow). **b** Corresponding lesions in invasive angiography. In addition, a left circumflex stenosis is present (not shown as an MDCT image).

stenoses influences the negative predictive value towards higher levels.

Even within the studies that were performed using 16-slice technology, it can be observed that faster rotation times and lower heart rates positively influence the diagnostic accuracy. Sixty-four-slice scanners with improved temporal and spatial resolution are expected to improve diagnostic accuracy while lowering the number of unevaluable segments (Figure 9.8), but comparisons to invasive angiography have not been published to date and this assumption remains to be proven in adequate clinical trials.

Clinical Implications

Coronary CT angiography does not have the same spatial or temporal resolution as invasive coronary angiography (Figure 9.9) and cannot be performed in all patients (e.g. those with arrhythmias). Furthermore, it is a purely diagnostic tool and does not provide the option for immediate interventional treatment. Thus, clinical application of CTA in patients with a high pretest likelihood for coronary artery disease is of limited value, such as in older individuals with typical chest pain. If the predicted necessity for an intervention is reasonably high, the patient should proceed directly to invasive angiography rather than CT. Also, routine "screening" of asymptomatic individuals by coronary CT angiography will not be beneficial, since treatment of an asymptomatic stenosis is generally not expected to alter the patient's prognosis.

However, many patients are symptomatic with atypical chest pain and have positive or equivocal stress test results, so that invasive coronary angiography is deemed necessary to rule out the unlikely presence of stenoses. Such patients with low or intermediate pretest likelihood are, for

Table 9.4. Diagnostic accuracy of 16-slice MDCT for the detection of coronary artery stenoses

Reference	Number of Patients	Gantry rotation time	Sensitivity (%)	Specificity (%)	Non-Interpretable (%)	Analysis
Nieman et al. [33]	59	420 ms	95	86	7%	Per-artery analysis, all segments >2.0 mm
Ropers et al. [34]	77	420 ms	93	92	12%	Per-artery analysis, all segments >1.5 mm
Mollet et al. [36]	128	420 ms	92	95	–	Per-segment analysis, all segments >2.0 mm
Martuscelli et al. [37]	64	500 ms	89	98	16%	Per-artery analysis, all segments >1.5 mm
Hoffmann et al. [38]	33	420 ms	63	96	–	Per-segment analysis, all segments
	33	420 ms	89	95	–	Per-segment analysis, prox. and mid segments
Kuettner et al. [39]	72	375 ms	82	98	7%	Per-segment analysis all segments
Mollet et al. [40]	51	375 ms	95	98	–	Per-artery analysis, all segments >2.0 mm
Schujif et al. [41]	51	400 ms	98	97	6%	Per-segment analysis, all segments[a]

[a] This study includes some patients with bypass grafts and stents which were not included in this evaluation.

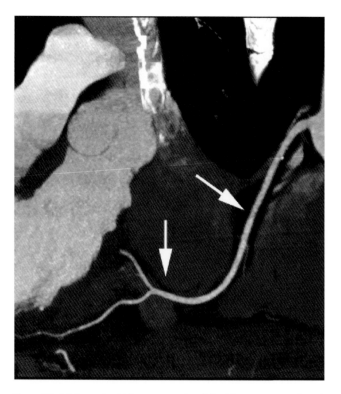

Figure 9.8. A 2-D curved multiplanar reconstruction of the right coronary artery (arrows) obtained by 64-slice MDCT, with a rotation time of 330 ms, and 64 × 0.6 mm collimation.

coronary stenoses and avoid the need for invasive angiography. However, appropriately designed clinical studies will have to verify this hypothesis and identify patient groups that will have clinical benefit from coronary CT angiography to rule out the presence of coronary artery stenoses.

CT angiography also has the potential to provide information that is complementary to invasive angiography. One smaller study has shown that in patients with chronic total occlusion, a challenging subset of patients referred for interventional treatment, occlusion length and degree of calcification as assessed by CT are more accurate predictors of interventional success than are angiographic parameters [43]. Similarly, it is conceivable that CT angiography may provide information that is valuable prior to interventional treatment of bifurcation lesions or other challenging subsets of coronary stenoses by evaluating plaque burden, extent of calcification, and by viewing the 3-D anatomy of the vessels. These assumptions, however, need to be proven and would only apply to a relatively small number of patients.

Because of the 3-D nature of the tomographic dataset, CT coronary angiography is the preferred modality to investigate patients with known or suspected congenital coronary artery anomalies (Figure 9.10). Several authors have convincingly shown that MDCT can identify both the origin and the often complex course of anomalous coronary vessels [44–46].

In a number of smaller studies, it has been shown that CT and EBT angiography can provide clinically relevant information in patients with Kawasaki syndrome by demonstration of calcification, coronary stenoses, and coronary aneurysms [47–49].

example, younger men and women with atypical chest pain [42]. In these patient groups, non-invasive coronary visualization by CT potentially can be a beneficial tool for further evaluation since it can reliably exclude significant

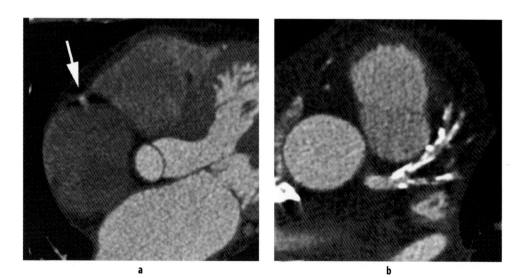

a   b

Figure 9.9. Typical artifacts which may impair evaluability of coronary artery segments concerning the detection of stenoses. **a** Motion artifact of the right coronary artery causes a "blurry" appearance of the vessel cross-section (arrow). **b** Severe calcification in the proximal left anterior descending coronary artery. Both images acquired by 16-slice MDCT.

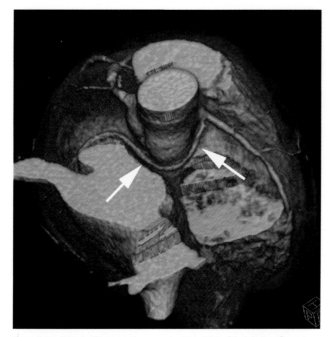

Figure 9.10. Patient with an anomalous coronary artery: Origin of the left circumflex coronary artery from the right coronary ostium and course distal to the aortic root toward the left coronary groove (arrows). The heart is seen from its posterior side.

Summary

Non-invasive CT angiography of the coronary arteries is a challenging and rapidly advancing technique. Electron beam tomography initially permitted the non-invasive visualization of coronary arteries and detection of stenoses. Multidetector CT provides very high spatial resolution and allows for excellent visualization of the coronary arteries. Hemodynamically significant stenoses can be detected and excluded with high accuracy. Current limitations of CT angiography include gantry rotation speed, arrhythmias, and the presence of severe coronary calcification. Continued technical progress is expected to overcome some of these limitations. The most likely beneficial clinical application for the use of CT coronary angiography will be to rule out the presence of relevant coronary artery stenoses in symptomatic patients with a low-to-intermediate likelihood of coronary artery stenoses. Sufficiently large outcome studies will ultimately have to define the most beneficial applications of CT coronary angiography and compare CTA to traditional diagnostic methods.

References

1. Nieman K, Rensing BJ, van Geuns RJM, et al. Non-invasive coronary angiography with multislice spiral computed tomography: impact of heart rate Heart 2002;88:470–474.
2. Giesler T, Baum U, Ropers D, et al. Noninvasive visualization of coronary arteries using contrast-enhanced multidetector CT: influence of heart rate on image quality and stenosis detection. AJR Am J Roentgenol 2002;179:911–916.
3. Schroeder S, Kopp AF, Kuettner A, et al. Influence of heart rate on vessel visibility in noninvasive coronary angiography using new multislice computed tomography: experience in 94 patients. Clin Imaging 2002;26:106–111.
4. Hoffmann MH, Shi H, Manzke R, et al. Noninvasive coronary angiography with 16-detector row CT: effect of heart rate. Radiology 2005; 234:86–97.
5. Herzog C, Abolmaali N, Balzer JO, et al. Heart-rate-adapted image reconstruction in multidetector-row cardiac CT: influence of physiological and technical prerequisite on image quality. Eur Radiol 2002;12:2670–2678.
6. Jakobs TF, Becker CR, Ohnesorge B, et al. Multislice helical CT of the heart with retrospective ECG gating: reduction of radiation exposure by ECG-controlled tube current modulation. Eur Radiol 2002;12:1081–1086.
7. Cademartiri F, Nieman K, van der Lugt A, Raaijmakers RMT, de Feyter P, Krestin GP. Intravenous contrast material administration at 16-detector row helical CT coronary angiography: test bolus versus bolus-tracking technique. Radiology 2004;233:817–823.
8. Cademartiri F, Mollet N, Lemos PA, et al. Standard versus user-interactive assessment of significant coronary stenoses with multislice computed tomography coronary angiography. Am J Cardiol 2004;94:1590–1593.
9. Moshage W, Achenbach S, Seese B, Bachmann K, Kirchgeorg M. Coronary artery stenoses: three-dimensional imaging with electrocardiographically triggered, contrast agent-enhanced, electron beam CT. Radiology 1995;196:707–714.
10. Nakanishi T, Ito K, Imazu M, Yamakido M. Evaluation of coronary artery stenoses using electron-beam CT and multiplanar reformation. J Comp Assist Tomogr 1997;21:121–127.
11. Schmermund A, Rensing BJ, Sheedy PF, et al. Intravenous electron-beam computed tomographic coronary angiography for segmental analysis of coronary artery stenoses. J Am Coll Cardiol 1998; 31:1547–1554.
12. Reddy GP, Chernoff DM, Adams JR, et al. Coronary artery stenoses: assessment with contrast-enhanced electron-beam CT and axial reconstructions. Radiology 1998;208:167–172.
13. Rensing BJ, Bongaerts A, van Geuns RJ, et al. Intravenous coronary angiography by electron beam computed tomography. A clinical evaluation. Circulation 1998;98:2509–2512.
14. Achenbach S, Moshage W, Ropers D, et al. Value of electron-beam computed tomography for the detection of high-grade coronary artery stenoses and occlusions. N Engl J Med 1998;339: 1964–1667.
15. Budoff MJ, Oudiz RJ, Zalace CP, et al. Intravenous three-dimensional coronary angiography using contrast-enhanced electron beam computed tomography. Am J Cardiol 1999;83:840–845.
16. Achenbach S, Ropers D, Regenfus M, et al. Contrast-enhanced electron-beam CT to analyze the coronary arteries in patients after acute myocardial infarction. Heart 2000;84:489–493.
17. Leber AW, Knez A, Mukherjee R, et al. Usefulness of calcium scoring using electron beam computed tomography and noninvasive coronary angiography in patients with suspected coronary artery disease. Am J Cardiol 2001;88:219–223.
18. Ropers D, Regenfus M, Stilianakis N, et al. A direct comparison of noninvasive coronary angiography by electron beam tomography and navigator-echo-based magnetic resonance imaging for the detection of restenosis following coronary angioplasty. Invest Radiol 2002;37:386–392.
19. Nikolaou K, Huber A, Knez A, et al. Intraindividual comparison of contrast-enhanced electron-beam computed tomography and navigator-echo-based magnetic resonance imaging for noninvasive coronary artery angiography. Eur Radiol 2002;12:1663–1671.
20. Lu B, Shavelle DM, Mao S, et al. Improved accuracy of noninvasive electron beam coronary angiography. Invest Radiol 2004;39:73–79.

21. Becker CR, Knez A, Leber A, et al. Initial experiences with multislice detector spiral CT in diagnosis of arteriosclerosis of coronary vessels. Radiologe 2000;40:118–122.

22. Ohnesorge B, Flohr T, Becker C, et al. Cardiac imaging by means of electrocardiographically gated multisection spiral CT: initial experience. Radiology 2000;217:564–571.

23. Achenbach S, Ulzheimer S, Baum U, et al. Noninvasive coronary angiography by retrospectively ECG-gated multislice spiral CT. Circulation 2000;102:2823–2828.

24. Nieman K, Oudkerk M, Rensing BJ, et al. Coronary angiography with multi-slice computed tomography. Lancet 2001;357:599–603.

25. Achenbach S, Giesler T, Ropers D, et al. Detection of coronary artery stenoses by contrast-enhanced, retrospectively ECG-gated, multi-slice spiral CT. Circulation 2001;103:2535–2538.

26. Knez A, Becker CR, Leber A, et al. Usefulness of multislice spiral computed tomography angiography for determination of coronary artery stenoses. Am J Cardiol 2001;88:1191–1194.

27. Herzog C, Abolmaali N, Balzer JO, et al. Heart-rate-adapted image reconstruction in multidetector-row cardiac CT: influence of physiological and technical prerequisite on image quality. Eur Radiol 2002;12:1670–1678.

28. Kopp AF, Schroeder S, Kuettner A, et al. Non-invasive coronary angiography with high resolution multidetector-row computed tomography. Results in 102 patients. Eur Heart J 2002;23:1714–1725.

29. Nieman K, Rensing BJ, van Geuns RJ, et al. Usefulness of multislice computed tomography for detecting obstructive coronary artery disease. Am J Cardiol 2002;89:913–918.

30. Becker CR, Knez A, Leber A, et al. Detection of coronary artery stenoses with multislice helical CT angiography. J Comp Assist Tomogr 2002;26:250–255.

31. Morgan-Hughes GJ, Marshall AJ, Roobottom CA. Multislice computed tomography coronary angiography: Experience in a UK centre. Clin Radiol 2003;58:378–383.

32. Sato Y, Matsumoto N, Kato M, et al. Noninvasive assessment of coronary artery disease by multislice spiral computed tomography using a new retrospectively ECG-gated image reconstruction technique. Comparison with angiographic results. Circ J 2003;67:401–405.

33. Nieman K, Cademartiri F, Lemos PA, et al. Reliable noninvasive coronary angiography with fast submillimeter multislice spiral computed tomography. Circulation 2002;106:2051–2054.

34. Ropers D, Baum U, Pohle K, et al. Detection of coronary artery stenoses with thin-slice multi-detector row spiral computed tomography and multiplanar reconstruction. Circulation 2003;107:664–666.

35. Kuettner A, Trabold T, Schroeder S, et al. Noninvasive detection of coronary lesions using 16-detector multislice spiral computed tomography technology. Initial Clinical Results. J Am Coll Cardiol 2004;44:1230–1237.

36. Mollet NR, Cademartiri F, Nieman K, et al. Multislice spiral computed tomography coronary angiography in patients with stable angina pectoris. J Am Coll Cardiol 2004;43:2265–2270.

37. Martuscelli E, Romagnoli A, D'Eliseo A, et al. Accuracy of thin-slice computed tomography in the detection of coronary stenoses. Eur Heart J 2004;25:1043–1048.

38. Hoffmann U, Moselewski F, Cury RC, et al. Predictive value of 16-slice multidetector spiral computed tomography to detect significant obstructive coronary artery disease in patients at high risk for coronary disease. Patient versus segment-based analysis. Circulation 2004;110:2638–2643.

39. Kuettner A, Beck T, Drosch T, et al. Diagnostic accuracy of non-invasive coronary imaging using 16-detector slice spiral computed tomography with 188 ms temporal resolution. J Am Coll Cardiol 2005;45:123–127.

40. Mollet NR, Cademartiri F, Krestin GP, et al. Improved diagnostic accuracy with 16-row multi-slice computed tomography coronary angiography. J Am Coll Cardiol 2005;45:128–132.

41. Schuijf JD, Bax JJ, Salm LP, et al. Noninvasive coronary imaging and assessment of left ventricular function using 16-slice computed tomography. Am J Cardiol 2005;95:571–574.

42. Williams SV, Fihn SD, Gibbons RJ; American College of Cardiology; American Heart Association; American College of Physicians-American Society of Internal Medicine. Guidelines for the management of patients with chronic stable angina: diagnosis and risk stratification. Ann Intern Med 2001;135:530–547.

43. Mollet NR, Hoye A, Lemos PA, et al. Value of preprocedure multislice computed tomographic coronary angiography to predict the outcome of percutaneous recanalization of chronic total occlusions. Am J Cardiol 2005;95:240–243.

44. Ropers D, Moshage W, Daniel WG, et al. Visualization of coronary artery anomalies and their course by contrast-enhanced electron beam tomography and three-dimensional reconstruction. Am J Cardiol 2001;87:193–197.

45. Deibler AR, Kuzo RS, Vohringer M, et al. Imaging of congenital coronary anomalies with multislice computed tomography. Mayo Clin Proc 2004;79:1017–1023.

46. Lessick J, Kumar G, Beyar R, Lorber A, Engel A. Anomalous origin of a posterior descending artery from the right pulmonary artery: report of a rare case diagnosed by multidetector computed tomography angiography. J Comput Assist Tomogr 2004;28:857–859.

47. Tomita H. Intravascular ultrasound and electron beam tomography of late developing coronary artery aneurysms after Kawasaki disease. Catheter Cardiovasc Interv 1999;47:114–115.

48. Sato Y, Kato M, Inoue F, et al. Detection of coronary artery aneurysms, stenoses and occlusions by multislice spiral computed tomography in adolescents with Kawasaki disease. Circ J 2003;67:427–430.

49. Kanamaru H, Sato Y, Takayama T, et al. Assessment of coronary artery abnormalities by multislice spiral computed tomography in adolescents and young adults with Kawasaki disease. Am J Cardiol 2005;95:522–525.

10

Coronary Angiography after Revascularization

Axel Schmermund, Stefan Möhlenkamp, Thomas Schlosser, and Raimund Erbel

Background

As a result of the high prevalence of coronary artery disease in the Western world and – increasingly – in the developing countries, coronary artery revascularization, albeit complex and expensive, is one of the most frequent medical procedures. It is estimated that currently, worldwide approximately 800,000 patients undergo bypass surgery annually [1], and >1.5 million percutaneous interventions are performed. With the increasing success of these procedures and improved long-term results, it is no longer current practice to perform routine invasive follow-up examination after revascularization. Only patients with evidence of recurrent ischemia undergo coronary angiography. However, the decision to perform or withhold coronary angiography can be exceedingly difficult in patients who have a history of coronary artery revascularization. Commonly, the fact that coronary artery disease has been previously established will lead many physicians to liberally order invasive coronary angiography if their patients experience symptoms faintly reminiscent of angina pectoris. In this setting, a non-invasive method for obtaining reliable information on coronary artery anatomy would be of great value.

Venous Grafts

Anatomy and Natural History

Venous bypass grafts still represent the majority of all grafts used for bypass surgery. Due to differences in anatomy and surgical techniques, their patency rates are inferior to internal mammary artery grafts [1,2]. Three modes of venous bypass graft degeneration have been described which occur at different time points after surgery. Within hours to weeks after surgery, technical deficiencies and thrombotic activation lead to early thrombotic occlusion in approximately 5–10% of the grafts [3].

Over the course of the following year, intimal hyperplasia and thrombosis appear to be the major mechanisms, accounting for an overall occlusion rate of 10–15% within the first year [3,4]. Finally, after the first year, mechanisms known from native coronary artery atherosclerosis predominate. Bypass attrition between postoperative years 1 and 5 appears to be minimal. After year 5, atherothrombotic occlusion of venous grafts accounts for a reduced patency rate. It has traditionally been estimated to range between 40% and 60% at 10–12 years [3,5]. However, recent data from the Veteran Affairs Cooperative Study indicate that venous grafts that are open 1 week after surgery have a patency rate of 68% after 10 years [1]. The presence of angiographic stenoses between 50% and 99% of graft diameter appears to be 17–22% at 10 years [1].

Non-invasive CT Examination

Venous bypass grafts are typically larger in diameter than the native large epicardial coronary arteries (approximately 4–10 mm versus 2–5 mm), and they are less subjected to cardiac motion. Accordingly, even with older-generation ("non-cardiac") CT machines, investigators examined contrast enhancement along the course of the graft to establish bypass patency [6–12]. Along with the technical developments, the accuracy reported with this approach increased. However, due to the inherent limitations of non-gated scanning with relatively long acquisition times, overall diagnostic accuracy regarding bypass graft patency remained at approximately 90%, with better results for (larger) vein grafts than for the arterial grafts. It was not possible to identify potential non-occlusive high-grade bypass body stenoses, the distal anastomosis of the grafts, or the native coronary arterial run-off.

As might be expected, the advent of electron beam computed tomography (EBCT) as the first dedicated cardiac CT scanner led to new applications. In an experimental model of saphenous vein grafts from the left innominate to the left circumflex coronary artery in dogs, Rumberger et al.

examined the ability to measure coronary bypass flow velocity by analyzing contrast clearance curves generated from a region of interest in the ascending aorta and in the bypass graft [13]. A variable vascular occluder and infusions of adenosine were used to create different flow velocities in the grafted vessels. The CT study was designed to determine the time difference between peak contrast opacification in the aorta and the bypass graft. Compared with Doppler probe measurements, this parameter ("time difference between peak contrast opacification") was closely correlated with individual values of relative bypass flow velocity. However, this approach was not translated into clinical applications, probably owing to the complexity of the measurements.

A decade later, after the introduction of non-invasive coronary angiography, Achenbach et al. visualized coronary bypass grafts and provided three-dimensional (3-D) representations of the graft vessels [14]. Along with the technical development of CT scanners, various protocols for non-invasive CT angiography have since then been used as the principal method for evaluating bypass grafts. Achenbach et al. examined 25 patients with a total of 56 bypass grafts (55 venous grafts, 1 internal mammary artery) and a mean of 6.9 years after surgery [14]. All but one graft were single grafts with no sequential anastomosis. In one patient with congestive heart failure who had two bypass grafts, image interpretation was altogether impossible because of respiratory artifacts and low contrast enhancement. The remaining 54 grafts in 24 patients were analyzed regarding patency and presence of stenoses. Image quality was insufficient to allow for detection of stenoses in 5 grafts in 4 patients. Accordingly, a total of 54 grafts were analyzed regarding their patency, and 49 grafts were additionally analyzed regarding the detection of possible stenoses. All patients underwent selective coronary angiography to provide a standard diagnostic evaluation.

A total of 13 grafts (all venous) were occluded, which were all detected by EBCT. All other grafts were correctly identified as being patent. There were 5 high-grade stenoses in the venous grafts, which were all detected by EBCT. All of these stenoses were located along the body of the bypass graft (and not in the region of the distal anastomosis). EBCT identified one high-grade stenosis which was not confirmed by selective coronary angiography ("false positive"). Accordingly, sensitivity and specificity regarding bypass patency were 100%, respectively, and regarding stenosis detection in the bypass body were 100% and 97%, respectively. Obviously, the small number of stenoses and the exclusion from analysis of a total of 7 grafts in 5 patients must be considered when interpreting these results. However, reliable diagnosis of bypass patency appeared absolutely feasible, and EBCT bypass angiography was used in this respect for some years. As opposed to native coronary arteries, venous bypass grafts tend to develop an extensive thrombotic burden and occlude quite rapidly once a high-grade stenosis has formed. Accord-

ingly, the ability to detect venous bypass occlusion by using EBCT coronary bypass angiography has been helpful in a subset of patients with unspecific symptoms after bypass surgery and was further examined in subsequent reports [15–18].

Ha et al. specified that venous grafts with the right coronary artery as recipient vessel appeared to be more difficult regarding the detection of graft occlusion than the other vascular territories [15]. Lu et al. examined contrast time–density curves as a possible means to improve the accuracy of evaluating bypass occlusion [16,17]. They basically observed that this approach was less feasible than the conventional anatomic representation with 3-D display of the contrast-filled grafts.

The first generation of multidetector CT (MDCT) scanners with four detector rows was evaluated by Ropers et al. [19]. They examined 56 patients with a total of 162 venous and 20 internal mammary arterial grafts after a mean interval of 7.6 years after surgery. The standard method, selective coronary angiography, was performed 1–3 days after MDCT and revealed occlusion of 56 venous grafts and stenoses in 23 of the patent ones. MDCT images were acquired with a gantry rotation time of 500 ms. A total dose of 180 mL contrast was injected at a rate of 4 mL/s. Depending on heart rate, electrocardiographically gated image reconstruction intervals varied between 127 and 248 ms. A slice thickness of 1.2–1.4 mm was reconstructed. No additional beta blockers were given. Using this protocol, all of the 162 venous grafts could be evaluated regarding patency, but only 75% of the 106 patent grafts could be evaluated regarding the detection of stenoses. Reasons for inferior image quality included respiration and motion artifacts, arrhythmias, and insufficient contrast opacification.

In the report, no clear differentiation between venous and arterial grafts was made regarding the detection of bypass occlusion and stenoses. Because only 20 arterial grafts were included (out of a total number of 182 grafts), and only 2 arterial grafts were occluded and 2 had a high-grade stenosis, respectively, the results pertain mainly to venous grafts. Overall, 54 of 56 grafts were correctly diagnosed as being occluded, and 122 of 124 as being patent. Sensitivity and specificity were 97% and 98%, respectively [19]. In the 77 patent grafts judged to be evaluable regarding the presence of stenoses, 12 of 16 stenoses were correctly detected. In 5 grafts, stenoses were diagnosed which were not confirmed by selective angiography. Accordingly, sensitivity for stenosis detection was 75% (12/16), and specificity was 92% (56/61). Of note, 3 of the 4 false-negative and 3 of the 5 false-positive diagnoses were located in the region of the distal anastomosis.

Nieman et al. also used 4-row MDCT and a similar imaging and reconstruction protocol (also with no additional beta blockers) in their examination of 24 patients with a total of 23 venous grafts [20]. The majority of the venous grafts had 2 or more sequential anastomoses, yielding a total of 60 graft segments. Surgery had been performed a mean of 9.6 years before the study. Selective angiography showed 17 venous grafts to be occluded and 6 to be stenosed. An analysis of interobserver variability for evaluation of the MDCT images was included. The two observers agreed that the vast majority (95–100%) of the venous grafts was assessable. Sensitivity and specificity for diagnosing graft occlusion were 100%, respectively. Assessability of bypass stenoses was limited to 90–95%, depending on the observer. There were only 6 stenoses in the patent venous graft segments. Depending on the observer and his judgment of assessability, 3–5 of these 6 stenoses were detected. Specificity was reported to be in the range of 90% [20].

The introduction of 16-slice MDCT with shorter rotation times and reduced slice thickness represented a major advance for non-invasive coronary imaging. Because of the dynamic technical development, scientific evaluation of the merits and limitations of the different scanner generations is becoming increasingly difficult. Currently, only two reports have evaluated 16-slice MDCT for examining bypass grafts [21,22]. These reports used the first generation of 16-slice scanners with application of 12–16 detector rows and a rotation time of 420–500 ms. At the time of this writing, the latest scanner generations have up to 64 detector rows and a gantry rotation time of 330 ms. This only underlines the importance of actual data, as the technology is constantly evolving.

Schlosser et al. examined 51 consecutive patients a mean of 5.5 years after surgery [21]. As opposed to the previous 4-slice MDCT studies, a reconstruction increment of only 0.5 mm was chosen, in theory allowing for improved through-plane spatial resolution. Also, patients with a heart rate ≥70 beats/min received an intravenous injection of a short-acting beta blocker (esmolol) shortly before the scan. Nevertheless, 3 patients were excluded from the analysis because they did not achieve a sufficient heart rate reduction (<70 beats/min) or had severe arrhythmic artifacts. The remaining 48 patients had 91 venous grafts and 40 internal mammary artery (IMA) grafts. Selective angiography demonstrated occlusion of 18 venous grafts and a significant stenosis in 2 grafts. Sensitivity and specificity regarding the detection of venous graft occlusion were both 100%, respectively. The 2 venous graft stenoses were correctly detected by 16-slice MDCT, even though one was an in-stent restenosis. However, in 5 venous grafts (all coursing to the right coronary artery), stenoses were incorrectly identified ("false positive"). In formal analysis, this would yield a sensitivity of 100% and a specificity of 93% for stenosis detection. Of note, 29% of the distal anastomoses could not be evaluated, in particular with the right coronary artery as recipient vessel. The major mechanisms identified by the authors were small vessel diameter, poor opacification, and/or cardiac motion artifacts. Figure 10.1 shows the appearance of venous (and one arterial) bypass grafts.

In a retrospective analysis, Dewey et al. confirmed the ability of 16-slice MDCT to identify venous bypass graft occlusion [22]. In the MDCT database, 27 patients were

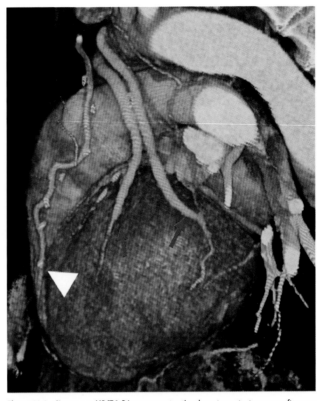

Figure 10.1. Sixteen-row MDCT 3-D image reconstruction shows two patent venous grafts coursing to a left diagonal (left arrow) and an obtuse marginal branch (right arrow) and a left internal mammary arterial graft with the left anterior descending coronary artery as the recipient vessel (arrowhead).

identified who had previously undergone bypass surgery and had 55 venous and 20 arterial grafts. Most, but not all, patients had also undergone selective coronary angiography. The patients were not given additional beta blockers. As far as is possible to judge from selective angiography in the majority of the patients and clinical information, 15 occluded bypass grafts and 2 stenoses were correctly identified, and 1 false-positive stenosis was observed in a venous graft.

Summary of Diagnostic Accuracy for Venous Bypass Graft Evaluation

Table 10.1 summarizes the data on venous bypass graft evaluation by EBCT and MDCT. The latest generation of 16-slice MDCT scanners in particular appear to provide reliable detection of venous graft occlusion. Recent published reports [21,22] and preliminary studies have observed that their accuracy in diagnosing venous graft occlusion is comparable to that of selective coronary angiography. There are not enough data available on the ability to identify stenoses. Whereas the bypass body appears readily assessable, the region of the distal anastomosis (insertion site) remains problematic. In clinical practice, patients with unspecific symptoms and an intermediate

Table 10.1. Selected results of CT examination of venous bypass grafts

| First author, CT scanner | Number of bypass grafts | Bypass patency | | Bypass stenosis detection | | Not evaluable regarding stenoses (%) |
		Sensitivity (%)	Specificity (%)	Sensitivity (%)	Specificity (%)	
Achenbach 1997, EBCT (14)	55	100	100	100	97	9
Ha 1999, EBCT (15)	57	92	91	–	–	–
Ropers 2001,[a] 4-row MDCT (19)	162	97	98	75	92	25
Nieman 2003,[b] 4-row MDCT (20)	23	100	100	60–83	90	5–10
Schlosser 2004,[c] 16-row MDCT (21)	91	100	100	100	93	29

[a] Results include analysis of 20 arterial grafts.
[b] Results obtained from analysis of two independent observers.
[c] Three patients were excluded from the analysis right away because of high heart rate or arrhythmic artefacts.

probability of venous bypass deterioration might derive benefit from MDCT (Figures 10.2 and 10.3). However, to be clinically useful in more than just a few selected cases, it would be necessary to achieve a valid evaluation not only of the bypass body, but also of the distal anastomosis. Whereas one recent, 16-slice MDCT-based report detailed that only 74% of distal anastomoses were assessable [21], another found 100% to be assessable [22]. Another concern relates to native coronary artery disease whose progression may be underlying the recurrent symptoms in a minority of patients with bypass grafts. Because of the complex and advanced disease pattern, frequent heavy calcification, and relative importance of small diameter native vessels in patients with coronary bypass grafts, comprehensive CT diagnosis may be difficult. In their study using 4-row MDCT, Nieman et al. observed that >30% of native coronary arteries were not assessable, and overall sensitivity for stenosis detection was in the order of only 53–70% [20]. Taken as a whole, the advances in temporal and spatial resolution have enabled reliable evaluation of the venous bypass body, including the detection of stenoses. However, because of diagnostic limitations in the anastomosis region and, in particular, the native vessels, clinical applicability will remain limited in the foreseeable future.

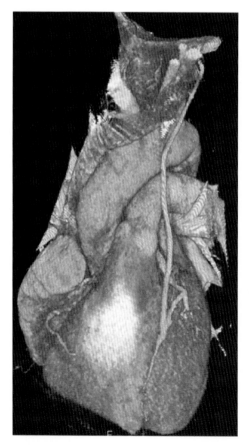

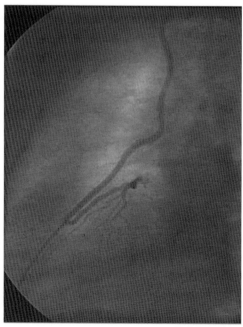

Figure 10.2. Sixteen-row MDCT 3-D image reconstruction shows a patent left internal mammary graft to the left anterior descending coronary artery and the corresponding selective angiogram.

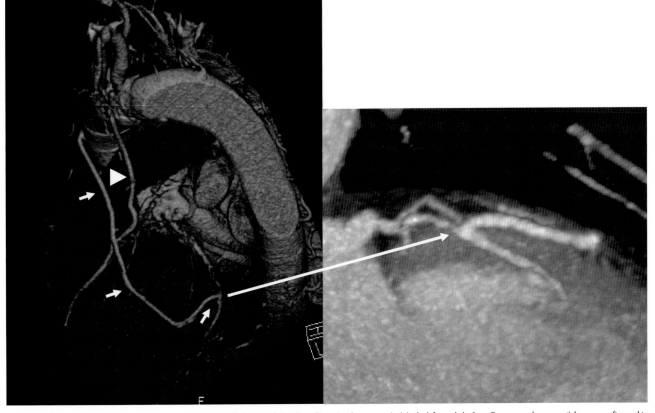

Figure 10.3. Patent bypass grafts imaged by a 64-row MDCT scanner (volume rendering three-dimensional reconstruction). In the left panel, the 3 small arrows mark a sequential venous graft sewed to a small diagonal branch and a larger marginal branch of the left circumflex coronary artery. The arrowhead marks the internal thoracic artery graft to the left anterior descending coronary artery. The right panel shows a maximum intensity projection image of the distal anastomosis of the venous graft with the marginal branch, clearly demonstrating non-obstructed flow despite the relatively small vessel diameter and the fast-moving location between left atrium and left ventricle. Please note that it would be difficult to evaluate stenoses in the native vessels in this patient.

Imaging Protocols

Non-invasive CT-based bypass graft evaluation should only be done in patients with stable sinus rhythm. Therefore most experts agree that beta blockade should be undertaken with the aim of reaching heart rates ≤60 beats/min [23]. Although the most recent scanner generations may be less susceptible to motion artifacts, practical experience dictates that this approach yields superior visibility of coronary artery segments. Many experts also recommend the administration of oral or intravenous nitrates for vasodilation immediately prior to the scan.

Specific scanning protocols with the various scanners are detailed in Chapter 4. Willmann et al. examined the influence of the reconstruction interval on image quality using a 4-slice MDCT scanner for the evaluation of bypass vessels [24]. Whereas the reconstruction interval appeared to be of minor importance for evaluating the proximal portion of the bypass vessels, significant differences in image quality between the different reconstruction times were seen for the bypass body and distal anastomosis. Consistent with observations in the native coronary arteries, these bypass segments appeared to be best depicted at a reconstruction interval between 50% and 70% of the R-R interval [24]. If

possible, submillimeter collimation should be used for MDCT data acquisition, and slice thickness should be reconstructed at small increments (≤1 mm). With the latest scanner generations (64-detector scanners), it appears useful to inject the contrast media at a higher rate of approximately 5 mL/s. Because of the short scanning times, the total amount of contrast can be reduced to <80 mL.

Arterial Grafts

Anatomy and Natural History

The left IMA is most often used in arterial grafts. Arterial vessels are by design much better adapted to systemic blood pressure values and shear stress than venous vessels, and this translates into improved patency rates [1,2]. IMA grafts patent at 1 week after surgery had a 10-year patency rate of 88% in the Veterans Affairs Cooperative Study [1]. As with venous grafts, recipient vessel location and status influence graft survival. Survival is best for grafts to the left anterior descending coronary artery and a native vessel diameter ≥2 mm [1]. Interestingly, IMA grafts sewn to a recipient vessel with <50% diameter stenosis may have a very high rate of occlusion, probably due to competing flow through the native vessel [25].

Non-invasive CT Examination

Compared with venous grafts, fewer data are available on arterial grafts, most likely because they are grafted less frequently. CT evaluation is hampered by a relatively small diameter and metal clips around the IMA graft. In a study using EBCT which examined a large number of arterial grafts ($n = 135$), Lu et al. only had to exclude 7% because of inferior image quality [16]. Only 2 of these grafts were occluded. Although the 4-row MDCT study by Ropers et al. concentrated on venous grafts, 20 arterial grafts were also included [19]. Of the 18 patent arterial grafts, 5 could not be evaluated in further detail because of metal clips and small lumen diameter.

Nieman et al., in their 4-row MDCT study, specifically examined arterial versus venous graft results [20]. In 24 patients, 18 arterial grafts had been used, with some having up to 5 sequential anastomoses, resulting in a total of 26 arterial graft segments. Selective angiography showed 5 arterial segment occlusions and 1 stenosis. The two observers who independently interpreted the studies reported that only 58–73% of the arterial graft segments were assessable. With this limitation, sensitivity and specificity for diagnosing IMA graft occlusion were 75–100% and 80–100%, respectively. Of the remaining 18 patent arterial graft segments, 5 or 6 – depending on the observer – could not be assessed regarding the presence of high-grade stenoses. One observer detected the only high-grade stenosis that was present, the other did not.

Marano et al. examined 57 patients with a total of 122 bypass grafts using 4-row MDCT [26]. As opposed to the other reports, the majority of the grafts ($n = 95$) were arterial. Most of these were IMA grafts (left IMA, $n = 57$; right IMA, $n = 15$), but there were also 15 radial arteries and 8 right gastro-epiploic arteries. Selective angiography demonstrated occlusion of 17 arterial grafts. MDCT evaluation comprised all arterial grafts and yielded a sensitivity of 100% and specificity of 99% regarding the detection of graft occlusion. Concerning stenoses in the patent arterial grafts, 24 (31%) of 78 were judged to be non-assessable. In the remaining grafts, 8 of 10 stenoses were correctly identified, whereas 2 stenoses in the region of the distal anastomosis were not detected ("false negative"). In 2 grafts, false-positive results were seen, in one of these cases again in the region of the anastomosis. Of note, complete evaluation of all bypass grafts with MDCT was feasible in 35 of 57 patients (61%). Patients whose grafts were all assessable had a lower heart rate (60 ± 11 beats/min) than patients with non-assessable grafts (72 ± 13 beats/min).

Using 16-row MDCT, Schlosser et al. found that all of 40 IMA grafts could be assessed regarding patency [21]. All

of 3 occluded grafts were correctly detected. There was one stenosis in the distal anastomosis which was missed by MDCT. In another study employing 16-row MDCT, Dewey et al. also reported assessability of all 20 arterial grafts [22], without giving more detailed information in comparison with selective angiography.

Summary of Diagnostic Accuracy for Arterial Bypass Graft Evaluation

Although it is more difficult to obtain good images of the smaller-diameter arterial grafts, recent studies have reported 100% visibility. Accordingly, diagnosis of graft occlusion appears to be feasible. However, few data are available regarding stenosis detection. Stenoses tend to be located in the region of the anastomosis with the recipient vessel. The anecdotal evidence we have suggests that reliable detection of stenoses in this area is not possible with the current generation of scanners. Small vessel diameter, metal clip artifacts, and cardiac motion account for the non-diagnostic image quality. It remains to be seen if these issues can be overcome by further improvements in spatial resolution.

Coronary Stents

The vast majority of coronary interventions are currently performed in association with placement of a coronary stent to provide scaffolding of the vessel wall [27] (Figures 10.4 and 10.5). Most coronary stents are slotted tubes made of stainless steel. Such stents have been demonstrated to result in less acute complications, increased patency rates, and reduced restenosis compared with conventional balloon angioplasty [27]. Long-term results of coronary stenting not only depend on the characteristics of the materials and stent design, but importantly also on the clinical scenario (unstable versus stable patient), concomitant medical therapy, coronary anatomy, and specific lesion morphology. Whereas conventional bare metal stents are typically associated with clinically symptomatic restenosis in 20–30% of all patients, stents with active drug coating embedded in a polymer on the surface of the metal struts have a clinical restenosis rate of approximately 12% [28]. Stent strut thickness may vary between 50 and 140 μm. Some stents have a closed cell design with comparably greater metal-to-surface ratio than stents with an open cell design. The weight of stents with common dimensions ranges from 8 to 16 mg. Further, some stents have radio-opaque markers attached at the extreme portions to allow for better fluoroscopic visibility. These factors account for substantial differences in the appearance of different stents when evaluated by cardiac CT.

CT-based assessment of metal stents in large vessels with little motion such as the aorta and the renal and iliac arter-

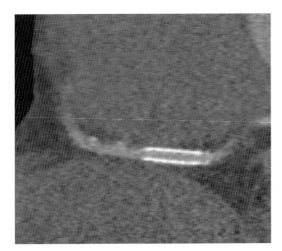

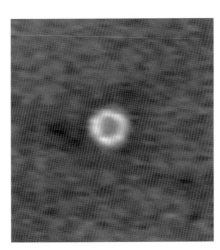

Figure 10.4. Patent stent in the distal right coronary artery in vivo.

ies has demonstrated the potential to obtain images with diagnostic quality in the coronary arteries. However, coronary stents usually measure 2.5–4 mm in diameter and are constantly subjected to cardiac motion. Whereas EBCT and the recent MDCT scanner generations have the ability to eliminate motion artifacts in most patients, the small stent diameter remains problematic. Virtually all coronary stents are made of metal and produce typical "blooming" artifacts. In combination with partial volume effects, this leads to decreased visibility of the stent lumen and underestimation of its diameter while at the same time the outer diameter is overestimated. Detailed analysis of the inner-stent lumen is necessary to detect various degrees of intimal hyperplasia, the major mechanism of in-stent restenosis.

Because of the above noted limitations regarding the assessment of coronary stent morphology, early EBCT studies used time–density curve analysis in regions of interest distal to the stent and in part compared these curves with the pattern in the aorta [29–32]. See Figure 4.8 for an example of flow rate analysis for stent patency. Also, 3-D reconstructions were done to allow for visualization of the coronary artery segments in the proximity of the stents [32]. Variable results regarding assessability of stented coronary artery segments and diagnostic accuracy were reported in these studies. Nevertheless, it can be stated in summary that only complete stent occlusion could be reliably detected, whereas high-grade and even subtotal stenoses were frequently not identified. This can be easily explained by the observation that even vessels with subtotal stenosis often display unimpeded contrast flow. Further, retrograde filling of an occluded vessel via collaterals is poten-

tially problematic, if several cardiac cycles are needed to generate time–density curves with low temporal resolution.

In vitro studies performed with different scanner generations have established the basic principles and issues of direct coronary stent imaging [30,33–38]. Clearly, the best possible spatial resolution is necessary [34–38]. Usually, the visible artifacts include blooming ("thickening") of the stent struts with an apparent reduction of the visible stent lumen, increased attenuation values inside the stent lumen, and beamlike artifacts in the vicinity of the stent [33]. The density of the stents is inhomogeneous and depends on the distribution of the struts. Maximum values range from 600 to >1500 Hounsfield units (HU) [35]. Inside the lumen, the CT artifacts lead to increases of attenuation by up to 250 HU [34]. This effect appears much less pronounced if submillimeter collimation and a sharp reconstruction kernel can be used, in which case increases of only approximately 20 HU are observed [34]. In the presence of a dedicated sharp kernel, an edge-preserving filter algorithm may be necessary [34,38].

In the motionless phantom, artificial stenoses could be reliably detected within the stents by using 16-row MDCT and a sharp reconstruction kernel [34]. Other phantom studies reported the different appearance of various stent designs [35,36]. Again, the use of a sharp reconstruction kernel appeared important. The authors pointed out that due to direct artifact reduction, stents with as little metal as possible would importantly contribute to improved image quality, independent of CT scanner characteristics [35,36].

Mahnken et al. recently used a prototype of a novel flat-panel detector CT to evaluate a static stent phantom [37]. Compared with a 16-row MDCT, they observed an impres-

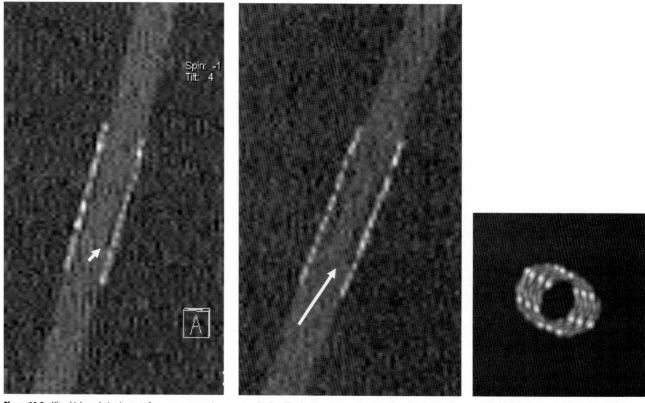

Figure 10.5. Ultra-high resolution images of a coronary stent using current multi-slice CT technology (64-row Somatom Sensation Cardiac, Siemens Medical Solutions, Germany). The 2 left panel pictures show the stent mounted on a vessel model placed in a phantom with realistic attenuation values. The short arrow marks an artificial 30% in-stent restenosis (produced within the stented vessel model), the longer arrow a 50% restenosis in the same setting. The right panel shows a three-dimensional reconstruction of the stent.

sive image quality almost free of artifacts such as the blooming phenomenon and the artificial stent lumen decrease (Figure 10.5). Although these CT machines are far from clinical applicability, such studies demonstrate that even the small "heavy metal" stents in the coronary arteries can potentially be imaged with diagnostic quality.

In an in vivo study, Hong et al. evaluated the ability to assess the in-stent lumen using 16-row MDCT [39]. They examined 19 patients who had undergone placement of a total of 26 stents 1–3 weeks before the CT study. There was no clinical evidence of early in-stent restenosis. The performance of a sharp compared with a medium-smooth reconstruction kernel was analyzed. During the CT study, heart rate ranged between 41 and 98 beats/min. Sufficient image quality was found in 14 patients with a total of 20 stents. The sharp reconstruction kernel resulted in significantly improved image quality compared with the medium-smooth kernel. Mean stent strut density measured 649 HU, and mean in-stent lumen density 342 HU. A close correlation was observed between contrast enhancement in the stent lumen and in the neighboring unstented segments, suggesting the ability to predict stent patency [39]. Use of the sharp reconstruction kernel resulted in less underestimation of the stent lumen diameter than use of the medium-smooth kernel (−16% versus −27%). Figure 10.4 shows an in vivo image of a patent stent in the distal right coronary artery (64-slice MDCT).

Seifarth et al. analyzed image quality and artifacts in vivo in 10 patients examined by using a 16-row MDCT scanner, and they compared different reconstruction kernels [38]. The patients had received a total of 15 coronary stents with a diameter between 2.75 and 4.0 mm. They were examined within 10 days following stent implantation, and there were no in-stent restenoses. A medium-smooth kernel resulted in a mean visible stent lumen of 1.93 ± 0.50 mm, whereas a sharp kernel and special filter algorithm yielded 2.16 ± 0.51 mm. This corresponded to an artificial stent lumen reduction of 37% and 29%, respectively. Compared with the aorta, intraluminal attenuation within the stent was increased by 111 HU as compared with only 60 HU when using the sharp kernel. Accordingly, dedicated reconstruction algorithms were able to improve image quality.

An early study assessed the ability to detect in-stent restenoses by using 4-row MDCT [40]. Twenty patients with a total number of 32 stents were examined at a mean interval of 9.6 ± 4.2 months after stent implantation. Invasive coronary angiography demonstrated significant (>50%) restenosis in 5 (16%) stents. Using MDCT, it was impossible to directly visualize the stent lumen. Only the coronary artery segments proximal and distal to the stent could be assessed. This allowed accurate identification of patent stents in 18 patients and of total stent occlusion in 2 patients. Only stent patency could be evaluated, and 3 high-grade non-occlusive stenoses were not detected.

The ability to identify coronary stent patency was also reported in a number of case reports using 4-row, 8-row, and 16-row MDTC [41–44]. Using 16-row MDCT, neo-intimal hyperplasia leading to non-significant in-stent restenosis was detected in a left main coronary stent [45]. Schuijf et al. examined 22 patients with a total of 68 stents by using 16-row MDCT [46]. Most stents had been only recently implanted, but 23 had been implanted >1 month before the study. The data of 1 patient were lost, and 15 of the 65 remaining stents (23%) were judged to have insufficient image quality to assess stent patency. The vast majority of non-assessable stents had a diameter ≤3 mm. In the stents judged to be assessable, restenosis was correctly ruled out in 41, and 7 stents with restenosis were correctly identified. Two restenotic stents were not identified. In a per-vessel analysis of 29 (81%) of the stented major coronary arteries, all 3 vessels with high-grade restenosis were correctly identified, and the 26 remaining vessels with no in-stent restenosis were also correctly classified.

Gilard et al. investigated the ability of 16-slice MDCT to detect restenosis in 29 consecutive patients who had undergone left main coronary artery stenting a mean of 6 months before the MDCT examination [47]. The final mean stent diameter was 3.9 mm, corresponding to a large lumen compared with usual coronary stents. In 4 patients, a restenosis (defined as >50% diameter stenosis) was identified by selective coronary angiography. The mean heart rate of the patients at the time of this examination was 66 beats/min, and no additional beta blockers were given. MDCT detected all stents and provided for visualization of the lumen in 27 patients (93%). MDCT detected neointimal proliferation in 7 patients. Six patients were classified as having >50% restenosis. Accordingly, all 4 restenoses were correctly identified. Sensitivity was 100%, and specificity 92%. The authors concluded that with the exception of arrhythmic or heavily calcified segments, MDCT might provide a non-invasive alternative in the follow-up after left main stent implantation.

Summary of Diagnostic Accuracy for Coronary Stent Evaluation

Because of the metal artefacts, MDCT does not enable reliable visualization of the coronary stent lumen. Stents with a comparably large diameter may in some patients allow for diagnostic images (Figure 10.6). However, no definite data are available, in part because restenosis is relatively rare in large stents, and the technical development of the CT scanners is continuously evolving. Most coronary stents measure 3 mm in diameter and have relatively dense metal struts. With "blooming" and related artefacts, their lumen appears artificially small, precluding a reliable analysis. Thus, there are currently no clinical applications for MDCT imaging of coronary stents. However, preliminary clinical data and, in particular, improvements in spatial resolution allow for an optimistic perspective.

Facilitation of Invasive Angiography

Some reports have analyzed the possible impact of coronary artery calcification, determined by EBCT, on restenosis after coronary intervention [48–50]. In these studies, an increased amount of focal calcification appeared to be associated with increased rates of restenosis, irrespective of whether stent implantation was done or simply angioplasty. Clinical expe-

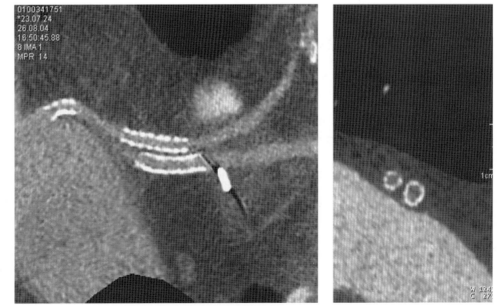

Figure 10.6. Images of three stents in venous coronary bypass grafts obtained by using 64-slice MDCT. The stent lumen appears to be clearly visualized, with no apparent restenosis. The stent diameter is 4.0–4.5 mm. A surgical metal clip causes some beam hardening artifacts, whereas the stents themselves cause few visual artifacts. (Images courtesy of Dr Stephan Achenbach, University of Erlangen-Nürnberg.)

rience and intravascular ultrasound data indicate that if intervention is possible with a good primary result, calcification does not lead to more frequent restenosis [51]. Heavy calcification detected by EBCT might indicate procedural difficulties and could be interpreted as a warning sign before coronary intervention. However, although a threshold amount of calcification has been suggested as predictive of restenosis [50], it is not known what amount of calcification will make plain angioplasty impossible and call for the use of additional techniques such as rotablation.

One might imagine that CT coronary angiography could help in planning interventions. Plaque volume, lesion length, degree of calcification, localization of side branches, and estimates of vessel diameter might all be helpful. On the other hand, such information is also provided by selective angiography immediately before the intervention, and an experienced operator will probably feel comfortable with it. A recent report analyzed the ability of MDCT to predict procedural failure in chronic total coronary occlusions by the combined use of diagnostic selective angiography and MDCT angiography [52]. Multivariate analysis identified a blunt stump (by conventional angiography), occlusion length >15 mm, and severe calcification (by MDCT) as independent predictors of procedural failure. Along these lines, it may be useful for a surgeon planning to graft a bypass to an occluded vessel to see if the periphery of this vessel is perfused via collaterals or, if that is not the case, if the vessel diameter appears large enough to employ surgical techniques for plaque and thrombus removal. Finally, anecdotal evidence suggests that MDCT coronary angiography can help to find bypass vessels which are grafted to the aorta in an unusual position and are difficult to find selectively.

References

1. Goldman S, Zadina K, Moritz T, et al.; VA Cooperative Study Group #207/297/364. Long-term patency of saphenous vein and left internal mammary artery grafts after coronary artery bypass surgery: results from a Department of Veterans Affairs Cooperative Study. J Am Coll Cardiol 2004;44:2149–2156.
2. Schwartz L, Kip KE, Frye RL, Alderman EL, Schaff HV, Detre KM; Bypass Angioplasty Revascularization Investigation. Coronary bypass graft patency in patients with diabetes in the Bypass Angioplasty Revascularization Investigation (BARI). Circulation 2002;106:2652–2658.
3. Lytle BW, Loop FD, Cosgrove DM, Ratliff NB, Easley K, Taylor PC. Long-term (5 to 12 years) serial studies of internal mammary artery and saphenous vein coronary bypass grafts. J Thorac Cardiovasc Surg 1985;89:248–258.
4. Shi Y, O'Brien JE Jr, Mannion JD, et al. Remodeling of autologous saphenous vein grafts. The role of perivascular myofibroblasts. Circulation 1997;95:2684–2693.
5. Fitzgibbon GM, Kafka HP, Leach AJ, Keon WJ, Hooper GD, Burton JR. Coronary bypass graft fate and patient outcome: angiographic follow-up of 5,065 grafts related to survival and reoperation in 1,388 patients during 25 years. J Am Coll Cardiol 1996;28:616–626.
6. Brundage BH, Lipton MJ, Herfkens RJ, et al. Detection of patent coronary bypass grafts by computed tomography. A preliminary report. Circulation 1980;61:826–831.
7. Daniel WG, Dohring W, Stender HS, Lichtlen PR. Value and limitations of computed tomography in assessing aortocoronary bypass graft patency. Circulation 1983;67:983–987.
8. McKay CR, Brundage BH, Ullyot DJ, Turley K, Lipton MJ, Ebert PA. Evaluation of early postoperative coronary artery bypass graft patency by contrast-enhanced computed tomography. J Am Coll Cardiol 1983;2:312–317.
9. Bateman TM, Gray RJ, Whiting JS, et al. Prospective evaluation of ultrafast cardiac computed tomography for determination of coronary bypass graft patency. Circulation 1987;75:1018–1024.
10. Stanford W, Brundage BH, MacMillan R, et al. Sensitivity and specificity of assessing coronary bypass graft patency with ultrafast computed tomography: results of a multicenter study. J Am Coll Cardiol 1988;12:1–7.
11. Engelmann MG, von Smekal A, Knez A, et al. Accuracy of spiral computed tomography for identifying arterial and venous coronary graft patency. Am J Cardiol 1997;80:569–574.
12. Tello R, Hartnell GG, Costello P, Ecker CP. Coronary artery bypass graft flow: qualitative evaluation with cine single-detector row CT and comparison with findings at angiography. Radiology 2002;224:913–918.
13. Rumberger JA, Feiring AJ, Hiratzka LF, et al. Quantification of coronary artery bypass flow reserve in dogs using cine-computed tomography. Circ Res 1987;61(5 Pt 2):II117–123.
14. Achenbach S, Moshage W, Ropers D, Nossen J, Bachmann K. Noninvasive, three-dimensional visualization of coronary artery bypass grafts by electron beam tomography. Am J Cardiol 1997;79:856–861.
15. Ha JW, Cho SY, Shim WH, et al. Noninvasive evaluation of coronary artery bypass graft patency using three-dimensional angiography obtained with contrast-enhanced electron beam CT. AJR Am J Roentgenol 1999;172:1055–1059.
16. Lu B, Dai RP, Jing BL, et al. Evaluation of coronary artery bypass graft patency using three-dimensional reconstruction and flow study on electron beam tomography. J Comput Assist Tomogr 2000;24:663–670.
17. Lu B, Dai RP, Zhuang N, Budoff MJ. Noninvasive assessment of coronary artery bypass graft patency and flow characteristics by electron-beam tomography. J Invasive Cardiol 2002;14:19–24.
18. Yamakami S, Toyama J, Okamoto M, et al. Noninvasive detection of coronary artery bypass graft patency by intravenous electron beam computed tomographic angiography. Jpn Heart J 2003;44:811–822.
19. Ropers D, Ulzheimer S, Wenkel E, et al. Investigation of aortocoronary artery bypass grafts by multislice spiral computed tomography with electrocardiographic-gated image reconstruction. Am J Cardiol 2001;88:792–795.
20. Nieman K, Pattynama PMT, Rensing BJ, van Geuns RJM, de Feyter PJ. Evaluation of patients after coronary artery bypass surgery: CT angiographic assessment of grafts and coronary arteries. Radiology 2003;229:749–756.
21. Schlosser T, Konorza T, Hunold P, Kuhl H, Schmermund A, Barkhausen J. Noninvasive visualization of coronary artery bypass grafts using 16-detector row computed tomography. J Am Coll Cardiol 2004;44:1224–1229.
22. Dewey M, Lembcke A, Enzweiler C, Hamm B, Rogalla P. Isotropic half-millimeter angiography of coronary artery bypass grafts with 16-slice computed tomography. Ann Thorac Surg 2004;77:800–804.
23. Nieman K, Rensing BJ, van Geuns RJ, et al. Non-invasive coronary angiography with multislice spiral computed tomography: impact of heart rate. Heart 2002;88:470–474.
24. Willmann JK, Weishaupt D, Kobza R, et al. Coronary artery bypass grafts: ECG-gated multi-detector row CT angiography – influence of image reconstruction interval on graft visibility. Radiology 2004;232:568–577.
25. Berger A, MacCarthy PA, Siebert U, et al. Long-term patency of internal mammary artery bypass grafts. Relationship with preoperative severity of the native coronary artery stenosis. Circulation 2004;110(suppl II):II-36–II-40.

26. Marano R, Storto ML, Maddestra N, Bonomo L. Non-invasive assessment of coronary artery bypass graft with retrospectively ECG-gated four-row multi-detector spiral computed tomography. Eur Radiol 2004;14:1353–1362.

27. Colombo A, Stankovic G, Moses JW. Selection of coronary stents. J Am Coll Cardiol 2002;40:1021–1033.

28. Lemos PA, Serruys PW, van Domburg RT, et al. Unrestricted utilization of sirolimus-eluting stents compared with conventional bare stent implantation in the "real world": the Rapamycin-Eluting Stent Evaluated At Rotterdam Cardiology Hospital (RESEARCH) registry. Circulation 2004;109:190–195.

29. Schmermund A, Haude M, Baumgart D, et al. Non-invasive assessment of coronary Palmaz-Schatz stents with contrast enhanced electron beam computed tomography. Eur Heart J 1996;17:1546–1553.

30. Möhlenkamp S, Pump H, Baumgart D, et al. Minimally invasive evaluation of coronary stents with electron beam computed tomography: In vivo and in vitro experience. Catheter Cardiovasc Interv 1999;48:39–47.

31. Pump H, Möhlenkamp S, Sehnert CA, et al. Coronary arterial stent patency: assessment with electron-beam CT. Radiology 2000;214:447–452.

32. Knollmann FD, Möller J, Gebert A, Bethge C, Felix R. Assessment of coronary artery stent patency by electron-beam CT. Eur Radiol 2004;14:1341–1347.

33. Maintz D, Juergens KU, Wichter T, Grude M, Heindel W, Fischbach R. Imaging of coronary artery stents using multislice computed tomography: in vitro evaluation. Eur Radiol 2003;13:830–835.

34. Maintz D, Seifarth H, Flohr T et al. Improved coronary artery stent visualization and in-stent stenosis detection using 16-slice computed-tomography and dedicated image reconstruction technique. Invest Radiol 2003;38:790–795.

35. Nieman K, Cademartiri F, Raaijmakers R, Pattynama P, de Feyter P. Noninvasive angiographic evaluation of coronary stents with multislice spiral computed tomography. Herz 2003;28:136–142.

36. Mahnken AH, Buecker A, Wildberger JE, et al. Coronary artery stents in multislice computed tomography: in vitro artifact evaluation. Invest Radiol 2004;39:27–33.

37. Mahnken AH, Seyfarth T, Flohr T, et al. Flat-panel detector computed tomography for the assessment of coronary artery stents: phantom study in comparison with 16-slice spiral computed tomography. Invest Radiol 2005;40:8–13.

38. Seifarth H, Raupach R, Schaller S, et al. Assessment of coronary artery stents using 16-slice MDCT angiography: evaluation of a dedicated reconstruction kernel and a noise reduction filter. Eur Radiol 2005 [Epub ahead of print].

39. Hong C, Chrysant GS, Woodard PK, Bae KT. Coronary artery stent patency assessed with in-stent contrast enhancement measured at multi-detector row CT angiography: Initial experience. Radiology 2004;233:286–291.

40. Krüger S, Mahnken AH, Sinha AM, et al. Multislice spiral computed tomography for the detection of coronary stent restenosis and patency. Int J Cardiol 2003;89:167–172.

41. Nieman K, Ligthart JMR, Serruys PW, de Feyter PJ. Left main rapamycin-coated stent: invasive versus noninvasive angiographic follow-up. Circulation 2002;105:e130–e131.

42. Shaohong Z, Yongkang N, Zulong C, Hong Z, Li Y. Imaging of coronary stent by multislice helical computed tomography. Circulation 2002;106:637–638.

43. Funabashi N, Komiyama N, Yanagawa N, Mayama T, Yoshida K, Komuro I. Coronary artery patency after metallic stent implantation evaluated by multislice computed tomography. Circulation 2003;107:147–148.

44. Schuijf JD, Bax JJ, Jukema JW, et al. Coronary stent imaging with multidetector row computed tomography. Int J Cardiovasc Imaging 2004;20:341–344.

45. Mollet NR, Cademartiri F. In-stent neointimal hyperplasia with 16-row multislice computed tomography coronary angiography. Circulation 2004;110:e514.

46. Schuijf JD, Bax JJ, Jukema JW, et al. Feasibility of assessment of coronary stent patency using 16-slice computed tomography. Am J Cardiol 2004;94:427–430.

47. Gilard M, Cornily JC, Rioufol G, et al. Noninvasive assessment of left main coronary stent patency with 16-slice computed tomography. Am J Cardiol 2005;95:110–112.

48. Stanford W, Travis ME, Thompson BH, Reiners TJ, Hasson RR, Winniford MD. Electron-beam computed tomographic detection of coronary calcification in patients undergoing percutaneous transluminal coronary angioplasty: predictability of restenosis. A preliminary report. Am J Card Imaging 1995;9:257–260.

49. Takahashi M, Takamoto T, Aizawa T, Shimada H. Severity of coronary artery calcification detected by electron beam computed tomography is related to the risk of restenosis after percutaneous transluminal coronary angioplasty. Intern Med 1997;36:255–262.

50. Sinitsyn V, Belkind M, Matchin Y, Lyakishev A, Naumov V, Ternovoy S. Relationships between coronary calcification detected at electron beam computed tomography and percutaneous transluminal coronary angioplasty results in coronary artery disease patients. Eur Radiol 2003;13:62–67.

51. Mintz GS, Popma JJ, Pichard AD, et al. Intravascular ultrasound predictors of restenosis after percutaneous transcatheter coronary revascularization. J Am Coll Cardiol 1996;27:1678–1687.

52. Mollet NR, Hoye A, Lemos PA, et al. Value of preprocedure multislice computed tomographic coronary angiography to predict the outcome of percutaneous recanalization of chronic total occlusions. Am J Cardiol 2005;95:240–243.

11

An Interventionalist's Perspective: Diagnosis of Cardiovascular Disease by CT Imaging

Jeffrey M. Schussler

Introduction

Computed tomographic angiography of the coronary arteries (coronary CTA) is gaining increasing recognition as a possible diagnostic test of choice for the determination of the presence and severity of coronary atherosclerosis. Coronary CTA could be an extremely helpful test in determining which patients need to go to the cardiac catheterization laboratory, as it gives a "preview" of the coronary anatomy before catheters are ever placed inside the patient's body. Coronary CTA is the only non-invasive test that currently provides structural and anatomic information similar to traditional coronary angiography.

Coronary CTA offers a new and unique opportunity to directly evaluate coronary anatomy in an extremely safe, non-invasive way. As opposed to functional non-invasive tests which indirectly infer stenosis, coronary CTA allows for the evaluation of both the presence of disease as well as severity of stenoses prior to any invasive procedure.

In preliminary investigations, coronary CTA has shown a high degree of both specificity and sensitivity in the detection of atherosclerotic coronary disease. This is especially true for patients with risk factors for atherosclerosis, symptoms of chest pain. When newer generations of scanners were used, and when appropriate measures to assure a low heart rate during the scan were taken, the results were even more dramatic. Thus, with further technological improvement probably translating into even higher diagnostic accuracy and smaller numbers of unevaluable studies, coronary CTA can potentially eliminate the need for invasive cardiac catheterization in many patients without significant disease. In patients who are identified as requiring invasive evaluation, it may give a "preview" of coronary anatomy, suggesting possible catheter choices, and even alerting to the presence of left main disease.

This technique is very versatile. Possible indications would include the follow-up after percutaneous coronary interventions (PCI) to evaluate stent patency, and after coronary artery bypass grafting (CABG) to evaluate graft patency. All of this information can be extremely helpful in planning strategies for invasive evaluation and treatment of patients with coronary atherosclerosis.

Invasive Cardiac Catheterization

Invasive cardiac catheterization, the "gold standard" diagnostic technique for the evaluation of coronary artery disease (CAD), has been used for clinical evaluation of coronary stenosis since the 1960s [1–6]. Despite this, it has several well-known drawbacks. There is a certain degree of interobserver variation when describing degree of stenosis [7]. Quantitative coronary angiography (QCA), which is not used routinely in clinical practice, is helpful but does not eliminate this error [8,9]. In addition, small to moderate amounts of plaque can be both under-identified as well as underreported. Unfortunately, these relatively minor stenoses can be the cause of acute coronary syndromes and myocardial infarction [10].

Since coronary angiography allows for the definition of the lumen of the coronary only, the wall of the coronary artery remains non-visualized unless intravascular ultrasound is used [11,12]. This can lead to underestimation of plaque burden [13]. Not only is this problematic in identifying the presence of disease in patients with minimal disease, but it can create problems with underestimation of plaque burden in patients with more severe disease due to compensatory expansion of the coronary arteries [14–16].

There is also an inherent risk associated with invasive coronary angiography. Although generally considered safe, there is a finite risk of complication associated with invasive evaluation of the coronary arteries. This is due to both the need for directly engaging the artery as well as the obligate arterial access. The risk of major complications such as death is approximately 0.1% [17,18], with a combined risk of all major complications (e.g. stroke, renal failure, or major bleeding) of <2% [19,20]. Minor complications such as local pain, ecchymosis, or hematoma at the catheterization site can be higher [21]. Although these minor complications are not a risk to the patient's life, they are frequently a source of delayed discharge and patient dissatisfaction with the procedure. More rare complications include perforation of the coronary arteries, embolization, and infection [22–28].

Invasive coronary angiography is considered the "gold standard" for definitive evaluation of the coronary arteries in patients with chest pain [19,29,30]. As it is such a powerful tool, it has even been suggested that angiography should be the standard screening test of choice in patients with chest pain, and even in patients who are considered a low overall risk [29,30]. Angiography has been shown to be better able to detect the presence of atherosclerotic coronary disease than functional tests, reduces early returns to the emergency department, and has an overall higher level of patient satisfaction. Invasive angiography may even be the screening test of choice in the primary prevention of CAD [31]. However, due to the aforementioned risks, it is often used as second line in patients who have low-to-moderate presumed risk, or after performing functional testing.

Coronary CT Angiography – The Basics

Coronary CTA is a cross-sectional imaging method which yields a three-dimensional (3-D) dataset (Figures 11.1–11.3). It is based on traditional computed tomography, but using dedicated scanner technology with extremely

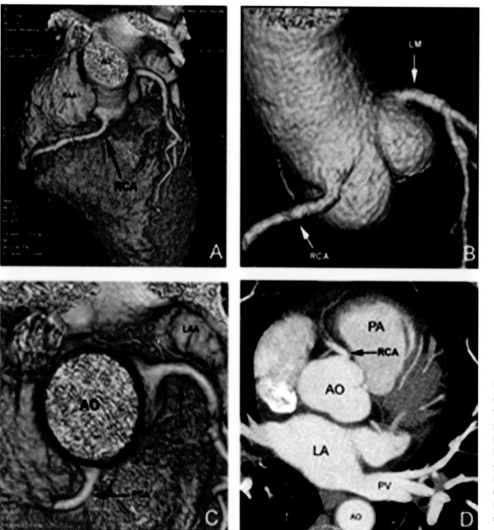

Figure 11.1. Anterior takeoff of the right coronary artery (RCA) seen by 3-D reconstruction (**A–C**) as well as axial images (**D**). In patients going for invasive coronary angiography, foreknowledge of an anterior RCA can be helpful in choice of diagnostic as well as guiding catheters. When viewed on the axial images, the takeoff of the RCA is at the "12 o'clock" position or even more "clockwise." LM = left main, RCA = right coronary artery, AO = aorta, PA = pulmonary artery, LA = left atrium, PV = pulmonary vein.

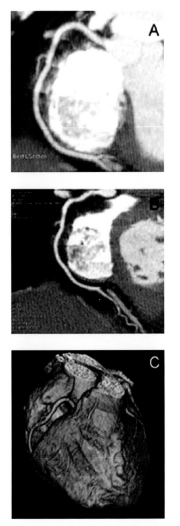

Figure 11.2. A normal coronary artery represented in three different imaging modalities. Oblique view (**A**) tends to maintain normal contours of the original artery. Multiplanar reformat (**B**) allows for a more complete view of the entire arterial lumen. Three-dimensional view (**C**) allows for visualization of the normal course of the artery in relation to the non-coronary structures, but does not give as much information about the coronary lumen.

fast acquisition times and the ability to gate image reconstruction to the cardiac cycle – achieved via the simultaneously recorded electrocardiogram. The methods of data acquisition, processing, and evaluation are described in detail in Chapters 3 and 4. It has to be pointed out that patient preparation, data acquisition, and data evaluation have to be performed with care and require some expertise in order to achieve optimal image quality and recognize artifacts which might otherwise lead to false-positive or false-negative results (Figures 11.4–11.7).

Uses

Given its ability to detect – and rule out – coronary artery stenoses (Figures 11.8 and 11.9), coronary CTA could take the place of invasive catheterization in most algorithms for detecting the presence of coronary disease. This applies for patients who are asymptomatic, who have had positive stress tests, or who have had chest pain. It could even be

used in the presence of unstable types of chest pain as a means of triage. Although coronary CTA can be used as a diagnostic tool prior to invasive procedures, it may also have potential utility in evaluation post angioplasty, stenting, or coronary bypass.

The greatest utility of coronary CTA is in patients with a low or moderate probability of coronary artery disease. Anecdotally, many physicians have had the experience of sending a low-risk patient for evaluation of chest pain. Functional testing is either inconclusive, or mildly positive, and so an invasive cardiac catheterization is planned. The patient has normal coronary arteries, but unfortunately has a retroperitoneal hematoma related to the catheterization site. Based on the preliminary data currently available it seems that coronary CTA will allow for evaluation of coronary disease prior to the patient even being in the cardiac catheterization laboratory.

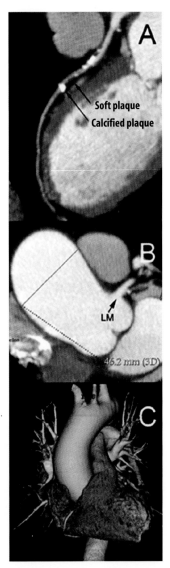

Figure 11.3. The volume of information obtained during CT imaging of the heart allows for detailed examination of the coronary arteries as well as non-coronary structures. This patient has significant plaque in the left anterior descending artery (**A**), but was also discovered to have dilation of the ascending aorta. This dilation was demonstrated on both oblique (**B**) and 3-D reconstruction (**C**). LM = left main.

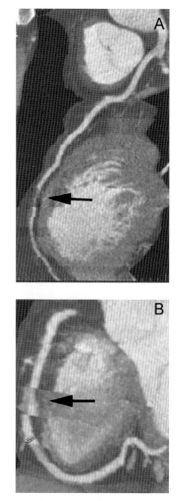

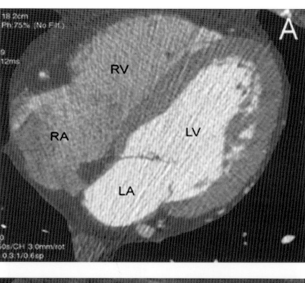

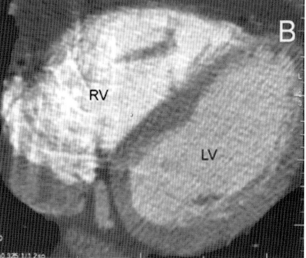

Figure 11.4. Heart rate irregularity causing artifact (arrows). A man in his mid 30s with occasional premature ventricular contractions (PVC). During acquisition of the CT scan, a PVC caused an artifact during the latter part of the scan, affecting the distal left anterior descending (**A**) and mid right coronary artery (**B**).

Figure 11.5. Axial image of the heart demonstrating differences in timing of the contrast bolus. A well-timed bolus (**A**) demonstrates almost no contrast in the right side of the heart. This compares to a scan which was performed too early (**B**), demonstrating the majority of the contrast bolus still on the right side of the heart. This usually results in poor opacification of the coronary arteries, and can cause artifact due to the large amount of contrast which remains in the right atrium.

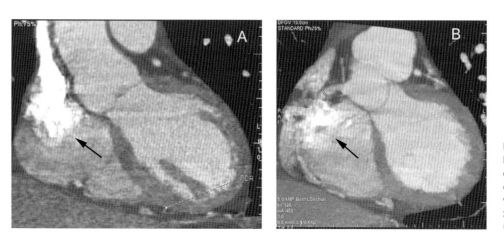

Figure 11.6. Due to poor timing, elevated levels of contrast remain in the right atrium during imaging of the heart (**A** – arrow). This creates a significant amount of scatter artifact, which obscures the visualization of the proximal portion of the right coronary artery (**B** – arrow).

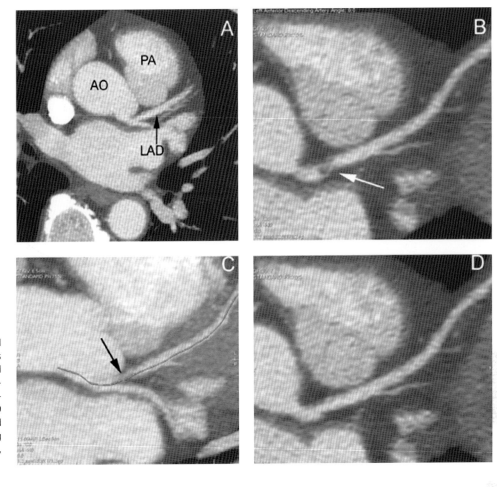

Figure 11.7. Tracking artifact in proximal left anterior descending (LAD). Axial views demonstrate a mild amount of non-calcified plaque in the proximal LAD (**A** – arrow). Multiplanar reformatted view (MPR) demonstrates a "pseudo-stenosis" of the proximal LAD (**B** – arrow). Centerline tracking (**C**) is biased towards one side of the artery lumen, creating the artifact. Once the centerline is corrected, the "stenosis" is no longer apparent (**D**).

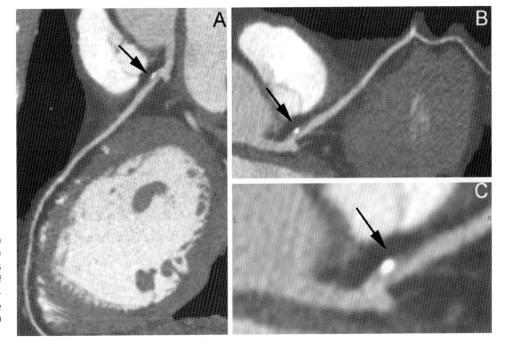

Figure 11.8. A high-grade lesion is seen (arrow) in the left anterior descending (LAD) (**A**). It is composed of both non-calcified as well as calcific plaque, and occupies >50% of the coronary lumen. Rotation of the multiplanar reformatted images demonstrates that the plaque extends from the ostium of the LAD into the distal left main (**B** and **C**).

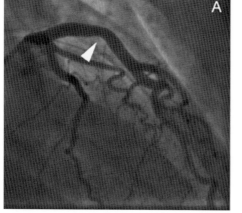
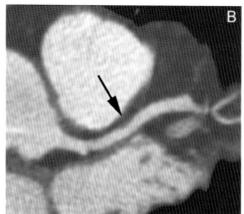

Figure 11.9. Essentially "normal" coronary angiogram in a 33-year-old woman. A "luminal irregularity" (**A** – white arrowhead) in the left anterior descending artery corresponds to a non-calcified plaque (**B** – black arrow) seen by CT coronary angiography.

Coronary Evaluation

Evaluation of the Coronaries Prior to Invasive Evaluation and Intervention

Non-invasive coronary angiography can be of great benefit to the patient and the physician before the patient is referred for invasive testing. With its high negative predictive value, it can be expected that coronary CTA has the ability to exclude the majority of patients who have no significant disease (Figure 11.9).

For patients who have been diagnosed by coronary CTA to have significant disease, there may be substantial information which can be helpful, prior to the invasive evaluation, in determining a strategy for treatment. Coronary CTA is sensitive and specific enough to determine which

arteries have high-grade lesions, and which have minimal disease, with relatively great confidence. This can mean the difference between planning an intervention in a single proximal vessel or in the expectation of a difficult multiple vessel intervention.

Sensitivity and Specificity of Coronary CTA

In multiple – albeit relatively small – studies, the sensitivity and specificity of coronary CTA to determine the presence of disease and the severity of stenosis has been extremely high (Table 11.1). It is notable that these studies typically compare the ability of CT to detect a >50% stenosis in an artery with that of QCA. Determining the exact percentage stenosis and correlating it with invasive evalu-

Table 11.1. Sensitivity and specificity of 16-slice scanners based on comparison to invasive angiography

Author	Year	Sensitivity (%)	Specificity (%)	Number of patients	Types of patients studied
Mollet et al. [32]	2005	95	98	51	Suspected CAD
Kuettner et al. [33]	2005	82	98	72	Suspected CAD
Schuijf et al. [34]	2005	98	97	45	Known or suspected CAD
Martuscelli et al. [35]	2004	89	98	64	Suspected CAD
Hoffmann et al. [36]	2004	63 (82)[a]	96 (93)[a]	33	Known CAD
Kuettner et al. [37]	2004	72 (98)[b]	97 (98)[b]	60	Suspected CAD
Martuscelli et al. [38]	2004	97	100	96	Evaluation of CAB conduits
Mollet et al. [39]	2004	92	95	128	Stable angina
Schlosser et al. [40]	2004	96	95	51	Evaluation of CAB conduits
Schuijf et al. [41][c]	2004	93	96	31	Hypertensive patients
Schuijf et al. [42][c]	2004	95	95	30	Type 2 diabetes
Burgstahler et al. [43]	2003	86	100	10	Evaluation of CAB conduits
Ropers et al. [44]	2003	92	93	77	Suspected CAD
Kopp et al [45]	2002	82	93	102	Suspected CAD
Nieman et al. [46]	2002	82	93	53	Suspected CAD

[a] Accuracy was improved if analysis was limited to segments with good image quality (83% of segments).

[b] Sensitivity and specificity improved when calcium score was used in conjunction to eliminate heavily calcified arteries from the pool of evaluated segments.

[c] These studies included some patients scanned with 4-slice technology.

ation is more difficult. This is not only because of the limitations of the resolution of current CT technology, but also due to the aforementioned difficulties in obtaining accurate evaluation of coronary stenosis by invasive means. That being said, coronary CTA remains a valuable tool in evaluating patients, both with and without symptoms, for the presence of coronary disease, and in making the determination as to whether or not further invasive testing is needed.

Plaque Evaluation

Coronary CT angiography has the unique ability to evaluate the wall of the artery as well as the coronary lumen. In comparison to invasive coronary angiography, which only allows for the definition of the lumen of the coronary, coronary CTA has the ability to visualize plaque and to roughly quantify its amount (Figures 11.10–11.13) [47,48]. It is well known that patients with minimal CAD may still have events due to plaque which is not fully defined by invasive coronary angiography. These types of non-stenotic plaques

are detectable by coronary CTA [48]. In the future, coronary CTA may thus allow for the possibility of early medical intervention and even monitoring of disease progression under therapy.

There is some correlation in plaque composition as defined by coronary CTA when compared to histopathologic examination [49]. Coronary CTA may thus be able to define unstable or vulnerable plaques [50–54] in a manner that has previously only been described by using intravascular ultrasound (IVUS) [55,56]. It may be possible in the future to evaluate plaques in a similar way by coronary CTA, giving the physician information predicting coronary events.

Similarly, remodeling of coronary atherosclerotic lesions can be appreciated in coronary CTA. As the plaque intrudes on the lumen of the artery, compensatory expansion of the artery occurs, which is seen on coronary CTA, but not by conventional angiography (Figure 11.14) [57–59]. In addition, CT may provide a means of estimating the total burden of disease [47,48,60].

Since the bolus of contrast in coronary CT angiography is not selective, it reaches all the arteries simultaneously.

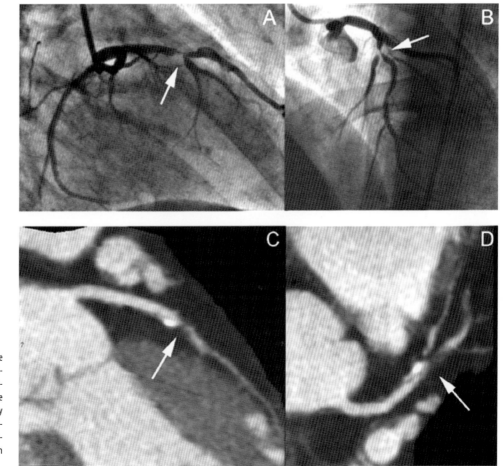

Figure 11.10. High-grade stenosis of the left anterior descending (arrow) seen by invasive (**A** and **B**) as well as CT coronary angiography (**C** and **D**). Note that while the degree of stenosis is obvious by invasive coronary angiography, the overall plaque burden, composition of plaque (both calcific and non-calcified), as well as compensatory expansion of the artery is seen with coronary CTA.

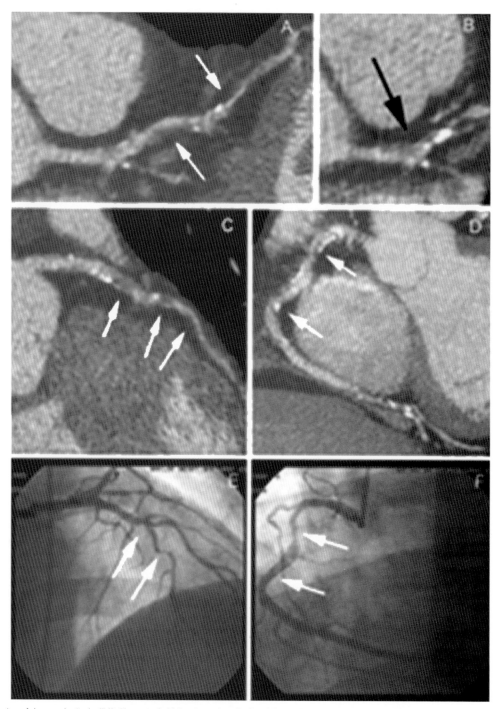

Figure 11.11. Comparison of plaque evaluation by CT (**A–D**) compared with invasive angiography (**E** and **F**). Note that plaque composition is readily apparent in CT coronary angiography, with calcified plaque (bright white) seen concurrently with non-calcified plaque (darker gray).

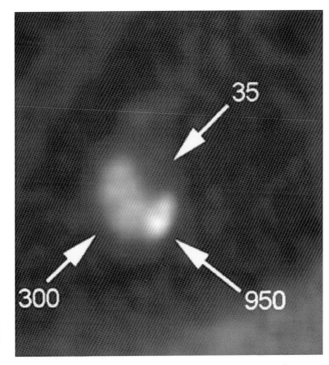

Figure 11.12. Cross-section of the proximal right coronary artery (RCA). Representative densities of different areas of this segment of the artery are demonstrated showing normal coronary lumen (~300 HU), non-calcified plaque (~35 HU), and calcified plaque (~950 HU).

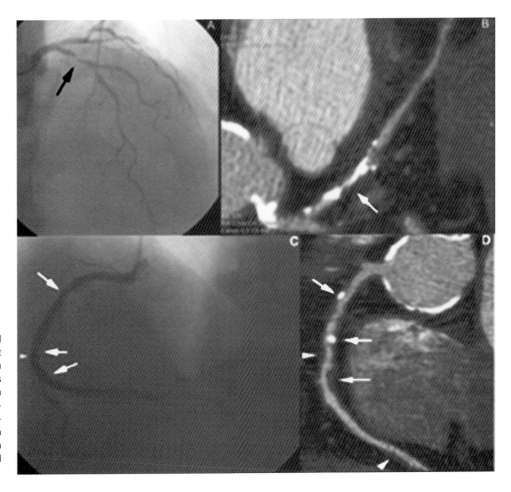

Figure 11.13. Diffusely diseased LAD and RCA in a patient who presented with chest pain. The LAD has a high-grade lesion seen on invasive angiography (**A** – arrow). This was clearly seen on coronary CTA (**B** – arrow) as an area of both calcification as well as a non-calcified plaque. The RCA has non-flow-limiting disease (**C** – arrows), which is much more clearly defined by coronary CTA (**D**) as a mixture of both non-calcified and calcified plaque.

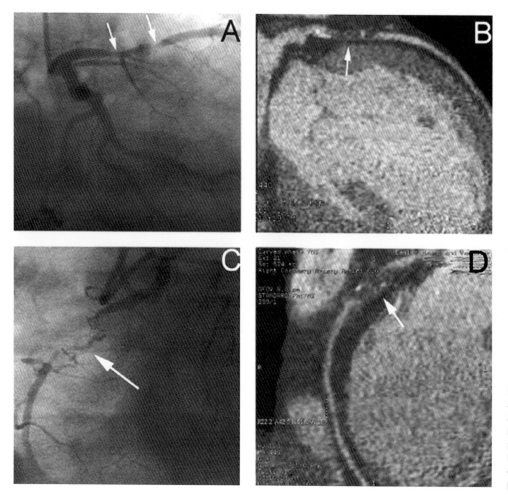

Figure 11.14. High-grade lesion in the left anterior descending, demonstrated by invasive angiography (**A**) and coronary CTA (**B**). The lesion has the same characteristics as a complete occlusion with bridging collaterals (**C** and **D**). There is paucity of contrast, compensatory expansion, and a large amount of non-calcified plaque.

Therefore, it is difficult (if not impossible) to differentiate between a high-grade occlusion and a complete occlusion with collateral filling (Figure 11.14). From a clinical standpoint, this is a moot point, as patients who have such a high burden of disease tend to be treated in a similar fashion. Invasive cardiac catheterization, usually the next step in this situation, can easily differentiate between the two.

Left Main Disease

Severe left main disease, a not uncommon cause of angina, is potentially dangerous if not known prior to diagnostic angiography. Placement of a catheter into a diseased left main coronary can cause dramatic reduction of coronary blood flow, and can even result in death during diagnostic angiography [61,62].

There have been several cases where we have determined that a patient had severe left main disease based on the CT coronary angiogram, and were better prepared to deal with the hemodynamic issues during cardiac catheterization (Figure 11.15). Coronary CTA may also be able to aid in the clarification of the severity of left main disease when invasive cardiac catheterization and intravascular ultrasound have not been helpful [63].

It is important to remember that CT cannot perform hemodynamic evaluation of lesion severity. "Damping" of pressure tracings during invasive catheterization is an important clue that an ostial or proximal stenosis is severe. CT cannot give this information, and so it is important to proceed to invasive evaluation if non-invasive angiography suggests an ostial left main stenosis. Using coronary CTA, what is typically observed with left main disease is a paucity of contrast at the left main ostium and the presence of significant amounts of plaque, either non-calcified or calcific. Narrowing of the ostium is seen on the axial data as well as the multiplanar reformatted (MPR) images, and this narrowing is seen in multiple views when the image is rotated. Since there is no catheter-induced spasm during

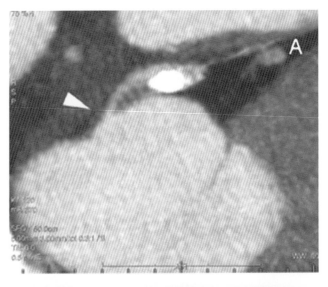

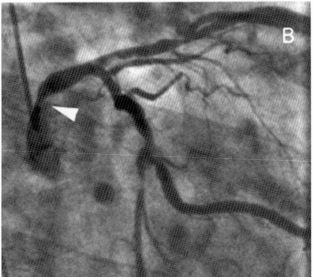

Figure 11.15. High-grade stenosis of the left main clearly seen by coronary CT angiography (coronary CTA) (**A** – arrowhead). The corresponding invasive coronary angiogram is seen (**B** – arrowhead) demonstrating a severe angiographic stenosis. There was immediate "damping" of the pressure tracing upon engagement of the 4-French diagnostic catheter. The non-invasive study was so dramatically abnormal that it prompted the operator to deliberately choose a smaller French-sized catheter, and have a balloon pump in the room before the invasive angiogram had started.

CT angiography, this can sometimes be used to clarify questionable disease during invasive angiography.

Post Intervention Evaluation by Coronary CTA

Post-PCI Evaluation

Although primarily thought of as a method for triaging patients who need to go on to invasive evaluation, coronary CTA may represent a significant breakthrough in the post-PCI evaluation. Imaging stents after placement is not as easy as imaging native coronary arteries, but it can be performed [64,65]. There is a significant amount of hardening artifact due to the scatter of X-rays by the metallic stents. It is important to use appropriate window and threshold levels to obtain adequate images. In-stent restenosis, a process that is brought on by smooth muscle cell migration and neointimal hyperplasia, has also been successfully evaluated by coronary CTA [66].

Post-bypass Evaluation

Another possible indication of coronary CTA is the evaluation of post-coronary artery bypass graft (CABG) patients who are having symptoms. Evaluation of bypass grafts by coronary CTA may be clinically useful, with a high degree of sensitivity for both patency and degree of graft stenosis [38,40,67–69].

In some respects, the imaging of bypass grafts is easier as there is less movement of the grafts, and there is greater contrast between the contrast in the grafts and the surrounding tissue. Visualization of grafts is often more easily performed using 3-D views, rather than axial or even MPR views (Figure 11.16).

Frequently, the area that needs to be imaged is larger, allowing more of the proximal grafts to be seen. It is important to alert the technologist that the study is to be performed with attention to bypass grafts so that more of the ascending aorta is visualized. This is necessary to visualize the proximal portion of venous conduits. In patients who have a relatively large amount of territory to scan, slice thickness may be increased to reduce breath-hold time. Imaging can be performed on conduits with metallic proximal connectors, but there tends to be some small amount of hardening artifact when many metallic clips are present [69].

In some instances, patients are referred with a history of bypass, but have no idea what types they had or which arteries were bypassed. In the catheterization laboratory, it can then be a challenging and time-consuming task to find all the grafts. Coronary CTA can be helpful, not only by delineating which grafts are patent, but by providing a "roadmap" as to the number of grafts, their origins, as well as the placement of the anastomoses prior to invasive angiography.

Even though evaluation of bypass grafts is relatively straightforward in coronary CTA, it has to be kept in mind that in most cases, the clinical situation will warrant evaluating not only the status of the patient's bypass grafts, but also that of the native coronary arteries – either distal to the bypass insertion site or of those coronary arteries that did not receive a bypass graft. Frequently, evaluation of native arteries in patients with bypass grafts tends to be difficult or even impossible because of the often pronounced calcification that occurs in the coronary arteries after bypass grafting. Newer scanner technology may overcome this limitation.

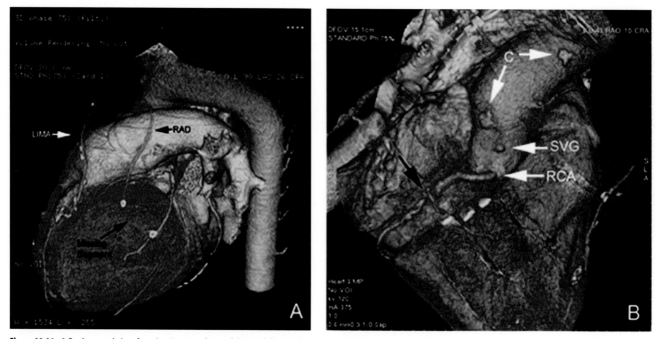

Figure 11.16. 3-D volume rendering of a patient 1 year post bypass. **A** A patent left internal mammary artery (LIMA) is seen. A radial graft (RAD) is anastomosed to a diagonal branch, and then is occluded from the diagonal to an obtuse marginal branch. **B** The saphenous vein graft (SVG) which originally was anastomosed to the right coronary artery (RCA) is occluded at its origin. Also visible are the cannula sites from the bypass surgery (C).

Unusual Circumstances Where Coronary CTA May Be Appropriate

Some patients are adamant about their refusal of invasive coronary evaluation, but may be willing to have a non-invasive evaluation. We have seen several occasions where patients who have had significant abnormalities on their stress tests, but who refused invasive catheterization, were more willing to undergo coronary CTA. Once this was performed, and a problem with significant coronary artery disease discovered, they were much more willing to then proceed with the invasive catheterization and intervention.

Patients with significant lower extremity peripheral vascular disease are often referred for preoperative evaluation. In some cases, they have such a large pretest probability of the presence of coronary disease that the physician in charge of their care has suggested that they proceed directly to invasive cardiac catheterization so that the presence of three-vessel or left main disease may be better defined. It is sometimes problematic to perform cardiac catheterization on these patients due to access problems, and so coronary CTA may be used to evaluate their overall burden of disease.

Clinical Use of CT Coronary Angiography

The identification of patients with coronary artery disease falls into two broad categories; those with and those without symptoms. Asymptomatic patients tend not to be

sent to the interventional cardiologist until stress testing suggests a strong likelihood of flow-limiting coronary disease. Symptomatic patients have a stronger likelihood of having invasive testing, regardless of whether they have positive functional tests. Coronary CTA may have the positive effect of reducing the number of normal or near-normal patients who end up having invasive testing, while on the other hand may expand the number of patients who are discovered to have significant coronary disease early in their clinical course.

Screening of Asymptomatic Patients

For many patients with a strong family history of coronary disease, or significant risk for developing premature coronary disease, it is very helpful to know if plaque exists, even though symptoms have not occurred. Primary prevention of atherosclerosis in patients with significant risk factors can be very expensive, and not necessarily risk free [70,71]. Some authors have even suggested that screening *invasive* coronary angiograms would not only be more cost-effective, but safer overall, as it would target those patients who had definitive disease rather than treating everyone in a "shotgun" type of tactic [31].

With half the population ultimately dying of a cardiovascular event, the prevalence of the disease process is obviously widespread. Primary prevention using medical therapy is a well established and cost-effective treatment for patients with significant risk factors [70–72]. In addition to the ability to exclude those patients who have no appreciable disease, thus allowing them to abstain from medical therapy, coronary CT imaging – most likely coronary calcium assessment – would have the added benefit of conclusively demonstrating plaque burden to the patient. For patients who are reluctant to start or remain on medicines, this can be a very powerful tool in enhancing compliance with medical therapy as well as lifestyle modification.

There is a great impetus to start medical treatment early, when the most impact can be achieved. Serum testing for high-risk markers such as C-reactive protein has been suggested as a way of identifying higher-risk asymptomatic individuals for statin therapy [73]. It has been hypothesized that coronary CTA may be an acceptable alternative to invasive coronary angiography in the screening of asymptomatic patients, if such is deemed reasonable. This would allow for the deferral of medical treatment for patients who have no demonstrated atherosclerotic disease burden, and early aggressive management for patients who demonstrate plaque.

This may be especially important in subgroups of people who have a strong family history, high number of risk factors, or who have critical or high-risk professions (e.g. airline pilots). Women are an especially vulnerable group. Women with significant coronary disease tend to present with a variety of atypical symptoms, and the focus in women's health has traditionally not been on cardiovascular mortality [74].

There has been much interest in the recent news that President Bill Clinton had passed stress tests only a few years before his need for coronary artery bypass surgery. The question was raised as to why, if he had normal tests, there was a complete lack of awareness by his physicians that he had coronary atherosclerosis. It was pointed out that Mr Clinton thought that he was relatively healthy as he was exercising and had lost weight, and had even gone so far as to stop his statin therapy several months before he found out about his need for bypass. In contrast, President George Bush has recently undergone "CT scanning" of his heart. He was told that he did have plaque, albeit minor, and was placed on statin therapy. It is conceivable that by early non-invasive evaluation, President Bush's physicians may have altered the course of his disease process.

Avoiding Invasive Cardiac Catheterization in "Normal" Patients

Up to 30% of patients who undergo invasive cardiac catheterization have "normal" coronary arteries [75,76]. Somewhat more disturbing is that patients who have been described as "normal" still have a small but significant chance that they will go on to have coronary events [77].

No physician would like cardiac catheterization performed on patients with normal coronary arteries. However, there has never been an accurate way to differentiate between significant and non-significant coronary

atherosclerosis based on the patient's symptoms [78], and functional testing is neither 100% sensitive nor 100% specific. One of the most significant benefits of coronary CTA is that it has a very high negative predictive value, and therefore may be a better way of determining if patients do or do not need further testing.

Patients with Chest Pain

When a patient with chest pain is referred to a cardiologist, there are usually two central questions being asked: Does the patient have coronary artery disease? If they do, how severe is it? Functional tests are readily accessible, relatively inexpensive, and very safe. They can provide insight into prognosis, but they are unable to directly answer those two questions, and must indirectly infer the patient's coronary anatomy. A negative stress test in a patient has good prognostic implications, but the referring physician and cardiologist are still left with the central question unanswered.

Outpatient Triage

Low Risk

For patients with chest pain who are judged to be "low" or "moderate" risk, the problem is 2-fold. First, the physician who is evaluating the patient would like reassurance that the patient does not have coronary disease which would need further invasive testing, and, second, the patient needs reassurance that they do not have disease that is potentially life-threatening. Stress testing is a valuable way of reassuring both the physician and the patient that there is good cardiac function, and that the prognosis of the patient over the next few years is good. Early invasive testing has the benefit of more reassurance to the patient, and results in fewer readmissions to the hospital for the same complaint [29].

Obviously, it is not standard care to perform routine invasive testing on low-risk patients. This may only be because the risk–benefit profile of such a strategy is not perceived as favorable. However, the idea of knowing the actual anatomy of the patient's coronary vasculature is certainly attractive for the physician, and can be reassuring to the patient. Although this has not been tested, coronary CTA may be able to take the place of invasive angiography in a similar manner.

Equivocal Stress Testing

Newer stress testing incorporates imaging modalities such as echocardiography or myocardial perfusion to add information to the traditional treadmill test. Although this has dramatically improved sensitivity and specificity of stress testing, there still remains the problem of what to do with patients who have high-risk markers (e.g. chest pain or dramatic electrocardiographic (ECG) changes) despite normal perfusion or wall motion.

It is not uncommon for patients who have good exercise capacity and normal wall motion to have ECG changes during peak exercise. The decision is whether or not to throw out this piece of data, with the understanding that the other portions of the stress test suggest a good overall prognosis. There are some patients who experience exertional chest pain during exercise testing, with otherwise normal findings (ECG, wall motion, or perfusion). Once again, although a normal functional capacity, normal wall motion, or normal perfusion gives a level of comfort when related to overall cardiovascular prognosis, it still leaves the underlying question unanswered. The sensitivity and specificity for the detection of coronary disease, whether in stress echocardiography [79,80] or nuclear perfusion, is not 100% [81].

Younger women who present with complaints of chest pain represent an interesting dilemma. Although cardiovascular disease is the number one cause of death in women, younger women who have symptoms of chest pain are often thought of as being in the "wrong group" to actually present with coronary disease. Risk stratifying these patients is fraught with difficulty as functional testing (even with an imaging component) has quite a low sensitivity and specificity [74].

Another common dilemma is the middle-aged patient who has good exercise capacity on the treadmill test, normal augmentation of ventricular function, but several millimeters of ST depression on the ECG at peak exercise. Many would consider the ECG to be falsely positive, and would ignore this piece of data in the face of good exercise capacity and normal left ventricular function. However, there are going to be patients with strong family history and multiple risk factors in whom it is prudent to evaluate further. In these patients, the next step would typically be invasive coronary angiography. In many of these cases, we are now performing coronary CTA instead of invasive catheterization. Based on their coronary CTA, they are going on to traditional angiography, or the evaluation of the patient is stopped altogether.

Inpatient Triage: An Unusual Circumstance

In the inpatient setting, it is somewhat unusual to think about non-invasive coronary angiography as a diagnostic test of choice for patients in whom there is a significant need for coronary evaluation. Invasive coronary angiography is readily available, safe, and relatively quick for patients who are already "in house." However, we have encountered several situations in which it was advantageous to have a coronary CTA performed rather than invasive coronary angiography.

Patients with bleeding diatheses may need coronary angiography, but represent a higher than normal risk for invasive evaluation. Patients with significant difficulty holding still for more than a few minutes may benefit from non-invasive coronary evaluation. There is occasionally the patient who develops symptoms on a Friday afternoon, and in whom early discharge would be preferable to a discharge late in the evening. All of these patients might benefit from coronary CTA.

Diabetic Patients

Diabetic patients represent a particularly high-risk subgroup for the development of early cardiovascular disease. They frequently present with unstable syndromes, and can develop aggressive coronary atherosclerosis at a very young age. When they do present with coronary syndromes, they are more likely to have poor overall outcomes and higher mortality [82].

In asymptomatic diabetic patients, it has been suggested that it would be not only medically advantageous but also cost-effective to screen for significant coronary artery disease using functional stress testing [83].

The evaluation of diabetics with standard stress testing is problematic, and sensitivity in the detection of disease is as low as 47% [84]. Screening with nuclear perfusion may improve the ability to triage diabetic patients who present with chest pain syndromes, but there is still a >50% admission rate to the hospital for diabetics who present with chest pain.

The ability of coronary CTA to evaluate the coronary vasculature and characterize non-calcified as well as calcific plaque may make it ideal to evaluate for coronary atherosclerosis in the diabetic patient in the future [85].

Future Directions for CT Coronary Angiography

The Quintuple "Rule Out"

A great deal of time, energy, and expense is expended on a daily basis in the evaluation of patients with chest pain who present to the emergency department. Currently, patients who are not obviously having a myocardial infarction, and who have negative initial markers, often are admitted to the hospital with a diagnosis of "unstable angina" and serial enzymes are obtained. Emergency triage in the future may consist of a coronary CTA to rule in or rule out the presence of coronary artery disease. The volume of information obtained during this type of scan would also potentially allow for evaluation of the presence of aortic dissection, pericardial effusion, pulmonary embolus, and pneumonic processes – sufficient volume coverage of the scan provided. This "quintuple rule out" may become a standard practice in the emergency department of the future.

Pre-surgical Evaluation

Current guidelines recommend routine invasive coronary evaluation for most patients who are scheduled to undergo open heart surgery for repair or replacement of regurgitant or stenotic valves. A segment of this population, such as patients with purely regurgitant valves, does not need concomitant coronary artery bypass surgery. It is possible that in the future, diagnosis with a combination of coronary CTA and echocardiography will be enough for the decision about valvular surgery to be made. Conceivably, coronary CTA technology could advance to the point whereby the decision to proceed with surgical revascularization could be made prior to any invasive tests being performed [86].

Prophylactic Treatment of "Vulnerable" Plaque

As described above, one of the strengths of coronary CTA is that it gives a significant amount of data about the composition of plaque, and may be helpful in identifying those plaques that are more unstable, and thereby prone to rupture and cause myocardial infarction or unstable coronary syndromes [47–54].

It has been theorized that one of the reasons that PCI has some difficulties with long-term prevention of future events is that although stenotic lesions are treated, more unstable plaques are left to cause future clinical problems. Several papers have suggested that a prophylactic "sealing" of these plaques using percutaneous techniques might be able to prevent those areas from causing coronary events in the future [87–90].

It may possible to use coronary CTA to identify those asymptomatic patients who have mild to moderate disease, but who have more vulnerable plaques. These patients could be targeted for this type of plaque stabilization, and potentially prevent future events.

Higher-resolution Scanners: 64-slices and Beyond

The greatest improvement that larger array scanners have is not improved resolution. Typically, the 32-, 40-, and 64-slice scanners do not have substantially smaller slice thicknesses, and therefore their spatial resolution is not a major improvement over current 16-slice scanners. Their greatest impact will be in the ability to perform a complete scan of the heart (or area of interest) in a much shorter time. Larger arrays of detectors will be able to image a larger area in a single cardiac cycle. This will theoretically allow for more diagnostic scans, and fewer patients who are unable to tolerate breath-holds of >10 seconds. Since the scan will be much shorter, the possibility of movement during the scanning time will be decreased, which will also reduce artifact.

In addition, since the coronary arterial tree would be imaged in such a short period of time, there could be significant reductions in the amount of contrast needed. However, this would require much more exact timing of the scan to coincide with the bolus of contrast arriving at the coronary arteries.

The ultimate goal for computed tomography of the coronary arteries is an array that is large enough to image the heart in its entirety in a single heartbeat. This would allow for the imaging of patients at much faster heart rates, and conceivably even those patients with significant arrhythmias.

Conclusion

Physicians should embrace non-invasive coronary angiography as a helpful addition to the armamentarium with which to diagnose and help combat cardiovascular disease. In selected patients, coronary CTA can be useful to rule out significant coronary artery or bypass graft stenoses and this helps avoid unnecessary invasive coronary angiograms. In the future, an important application may be in the anatomic definition of plaque burden and composition. Technical improvements will continue to broaden the spectrum of patients who may profit from computed tomographic imaging of the coronary arteries.

References

1. Weidner W, MacAlpin R, Hanafee W, Kattus A. Percutaneous transaxillary selective coronary angiography. Radiology 1965;85(4):652–657.
2. Selinger H. Selective coronary cine-angiography. W V Med J 1966;62(10):336–337.
3. Benchimol A, Tippit HC, Maia IG. The clinical value of selective coronary angiography. Ariz Med 1967;24(11):1067–1072.
4. Sketch MH. Selective cine coronary angiography in the diagnosis of ischemic heart disease. Chronicle 1967;30(5):151.
5. Spellberg RD, Unger I. The percutaneous femoral artery approach to selective coronary arteriography. Circulation 1967;36(5):730–733.
6. Bourassa MG, Lesperance J, Campeau L. Selective coronary arteriography by the percutaneous femoral artery approach. Am J Roentgenol Radium Ther Nucl Med 1969;107(2):377–383.
7. Banerjee S, Crook AM, Dawson JR, Timmis AD, Hemingway H. Magnitude and consequences of error in coronary angiography interpretation (the ACRE study). Am J Cardiol 2000;85(3):309–314.
8. Goldberg RK, Kleiman NS, Minor ST, Abukhalil J, Raizner AE. Comparison of quantitative coronary angiography to visual estimates of lesion severity pre and post PTCA. Am Heart J 1990;119(1):178–184.
9. Herrington DM, Siebes M, Walford GD. Sources of error in quantitative coronary angiography. Cathet Cardiovasc Diagn 1993;29(4):314–321.
10. Macieira-Coelho E, Cantinho G, da Costa BB, et al. Minimal residual coronary obstructions in patients who suffered a first myocardial infarction. A prospective study comparing coronary angiography and exercise thallium scintigraphy. Clin Cardiol 1993;16(12):879–882.
11. Nissen SE, Gurley JC. Application of intravascular ultrasound for detection and quantitation of coronary atherosclerosis. Int J Card Imaging 1991;6(3–4):165–177.
12. Topol EJ, Nissen SE. Our preoccupation with coronary luminology. The dissociation between clinical and angiographic findings in ischemic heart disease. Circulation 1995;92(8):2333–2342.

13. Arnett EN, Isner JM, Redwood DR, et al. Coronary artery narrowing in coronary heart disease: comparison of cineangiographic and necropsy findings. Ann Intern Med 1979;91(3):350–356.

14. Yamashita T, Colombo A, Tobis JM. Limitations of coronary angiography compared with intravascular ultrasound: implications for coronary interventions. Prog Cardiovasc Dis 1999;42(2):91–138.

15. Glagov S, Weisenberg E, Zarins CK, Stankunavicius R, Kolettis GJ. Compensatory enlargement of human atherosclerotic coronary arteries. N Engl J Med 1987;316(22):1371–1375.

16. Stiel GM, Stiel LS, Schofer J, Donath K, Mathey DG. Impact of compensatory enlargement of atherosclerotic coronary arteries on angiographic assessment of coronary artery disease. Circulation 1989;80(6):1603–1609.

17. Kennedy JW, Baxley WA, Bunnel IL, et al. Mortality related to cardiac catheterization and angiography. Cathet Cardiovasc Diagn 1982; 8(4):323–340.

18. Noto TJ Jr, Johnson LW, Krone R, et al. Cardiac catheterization 1990: a report of the Registry of the Society for Cardiac Angiography and Interventions (SCA&I). Cathet Cardiovasc Diagn 1991;24(2):75–83.

19. Scanlon PJ, Faxon DP, Audet AM, et al. ACC/AHA guidelines for coronary angiography. A report of the American College of Cardiology/American Heart Association Task Force on practice guidelines (Committee on Coronary Angiography). Developed in collaboration with the Society for Cardiac Angiography and Interventions. J Am Coll Cardiol 1999;33(6):1756–1824.

20. Heuser RR. Outpatient coronary angiography: indications, safety, and complication rates. Herz 1998;23(1):21–26.

21. Ammann P, Brunner-La Rocca HP, Angehrn W, Roelli H, Sagmeister M, Rickli H. Procedural complications following diagnostic coronary angiography are related to the operator's experience and the catheter size. Catheter Cardiovasc Interv 2003;59(1):13–18.

22. Abu-Ful A, Benharroch D, Henkin Y. Extraction of the radial artery during transradial coronary angiography: an unusual complication. J Invasive Cardiol 2003;15(6):351–352.

23. Fagih B, Beaudry Y. Pseudoaneurysm: a late complication of the transradial approach after coronary angiography. J Invasive Cardiol 2000;12(4):216–217.

24. Gellen B, Remp T, Mayer T, Milz P, Franz WM. Cortical blindness: a rare but dramatic complication following coronary angiography. Cardiology 2003;99(1):57–59.

25. Jain D, Kurz T, Katus HA, Richardt G. A unique complication during coronary angiography: peripheral embolism by selective right coronary engagement – a case report. Angiology 2001;52(7):493–499.

26. Liu JC, Cziperle DJ, Kleinman B, Loeb H. Coronary abscess: a complication of stenting. Catheter Cardiovasc Interv 2003;58(1):69–71.

27. Lubavin BV. Retroperitoneal hematoma as a complication of coronary angiography and stenting. Am J Emerg Med 2004;22(3):236–238.

28. Timurkaynak T, Ciftci H, Cemri M. Coronary artery perforation: a rare complication of coronary angiography. Acta Cardiol 2001;56(5): 323–325.

29. deFilippi CR, Rosanio S, Tocchi M, et al. Randomized comparison of a strategy of predischarge coronary angiography versus exercise testing in low-risk patients in a chest pain unit: in-hospital and long-term outcomes. J Am Coll Cardiol 2001;37(8):2042–2049.

30. Wyer PC. Predischarge coronary angiography was better than exercise testing for reducing hospital use after low-risk chest pain. ACP J Club 2002;136(1):8.

31. Gandelman G, Bodenheimer MM. Screening coronary arteriography in the primary prevention of coronary artery disease. Heart Dis 2003;5(5):335–344.

32. Mollet NR, Cademartiri F, Krestin GP, et al. Improved diagnostic accuracy with 16-row multi-slice computed tomography coronary angiography. J Am Coll Cardiol 2005;45:128–132.

33. Kuettner A, Beck T, Drosch T, et al. Diagnostic accuracy of non-invasive coronary imaging using 16-detector slice spiral computed tomography with 188 ms temporal resolution. J Am Coll Cardiol 2005;45:123–127.

34. Schuijf JD, Bax JJ, Salm LP, et al. Noninvasive coronary imaging and assessment of left ventricular function using 16-slice computed tomography. Am J Cardiol 2005;95:571–574.

35. Martuscelli E, Romagnoli A, D'Eliseo A, et al. Accuracy of thin-slice computed tomography in the detection of coronary stenoses. Eur Heart J 2004;25:1043–1048.

36. Hoffmann U, Moselewski F, Cury RC, et al. Predictive value of 16-slice multidetector spiral computed tomography to detect significant obstructive coronary artery disease in patients at high risk for coronary artery disease: patient-versus segment-based analysis. Circulation 2004;110(17):2638–2643.

37. Kuettner A, Trabold T, Schroeder S, et al. Noninvasive detection of coronary lesions using 16-detector multislice spiral computed tomography technology: initial clinical results. J Am Coll Cardiol 2004;44(6):1230–1237.

38. Martuscelli E, Romagnoli A, D'Eliseo A, et al. Evaluation of venous and arterial conduit patency by 16-slice spiral computed tomography. Circulation 2004;110(20):3234–3238.

39. Mollet NR, Cademartiri F, Nieman K, et al. Multislice spiral computed tomography coronary angiography in patients with stable angina pectoris. J Am Coll Cardiol 2004;43(12):2265–2270.

40. Schlosser T, Konorza T, Hunold P, Kuhl H, Schmermund A, Barkhausen J. Noninvasive visualization of coronary artery bypass grafts using 16-detector row computed tomography. J Am Coll Cardiol 2004;44(6):1224–1229.

41. Schuijf JD, Bax JJ, Jukema JW, et al. Noninvasive evaluation of the coronary arteries with multislice computed tomography in hypertensive patients. Hypertension 2004;45(2):227–232.

42. Schuijf JD, Bax JJ, Jukema JW, et al. Noninvasive angiography and assessment of left ventricular function using multislice computed tomography in patients with type 2 diabetes. Diabetes Care 2004; 27(12):2905–2910.

43. Burgstahler C, Kuettner A, Kopp AF, et al. Non-invasive evaluation of coronary artery bypass grafts using multi-slice computed tomography: initial clinical experience. Int J Cardiol 2003;90(2–3):275–280.

44. Ropers D, Baum U, Pohle K, et al. Detection of coronary artery stenoses with thin-slice multi-detector row spiral computed tomography and multiplanar reconstruction. Circulation 2003;107(5):664–666.

45. Kopp AF, Schroeder S, Kuettner A, et al. Non-invasive coronary angiography with high resolution multidetector-row computed tomography. Results in 102 patients. Eur Heart J 2002;23(21):1714–1725.

46. Nieman K, Rensing BJ, van Geuns RJ, et al. Usefulness of multislice computed tomography for detecting obstructive coronary artery disease. Am J Cardiol 2002;89(8):913–918.

47. Achenbach S, Moselewski F, Ropers D, et al. Detection of calcified and noncalcified coronary atherosclerotic plaque by contrast-enhanced, submillimeter multidetector spiral computed tomography: a segment-based comparison with intravascular ultrasound. Circulation 2004;109(1):14–17.

48. Leber AW, Knez A, Becker A, et al. Accuracy of multidetector spiral computed tomography in identifying and differentiating the composition of coronary atherosclerotic plaques: a comparative study with intracoronary ultrasound. J Am Coll Cardiol 2004;43(7): 1241–1247.

49. Schroeder S, Kuettner A, Leitritz M, et al. Reliability of differentiating human coronary plaque morphology using contrast-enhanced multislice spiral computed tomography: a comparison with histology. J Comput Assist Tomogr 2004;28(4):449–454.

50. Caussin C, Ohanessian A, Lancelin B, et al. Coronary plaque burden detected by multislice computed tomography after acute myocardial infarction with near-normal coronary arteries by angiography. Am J Cardiol 2003;92(7):849–852.

51. Inoue F, Sato Y, Matsumoto N, Tani S, Uchiyama T. Evaluation of plaque texture by means of multislice computed tomography in patients with acute coronary syndrome and stable angina. Circ J 2004;68(9):840–844.

52. Leber AW, Knez A, White CW, et al. Composition of coronary atherosclerotic plaques in patients with acute myocardial infarction and stable angina pectoris determined by contrast-enhanced multislice computed tomography. Am J Cardiol 2003;91(6):714–718.

53. Yuichi S, Takako I, Fumio I, et al. Detection of atherosclerotic coronary artery plaques by multislice spiral computed tomography in patients with acute coronary syndrome: report of 2 cases. Circ J 2004;68(3):263–266.

54. Arampatzis CA, Ligthart JM, Schaar JA, Nieman K, Serruys PW, de Feyter PJ. Images in cardiovascular medicine. Detection of a vulnerable coronary plaque: a treatment dilemma. Circulation 2003;108(5):e34–35.

55. Gyongyosi M, Yang P, Hassan A, et al. Intravascular ultrasound predictors of major adverse cardiac events in patients with unstable angina. Clin Cardiol 2000;23(7):507–515.

56. Rasheed Q, Nair RN, Sheehan HM, Hodgson JM. Coronary artery plaque morphology in stable angina and subsets of unstable angina: an in vivo intracoronary ultrasound study. Int J Card Imaging 1995;11(2):89–95.

57. Achenbach S, Ropers D, Hoffmann U, et al. Assessment of coronary remodeling in stenotic and nonstenotic coronary atherosclerotic lesions by multidetector spiral computed tomography. J Am Coll Cardiol 2004;43(5):842–847.

58. Imazeki T, Sato Y, Inoue F, et al. Evaluation of coronary artery remodeling in patients with acute coronary syndrome and stable angina by multislice computed tomography. Circ J 2004;68(11):1045–1050.

59. Schoenhagen P, Tuzcu EM, Stillman AE, et al. Non-invasive assessment of plaque morphology and remodeling in mildly stenotic coronary segments: comparison of 16-slice computed tomography and intravascular ultrasound. Coronary Artery Dis 2003;14: 459–462.

60. Achenbach S, Moshage W, Ropers D, Bachmann K. Comparison of vessel diameters in electron beam tomography and quantitative coronary angiography. Int J Card Imaging 1998;14(1):1–7; discussion 9.

61. Curtis MJ, Traboulsi M, Knudtson ML, Lester WM. Left main coronary artery dissection during cardiac catheterization. Can J Cardiol 1992;8(7):725–728.

62. Devlin G, Lazzam L, Schwartz L. Mortality related to diagnostic cardiac catheterization. The importance of left main coronary disease and catheter induced trauma. Int J Card Imaging 1997; 13(5):379–384; discussion 385–386.

63. Koos R, Mahnken AH, Sinha AM, Wildberger JE, Hoffmann R. ECG-gated multislice spiral computed tomography to clarify lesion severity in a case of left main stenosis. Multislice spiral computed tomography to clarify lesion severity. Int J Cardiovasc Imaging 2003;19(4):349–353.

64. Schuijf JD, Bax JJ, Jukema JW, et al. Feasibility of assessment of coronary stent patency using 16-slice computed tomography. Am J Cardiol 2004;94(4):427–430.

65. Gilard M, Cornily JC, Rioufol G, et al. Noninvasive assessment of left main coronary stent patency with 16-slice computed tomography. Am J Cardiol. 2005;95:110–112.

66. Mollet NR, Cademartiri F. Images in cardiovascular medicine. In-stent neointimal hyperplasia with 16-row multislice computed tomography coronary angiography. Circulation 2004;110(21):e514.

67. Rossi R, Chiurlia E, Ratti C, Ligabue G, Romagnoli R, Modena MG. Noninvasive assessment of coronary artery bypass graft patency by multislice computed tomography. Ital Heart J 2004;5(1):36–41.

68. Ropers D, Ulzheimer S, Wenkel E, et al. Investigation of aortocoronary artery bypass grafts by multislice spiral computed tomography with electrocardiographic-gated image reconstruction. Am J Cardiol 2001;88(7):792–795.

69. Schussler JM, Hamman BL. Multislice cardiac computed tomography of symmetry bypass connector. Heart 2004;90(12):1480.

70. Johannesson M. At what coronary risk level is it cost-effective to initiate cholesterol lowering drug treatment in primary prevention? Eur Heart J 2001;22(11):919–925.

71. Brandle M, Davidson MB, Schriger DL, Lorber B, Herman WH. Cost effectiveness of statin therapy for the primary prevention of major coronary events in individuals with type 2 diabetes. Diabetes Care 2003;26(6):1796–1801.

72. Hay JW, Yu WM, Ashraf T. Pharmacoeconomics of lipid-lowering agents for primary and secondary prevention of coronary artery disease. Pharmacoeconomics 1999;15(1):47–74.

73. Blake GJ, Ridker PM, Kuntz KM. Potential cost-effectiveness of C-reactive protein screening followed by targeted statin therapy for the primary prevention of cardiovascular disease among patients without overt hyperlipidemia. Am J Med 2003;114(6):485–494.

74. De S, Searles G, Haddad H. The prevalence of cardiac risk factors in women 45 years of age or younger undergoing angiography for evaluation of undiagnosed chest pain. Can J Cardiol 2002;18(9):945–948.

75. Ethevenot G, Westphal JC, Massin N, et al. [Normal coronary angiography. Have the indications changed during the 1980s?]. Arch Mal Coeur Vaiss 1997;90(7):905–910.

76. Christiaens L, Allal J, Martin Landragin I, et al. [Normal coronary angiography. Survival and functional status at 6 years]. Arch Mal Coeur Vaiss 2000;93(12):1515–1519.

77. Papanicolaou MN, Califf RM, Hlatky MA, et al. Prognostic implications of angiographically normal and insignificantly narrowed coronary arteries. Am J Cardiol 1986;58(13):1181–1187.

78. Mukerji V, Alpert MA, Hewett JE, Parker BM. Can patients with chest pain and normal coronary arteries be discriminated from those with coronary artery disease prior to coronary angiography? Angiology 1989;40(4 Pt 1):276–282.

79. Dolan MS, Riad K, El-Shafei A, et al. Effect of intravenous contrast for left ventricular opacification and border definition on sensitivity and specificity of dobutamine stress echocardiography compared with coronary angiography in technically difficult patients. Am Heart J 2001;142(5):908–915.

80. Afridi I, Quinones MA, Zoghbi WA, Cheirif J. Dobutamine stress echocardiography: sensitivity, specificity, and predictive value for future cardiac events. Am Heart J 1994;127(6):1510–1515.

81. Schwartz JG, Johnson RB, Aepfelbacher FC, et al. Sensitivity, specificity and accuracy of stress SPECT myocardial perfusion imaging for detection of coronary artery disease in the distribution of first-order branch vessels, using an anatomical matching of angiographic and perfusion data. Nucl Med Commun 2003;24(5):543–549.

82. Fava S, Azzopardi J, Agius-Muscat H. Outcome of unstable angina in patients with diabetes mellitus. Diabet Med 1997;14(3):209–213.

83. Hayashino Y, Nagata-Kobayashi S, Morimoto T, Maeda K, Shimbo T, Fukui T. Cost-effectiveness of screening for coronary artery disease in asymptomatic patients with type 2 diabetes and additional atherogenic risk factors. J Gen Intern Med 2004;19(12):1181–1191.

84. Lee DP, Fearon WF, Froelicher VF. Clinical utility of the exercise ECG in patients with diabetes and chest pain. Chest 2001;119(5):1576–1581.

85. Schussler JM, Dockery WD, Johnson KB, Rosenthal RL, Schumacher JR, Stoler RC. Images in cardiovascular medicine. Superiority of computed tomography coronary angiography over calcium scoring to accurately evaluate atherosclerotic disease in a 35-year-old man. Circulation 2004;109(23):e318–e319.

86. Pasowicz M, Klimeczek P, Wicher-Muniak E, et al. The use of coronary artery multislice spiral computed tomography (MSCT) to identify patients for surgical revascularisation. Acta Cardiol 2004;59(2): 221–222.

87. Meier B, Ramamurthy S. Plaque sealing by coronary angioplasty. Cathet Cardiovasc Diagn 1995;36(4):295–297.

88. Meier B. Plaque sealing or plumbing for coronary artery stenoses? Circulation 1997;96(6):2094–2095.

89. Mercado N, Maier W, Boersma E, et al. Clinical and angiographic outcome of patients with mild coronary lesions treated with balloon angioplasty or coronary stenting. Implications for mechanical plaque sealing. Eur Heart J 2003;24(6):541–551.

90. Meier B. Plaque sealing by coronary angioplasty. Heart 2004;90(12): 1395–1398.

12

CT Imaging of Non-calcific Atherosclerotic Plaque with Cardiac Computed Tomography

M. Leila Rasouli

Background

Atherosclerosis is a disease process affecting the vessel walls of coronary arteries [1]. Atherosclerotic plaque is comprised of three main components: (1) cholesterol, cholesteryl esters, and phospholipids; (2) connective tissue extracellular matrix; and (3) cells including smooth muscle cells and inflammatory cells such as T lymphocytes and monocyte-derived macrophages [2]. Varying degrees of these constituents give rise to different plaque morphologies. The so-called "vulnerable plaque" is composed of a large lipid core covered by a thin fibrous cap. It is highly prone to rupture or erosion, ultimately leading to acute coronary syndromes.

Coronary angiography has traditionally served as the principal imaging modality to evaluate coronary artery disease (CAD) [3]. However, both necropsy and coronary intravascular ultrasound (IVUS) studies have consistently shown that angiographically "normal" coronary artery segments may contain a significant amount of atherosclerotic plaque [4–7]. Furthermore, previous angiographic studies have shown that most myocardial infarctions (MI) often result from rupture of a vulnerable plaque in the absence of a significant luminal stenosis. These rupture-prone plaques, which are 7 times more likely to cause disruption than the more severe, extensive plaques, are not visible on two-dimensional X-ray angiography [8–10].

Intravascular ultrasound (IVUS), on the other hand, has traditionally allowed for a direct, 360º visualization of coronary atheroma within the vessel wall and identifies both plaque distribution and composition. The utility of coronary IVUS over angiography in recognizing these smaller plaques is offset by a higher procedural complication rate secondary to its more invasive nature, and increased costs (requiring additional catheters and dedicated equipment) [11]. In recent years, investigators have been studying effective identification of these early,

non-obstructive coronary plaques with minimally invasive imaging modalities such as multidetector computed tomography (MDCT) and electron beam computed tomography (EBCT). These non-invasive technologies hold promise as a diagnostic tool for risk stratification in patients as well as a means to monitor plaque stabilization in patients receiving therapy such as lipid-lowering medications.

This chapter provides an overview of the CT literature related to plaque morphology, summarizing the CT protocols in assessing atherosclerotic plaque, the accuracy of plaque characterization compared to IVUS, plaque configuration score determination, and a brief comparison to MRI scanning.

Intravascular Ultrasound

IVUS is an invasive method of detecting vessel wall plaque directly and is the gold standard for plaque characterization in CT comparative studies. IVUS utilizes the transmission and reception of high-frequency sound waves to delineate the coronary vessel wall into three components, the intima, media, and the adventitia. In diseased arteries, it provides real-time, tomographic imaging of atheroma. Depending on the cellular composition of the atherosclerotic plaque and its resultant echogenicity, atheroma is differentiated into at least three morphologies: (1) hypoechoic plaque is echolucent compared to the adventitia and represents soft plaque and high lipid content; (2) hyperechoic plaque is equal or greater in density to the adventitia, without calcification, and represents fibrous tissue; and (3) calcified atheroma (brighter than the surrounding adventitia and is accompanied by acoustic shadowing) [12]. In addition to elucidating vessel wall composition, IVUS has the ability to quantitate the extent and distribution of atherosclerosis in coronary arteries (Figure 12.1).

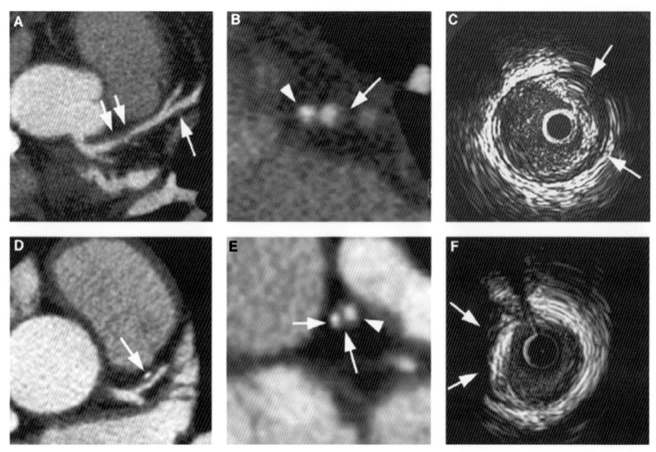

Figure 12.1. A Axial multidetector computed tomographic image demonstrates non-calcific plaque in proximal and mid left anterior descending (LAD). **B** Multiplanar reconstruction showing cross section of the LAD segment (arrow). Arrowhead depicts diagonal branch. **C** Intravascular ultrasound image showing non-calcified plaque in mid LAD (arrows). **D** Axial MDCT demonstrating partly calcified plaque in proximal LAD. **E** Multiplanar reconstruction of the MDCT demonstrating cross-section of proximal LAD with plaque (large arrow), including calcification (small arrow). **F** IVUS image demonstrating partly calcified plaque in proximal LAD (arrows). (Reproduced with permission from Lippincoff Williams & Wilkins [14].)

Multidetector Spiral Computed Tomography (MDCT) Protocol

Improved spatial and temporal image acquisition with sub-millimeter slice collimation has facilitated atherosclerotic plaque detection with MDCT. Several studies using contrast-enhanced spiral scanning and retrospective gating have documented the same general protocol. In summary, a test bolus of 20 mL of contrast medium and a chaser bolus of 20 mL of saline solution are injected through an 18-gauge antecubital intravenous catheter to determine circulation time. Then, a larger bolus ranging between 80 and 130 mL of contrast agent is injected intravenously at a rate ranging from 3.5 to 5 mL/s via a power injector. Once the signal density level in the ascending aorta reaches a predefined threshold of 100 Hounsfield units (HU), CT data acquisition and ECG tracing commences. CT parameters (for the 16-slice scanner) have been described as follows: detector collimation = 12 × 0.75 mm (1 mm collimation also utilized in some studies); tube voltage = 120 kV; tube current = 370–450 mAs during 55% of the cardiac cycle (diastole) and a reduction of the current by 80% during the remaining time of the R-R interval; gantry rotation = 400–500 ms. Images are reconstructed with acquisition times ranging from 130 to 250 ms in diastole 350–450 ms before the R wave using retrospective electrocardiogram gating. Slice thickness is 0.625–1.0 mm, with reconstruction slice increments of 0.5 mm. Heart rates need to be <60–65 beats/min to avoid motion artifacts; most commonly oral metoprolol is administered to patients with heart rates >65 [13–16].

Plaque analysis and tissue differentiation are conducted at the optimal image display setting; in general at a window between 600 and 900 HU and at a level between 40 and 250 HU. Plaque with density below the vessel contrast is defined as non-calcified plaque. Conversely, structures with densities above the adjacent vessel lumen are considered calcified [13]. Some studies have defined three levels of plaque: "soft" plaque – presumably lipid laden with lower densities, intermediate or presumably fibrous plaques, and calcific or high-density plaques (Figure 12.2).

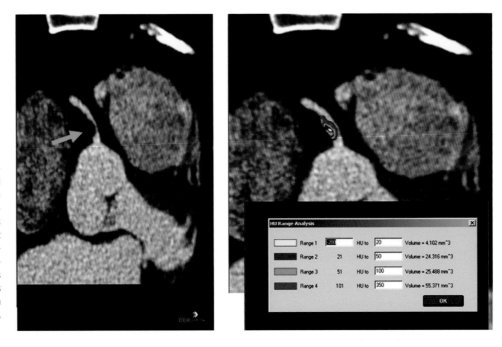

Figure 12.2. A contrast study demonstrating significant soft plaque in the proximal right coronary artery. The left image demonstrates the soft plaque on an axial two-dimensional image (arrow). The stenosis is approximately 80% in severity. The right image demonstrates the software to quantitate plaque, using different Hounsfield thresholds to determine lipid-laden plaque, fibrous plaque, contrast, and calcium. The thresholds can be changed in the program depending on the user. (Aquarius Workstation, TeraRecon, CA.)

Electron Beam Computed Tomography (EBCT) Protocols

Faster, higher-resolution imaging and soft tissue delineation with EBCT, especially with its newest iteration, e-Speed EBCT, has paved the way for soft plaque detection. Older EBCT studies utilized non-enhanced CT scan (no contrast agents), in a high-resolution mode with 100 ms scan time and 3 mm slice thickness, using single slice technique [17]. Up to 60 slices were obtained during a single breath-hold for approximately 45 seconds. Each slice was triggered to 80% of the R-R interval (in diastole). Results using this protocol in non-calcific plaque identification were encouraging, but still not sensitive enough for diagnostic purposes.

Contrast-enhanced electron beam angiography, utilizing e-Speed EBCT, incorporates an improved methodology for enhanced plaque characterization. All scans are performed in the high-resolution volume mode using 100 ms exposure time. A flow study is first performed to obtain circulation time (the time from the venous contrast injection to the peak visualization of the ascending aorta). Hence, a bolus of 15–20 mL of contrast agent is injected intravenously at 4 mL/s through an antecubital vein and 20 axial cross-sections of the chest are acquired in multislice mode.

The final contrast-enhanced coronary volume scan is performed with 1.5 mm collimation, 1.5 mm section thickness, and 1.5 mm table incrementation. Patients with heart rates <60 beats/min are given intravenous atropine, to decrease breath-hold. Non-ionic contrast is administered through an antecubital vein with an injection rate of 4 mL/s (100–120 mL per study). This is followed with a saline flush.

The total scan time is 25–45 seconds, rendering 50–70 slices, with thickness of the dataset equaling 75–105 mm. In axial images and three-dimensional reconstructions, all coronary arteries and side branches with a diameter of 1.5 mm are assessed. Plaque is defined as tissue thickening >1.0 mm^2 within or adjacent to the artery. Atheroma with greater density/brightness than the vessel lumen is considered calcific; that of equal density is defined as fibrous, and that with less density as soft plaque (Figure 12.3).

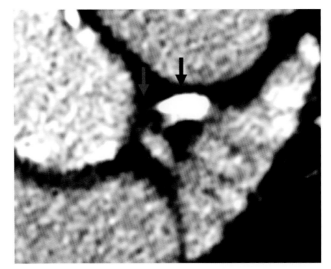

Figure 12.3. A patient with high-grade stenosis of the ostial LAD. The CT image clearly demonstrates a low-density plaque (seen as black on CT) in the ostium of the left anterior descending (red arrow). The proximal LAD also has a dense calcific lesion (black arrow). CT allows measurement of the density (Hounsfield units) and area of the plaque; however, area measurements tend to underestimate total plaque burden when compared to IVUS.

Table 12.1. Accuracy of MDCT and EBCT in plaque morphology identification

Study (first author)	Date	No. of patients	No. of segments	Hypoechoic (soft)	Sensitivity Hyperechoic (fibrous)	Calcific	Specificity
Leber	2004	37	875	78%	78%	95%	92%
Achenbach	2004	22	166	53%	a	94%	87–94%
Schoenhagen	2003	14	37	88–92%	a	88–92%	a
Schroeder	2001	15	34	b	b	b	b
Baumgart	1997	57	267	47%	a	97%	75–80%
Rasouli	2004	10	52	100%	50%	100%	83%

[a] Groups were divided into calcific and non-calcific plaque only.
[b] This study strictly evaluated MDCT density measurements of plaques detected by IVUS.

Accuracy of Plaque Detection by MDCT

Recent contrast-enhanced MDCT studies have shown that non-invasive scanning permits accurate detection and differentiation of coronary plaque, when compared to IVUS. Table 12.1 summarizes the results of six main studies comparing CT technology with IVUS in the detection of soft and hard atheroma. The first four studies incorporate MDCT as the non-invasive modality [13–16], while the last two represent data from EBCT studies [17,18].

Sensitivities for non-calcific (hypoechoic, soft) plaque detection by MDCT range from 53% to 92% with sample size of patients ranging from 14 to 37 patients. In one of the more robust MDCT studies, which evaluated 875 segments, sensitivity for hypoechoic, hyperechoic, and calcific plaques was 78%, 78%, and 95%, respectively. Specificity was a respectable 92% [13]. As expected, the sensitivities for detecting calcific atheroma were relatively higher than for non-calcific plaque in these studies, approximately 88–95%. Although the sample sizes are relatively small in these studies, they do demonstrate diagnostic accuracy in characterizing non-calcific atheroma. Limitations to the feasibility of utilizing MDCT for diagnostic purposes include the fact that motion artifact still exists. In the study by Leber et al. [13] optimal diagnostic image quality was not obtained for 15% of coronary vessels. The investigators also concede that non-calcific plaque visualization is limited by plaque and vessel size. The smaller plaques located in smaller coronary sections were not accurately characterized. In the study by Achenbach et al. [14], plaque volume was estimated by both MDCT and IVUS. They found MDCT substantially underestimated plaque volume per segment as compared with IVUS ($24 \pm 35\,mm^3$ versus $43 \pm 60\,mm^3$, $p < 0.001$).

Accuracy of Plaque Detection by EBCT

It is well documented that EBCT provides accurate non-invasive assessment of calcific coronary plaque and coronary artery stenosis [19–22]. However, the ability of EBCT to detect non-calcific coronary atheroma is not as well established. In an older non-contrast EBCT study, while the sensitivity for visualizing calcific plaque was very high (97%), soft plaque analysis was suboptimal with a sensitivity of only 47% [22].

Until recently, there were no data available on the assessment of coronary plaque composition using contrast-enhanced electron beam angiography. Recent data from Harbor-UCLA, utilizing e-Speed EBA, demonstrate accurate characterization of both calcific and soft atheroma, using IVUS as the gold standard. Overall accuracy in defining plaque morphology for EBA was 94% (49 of 52 lesions) [18]. Sensitivity for detecting soft and calcific plaques, respectively, was 100% for both types. Specificity was over 80% (Table 12.1). Figure 12.1 shows different plaque morphologies using IVUS and corresponding plaque images. The major limitation with EBA was detecting fibrous plaque; however, the sample size for fibrous plaque was $n = 2$ and therefore insufficient to make sweeping conclusions. These preliminary results show promise for EBA as a diagnostic tool for plaque detection and characterization (Figure 12.4).

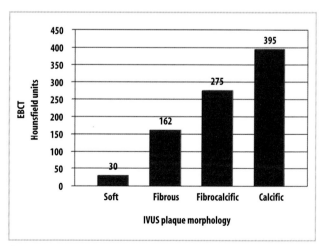

Figure 12.4. A comparison of plaque Hounsfield units measured on EBCT and the corresponding lesion classification by intravascular ultrasound. Low density (low Hounsfield unit measures) is consistent with soft or lipid-laden plaques on IVUS. Increasing Hounsfield units are correlated to fibrous, fibrocalcific, and calcific lesions. (Data derived from Rasouli et al. [18].)

Plaque Configuration Score Determination

A few CT studies have further attempted to classify plaque composition by density scores using Hounsfield unit values (Figures 12.2, 12.4, 12.5). Two MDCT studies and one EBA study have shown that mean CT density values for hypoechoic, hyperechoic, and calcified lesions are statistically different [13,16,18]. Mean CT density values for hypoechoic, hyperechoic, and calcific plaques in Leber et al. were 49 ± 22, 91 ± 22, and 391 ± 156, respectively, with p value <0.02. Similarly, in the Schroeder et al. investigation, those values were 14 ± 26, 91 ± 21, 419 ± 194, respectively, with p < 0.0001. In the only EBA study to evaluate plaque for density measurements, these values were 30 ± 33 for soft, 105 for fibrous, and 395 ± 230 for calcific plaque structures, p < 0.0001 [18]. These studies demonstrate that lesion echogenicity of IVUS correlates with CT density measurements in coronary atheroma. This indicates that CT attenuation reflects major plaque composition. Ultimately this could mean that low-attenuation plaques on CT would reveal atheroma with high lipid content, a precursor of vulnerable plaque. Some have even suggested evaluating lumen heterogeneity to assess low-density areas in the lumen on *non-contrast* studies, which may correlate with soft plaque (Figure 12.6).

Software to specifically quantitate soft plaque is now available. The software allows for detailed investigation of suspected soft plaques through the definition of a set of Hounsfield unit ranges, each of which is highlighted in a different color in an overlay on the CT image (Figures 12.2, 12.6). Hence, contrast-enhanced lumen can be depicted in one color, the fatty tissue around a vessel in another color, and the vessel wall in a third color, highlighting the subtle differences between these tissue types. A fourth color map can then be established for hypodense tissue, which may be indicative of a lipid-rich lesion or region. Through this technique, the morphology of the lesion can be more clearly depicted, with quantitative calculation of the volume within a CT image of each given Hounsfield unit range (corresponding to the different tissue types). Examples of this software (Aquarius Workstation, TeraRecon Inc, San Mateo, CA) is seen for contrast studies (Figure 12.2) and non-contrast studies (Figure 12.6).

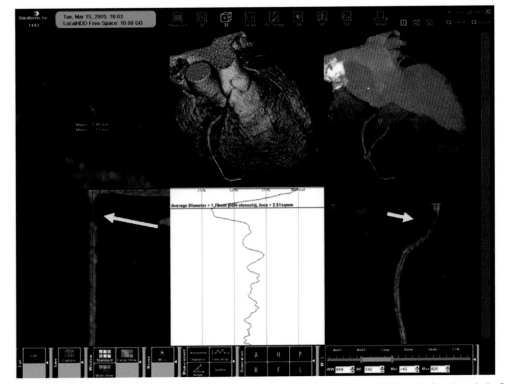

Figure 12.5. Patient with significant disease in the proximal right coronary artery (RCA). A large soft plaque is visualized (arrow), seen well with maximal intensity projection (lower right) and curved multiplanar (lower left). The volume-rendered image (top, middle) does not show the plaque or stenosis as well.

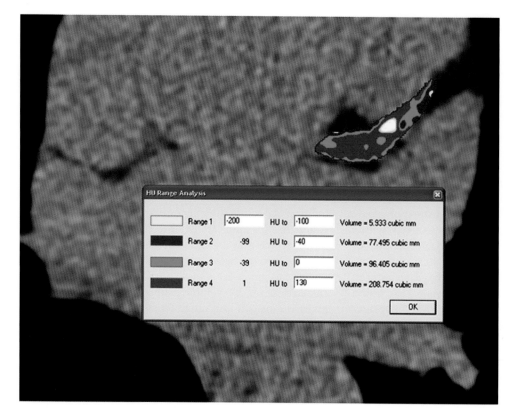

Figure 12.6. New software that automatically allocates color to the different densities in each pixel. This is a non-contrast study. This program allows for computer quantification (in cubic mm) the different plaque morphologies. The left main and proximal left anterior descending are depicted. The white area represents calcification, red depicts normal tissue, and blue and green depict low-density structures, mostly consistent with lipid-laden plaque on CT. (Aquarius Workstation, TeraRecon Inc, San Mateo, CA).

CT Versus MRI Scanning

MRI also represents a potential leading non-invasive imaging modality for atherosclerotic plaque identification. It incorporates biophysical and biochemical parameters such as chemical composition and concentration, water content, physical state, and molecular motion to differentiate plaque morphology [23]. Its advantage over CT lies in the fact that MR provides imaging without radiation exposure. However, this is offset by its limitations, which include low signal-to-noise ratio and lower spatial resolution (>1 mm) when compared to CT scanning. This leads to poorer image quality and less reproducibility [16].

Limitations

The limitations of soft plaque detection may be much more significant than a limited sensitivity or underestimation of plaque burden. The reproducibility of the measure has never been reported. There is no prognostic information to say whether soft plaque adds any information on top of risk factors, angiographic disease severity, or calcified plaque. Finally, this procedure requires both contrast and radiation, and the risks may outweigh the benefit in individual patients. All of this will need to be studied over the next few years, before soft plaque detection by CT or EBCT becomes routine.

CT studies are still needed to demonstrate the prognostic impact of non-calcified plaques. Additionally, study populations in CT studies have consisted of symptomatic people with high plaque burden. Plaque detection in asymptomatic, lower-risk individuals may be less accurate using non-invasive CT imaging. It is difficult to justify, however, performing IVUS on asymptomatic patients in order to draw firmer conclusions.

Future Directions

As the accuracy in the evaluation of soft plaque is improving with technological advancements in the CT realm, we are coming closer to defining the vulnerable plaque in a non-invasive manner. Reliable plaque identification by CT will become an important diagnostic tool for risk stratification in patients with known or suspected CAD. We may also come to rely on this modality to monitor plaque stabilization and potential regression in patients receiving therapy such as statins. Current reconstruction techniques that are most accurate to depict different densities are: two-dimensional axial images, and the maximal intensity and curved multiplanar reformatting techniques (Figures 12.5, 12.7). Given a total study time of 20–30 minutes, the requirement only for intravenous access, and no hospitalization or observation period after the study, CT angiography costs and morbidity are much lower than with

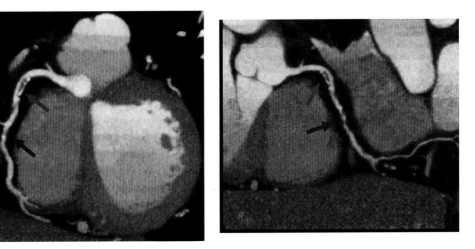

Figure 12.7. Three-dimensional reconstructions of a mixed fibrocalcific plaque (red arrows) and soft plaque (purple arrows) in the right coronary artery. The left image represents a maximal intensity projection, and the right image is created using curved multiplanar reformatting of the same coronary artery.

conventional angiography or IVUS. Of course, if the results are promising, soft plaque detection could potentially serve as a non-invasive imaging method to not only diagnose early unstable coronary plaques, but also to assess the response to medical therapy and therefore improve risk stratification for future cardiac events.

References

1. Fuster V, Fayad ZA, Badimon JJ. Acute coronary syndromes: biology. Lancet 1999;353(suppl):S115–119.
2. Libby P. Molecular basis of the acute coronary syndromes. Circulation 1995;91:2844–2850.
3. De Franco AC. Understanding the development and potential regression of atherosclerosis. Am J Cardiol 2001;88(suppl):7M–20M.
4. Roberts W, Jones AA. Quantitation of coronary arterial narrowing at necropsy in sudden coronary death. Am J Cardiol 1979;44:39–44.
5. Nissen SE, Gurley JC, Grines CL, et al. Intravascular ultrasound assessment of lumen size and wall morphology in normal subjects and patients with coronary artery disease. Circulation 1991;84:1087–1099.
6. Topol E, Nissen S. Our preoccupation with coronary luminology: the dissociation between clinical and angiographic findings in ischemic heart disease. Circulation 1995;92:2333–2342.
7. Mintz GS, Painter JA, Pichard AD, et al. Atherosclerosis in angiographically "normal" coronary artery reference segments: an intravascular ultrasound study with clinical correlations. J Am Coll Cardiol 1995;25:1479–1485.
8. Little WC, Constantinescu M, Applegate RJ, et al. Can coronary angiography predict the site of a subsequent myocardial infarction in patients with mild-to-moderate coronary artery disease? Circulation 1988;78:1157–1166.
9. Little WC, Downes TR, Applegate RJ. The underlying coronary lesion in myocardial infarction: implications for coronary angiography. Clin Cardiol 1991;14:868–874.
10. Falk E, Shah PK, Fuster V. Coronary plaque disruption. Circulation 1995;92:657–671.
11. Batkoff BW, Linker DT. Safety of intracoronary ultrasound: data from a Multicenter European Registry. Cathet Cardiovasc Diagn 1996;38:238–241.
12. Nissen SE, Yock P. Intravascular ultrasound: novel pathophysiological insights and current clinical applications. Circulation 2001;103:604–616.
13. Leber AW, Knez A, Becker A, et al. Accuracy of multidetector spiral computed tomography in identifying and differentiating the composition of coronary atherosclerotic plaques. J Am Coll Cardiol 2004;43:1241–1247.
14. Achenbach S, Moselewski F, Ropers D, et al. Detection of calcified and noncalcified coronary atherosclerotic plaque by contrast-enhanced, submillimeter multidetector spiral computed tomography. Circulation 2004;109:14–17.
15. Schoenhagen P, Tuzcu EM, Stillman AE, et al. Non-invasive assessment of plaque morphology and remodeling in mildly stenotic coronary segments: comparison of 16-slice compute tomography and intravascular ultrasound. Coron Artery Dis 2003;14:459–462.
16. Schroeder S, Kopp AF, Baumbach A, et al. Noninvasive detection and evaluation of atherosclerotic coronary plaques with multislice computed tomography. J Am Coll Cardiol 2001;37:1430–1435.
17. Dietrich B, Schmermund A, Guenter G, et al. Comparison of electron beam compute tomography with intracoronary ultrasound and coronary angiography for detection of coronary atherosclerosis. J Am Coll Cardiol 1997;30:57–64.
18. Rasouli ML, Shavelle DM, McKay C, French WJ, Budoff MJ. Electron Beam angiography in the assessment of coronary plaque morphology. Catheter Cardiovasc Interv 2004;62(1): abstract A-3.
19. Achenbach S, Moshage W, Ropers D, et al. Value of EBCT for the non-invasive detection of high-grade coronary artery stenoses and occlusions. N Engl J Med 1998;339:1964–1971.
20. Schmermund A, Rensing B, Sheedy P, et al. Intravenous EBCT coronary angiography for segmental analysis of coronary artery stenosis. J Am Coll Cardiol 1998;31:1547–1554.
21. Budoff MJ, Lu B, Shinbane JS, et al. Methodology for improved detection of coronary stenoses with computed tomographic angiography. Am Heart J 2004;148(6):1085–1090.
22. Baumgart D, Schmermund A, Guenter G, et al. Comparison of EBCT with intracoronary ultrasound and coronary angiography for detection of coronary atherosclerosis. J Am Coll Cardiol 1997;30:57–64.
23. Fayad ZA, Fuster V. Clinical imaging of the high-risk or vulnerable atherosclerotic plaque. Circ Res 2001;89:305–316.

13

Peripheral Angiography

Khurram Nasir and Matthew J. Budoff

Introduction

Since its clinical implementation in the early 1990s, single-detector computed tomography (SDCT) has revolutionized body imaging through the use of slip-ring technology and had a significant impact on the field on non-invasive diagnostic imaging [1,2]. It has experienced a revolution of its technology in the last decade by improving X-ray tube capabilities, gantry rotation, and interpretation algorithm performances, and as a result becoming a tool for large vessel assessment [1]. Development of multidetector CT angiography (MDCTA) in the late 1990s represented the most significant advancement in helical CT. The resulting faster gantry speed rotation time and increased table speed that are hallmarks of MDCT are particularly suited for CT angiography (CTA) [1,3–6]. This review will focus on the performance and diagnostic accuracy of SDCT as well MDCT angiography for imaging the peripheral vasculature, and will also discuss scanning protocols, contrast material issues, post-processing, strengths and limitations, comparison with other modalities and cost-effectiveness.

Peripheral Arterial Occlusive Disease

Recent epidemiological evidence indicates that peripheral arterial occlusive disease (PAOD) affects nearly 10% of men by 65 years of age, increasing to 20% of men and women ≥75 years. Peripheral vascular disease (PVD) is a condition in which the arteries that carry the blood to the lower extremities become narrowed or occluded causing ischemia in tissues, particularly the muscles [3]. Although PAOD is not a frequent primary cause of mortality, it is an adverse prognostic indicator among the elderly [2]. The most common cause of peripheral vascular disease is atherosclerosis, and is associated with presence of traditional cardiovascular disease (CVD) risk factors such as cigarette smoking, hypertension, and diabetes. The disease severity is reflected by the symptoms, ranging from the typical calf or buttock pain on exertion that is relieved by rest (claudication) to pain at rest. Those with intermittent claudication generally have a comparatively good prognosis, a relatively benign course, a low rate of amputation, and limited need for surgical intervention [7]. These patients may improve with conservative measures. In contrast, patients with limb-threatening ischemia have a much worse prognosis with a higher rate of amputation, particularly in those with diabetes [7]. A lower extremity intervention is a treatment option in these cases for which characterization of the lesion itself and the inflows to and outflows from the lesions is central in planning intervention [2]. Clinically significant lesions could be located anywhere between the aorta and the trio of lower leg vessels, the anterior tibial, peroneal, and posterior tibial arteries. The vessels proximal to the femoral arteries are considered inflow vessels, while those distal are "runoff." In general, it is important clinically to distinguish in atherosclerotic occlusive peripheral vascular disease between high-grade stenosis (usually >50%) and lower-grade stenosis (<50% narrowing), as well as whether it is a short- or long-segment lesion, respectively [1,2]. Although not absolute, these distinctions provide a framework for therapeutic considerations [2].

To date, lower extremity vascular studies have been largely been performed and interpreted by conventional angiograms. These techniques have also been modified by the introduction of digital subtraction imaging (DSA), which has significantly reduced the procedural time, improved post-processing and provided road mapping for interventional procedures. New dose-reduction techniques, such as pulsed fluoroscopy, have led to a relevant decrease in radiation exposure, both for the patient and for the radiologist [8]. However, the complications and patient discomfort associated with DSA have prompted the investigation of less invasive means of assessing the lower extremity arterial circulation. The development of imaging modalities such as ultrasonography (US), CT angiography (CTA), and magnetic resonance angiography (MRA) has provided the medical community with imaging modalities that may be used for non-invasive vascular imaging of peripheral vessels [8].

Diagnostic Value of CT Angiography for PAOD

SDCT angiography has mainly focused on the thoracic and abdominal aorta and its major branches [7]. On the other hand, the visualization of small branches and large vascular territories with SDCT such as lower extremities has been limited due to the limited volume coverage and spatial resolution [7,9,10].

Lawrence et al. (1995) described the first technique to image a portion of the lower extremity arterial system, from the inguinal ligament to the proximal calf, in six patients by using 1-second gantry rotation SDCT [11]. Two consecutive 60-second helical acquisitions with 5 mm collimation and a pitch of 1.0 (5 mm/s table speed) were used to cover 60 cm over a minimum of 129 seconds. Compared with catheter arteriography, CT angiography correctly depicted segmental occlusions and significant stenoses (>50%) in 26 of 28 arteries, yielding a sensitivity of 92.9%, a specificity of 96.2%, and an overall accuracy of 95.5% [11].

In 1996, Rieker et al., using SDCT angiography, demonstrated a complete coverage of lower extremities from the groin to the mid calf in a single helical acquisition with a single-detector scanner using a 5 mm collimation and a pitch of 2.0 [12]. Compared to conventional angiograms, sensitivities of 94–100% for arterial occlusions and 67–88% for stenoses of 75–99% were reported, with specificities ranging from 98% to 100% for occlusions and from 94% to 100% for severe stenoses, respectively. Interestingly, they also reported 9 stenoses distal to superficial femoral arterial occlusions, as well as 6 calf runoff arteries, identified at CT angiography but not at conventional digital subtraction angiography [12]. Although the results of this study were promising, the scan coverage was limited to 70 cm, and therefore the aortoiliac vessels and the distal calves were not evaluated. The major obstacle was the length of the vascular tree: a complete coverage of the arteries of lower extremities with a sufficient spatial resolution using a single volume data acquisition was not possible because of limited z-axis coverage [1,3].

In a similar fashion using sequential single-detector row helical CT, Raptopoulos and associates achieved sufficient vessel enhancement for assessing an extended vascular territory (range: celiac axis down to the femoral arteries) [13]. However, they used two sessions of helical scanning with a collimation of 3 and 5 mm, respectively, with two separate bolus injections of iodinated contrast agent. By substantially increasing the dose of contrast agent, they demonstrated a sensitivity of 94% and a specificity of 97% for the detection of severely stenotic (≥85% luminal narrowing) aortoiliac arterial segments [13].

Beregi et al. studied the popliteal arteries of 26 patients with suspected popliteal arterial disease [14]. Because the coverage was limited to the popliteal artery, 29–45-second single–detector row CT angiography was performed with 3–5 mm collimation and a pitch of 1.0–1.2. The results of this study demonstrated improved popliteal aneurysm detection with CT, when compared with the detection at conventional angiography (100% versus 61% sensitivity) [14].

Mesurolle et al. (2004) using a dual-slice helical CT evaluated 16 patients with PAOD who also underwent transcatheter angiography [15]. The average z-axis coverage was 820 mm from the celiac aorta to the proximal part of the legs. The investigators performed only one spiral set. The dual-slice helical CT was inconclusive in 6.2% of segments whereas angiography was inconclusive in 5%. The overall sensitivity of helical CT was 91% and specificity was 93%. Segmental analysis found a sensitivity of 43% in infrapopliteal arteries, and a specificity of 86% [15].

An important aspect of peripheral investigation as seen in DSA is the requirement of the entire range from the renal arteries down to the ankles, which is approximately 1200–1400 mm [4,6,7;9,10,16]. As observed in the above studies, with the SDCT, it is not possible to scan the complete volume of interest (from the abdominal aorta down to the ankle) in one scan [11,12]. However with the advent of multislice CT in 1998, CTA has experienced a considerable boost and is now available for routine use in most diagnostic settings. MDCT angiography provides three major advantages over SDCT angiography: shorter scanning durations associated with improved contrast medium efficiency, thinner sections of entire anatomic territories within a breath-hold, and greater longitudinal coverage [1,3]. With multislice CTA spatial resolution no longer poses a problem. At present, multislice CTA can be considered the imaging technique of choice for a vast number of vascular indications [17]. The use of MDCT scanners has resulted in increased speed of data acquisition with nearly isometric voxels, allowing the performance of CT angiography over wider anatomic areas with similar contrast dose, narrower effective slice thickness, and reduced reconstruction artifact than was possible with single-detector scanners [18]. In fact, the diagnostic accuracy of CT angiography has been proved superior to that of conventional arteriography in several applications [2]. In recent years a complete acquisition of lower extremity inflow and runoff has become a real possibility with MDCT angiography (MDCTA) [9]. Also spatial resolution by MDCTA not only differentiates between high-grade and low-grade stenoses in peripheral vasculature, but also improves characterization of the lesion, differentiating atheromatous from thrombotic occlusions [19].

Rubin et al. (2000) were the first to compare the utility of four- versus one-channel CT for evaluation of peripheral vasculature [20]. The imaging of the entire arterial supplies of the lower extremities in a single helical acquisition using 2.5 mm collimation and a table speed of

18.8 mm/s (3.2 mm-effective section thickness) was performed with the 4-slice MDCT in less than 70 seconds. Compared to SDCT, CT angiography with a 4-slice scanner was 2.6 times faster, scanning efficiency was 4.1 times greater, contrast efficiency was 2.5 times greater, dose of contrast material was nearly 47% less (97 mL versus 232 mL) without a significant change in aortic enhancement, and sections were 40% thinner (3.2 versus 5.3 mm) despite a 59% shorter scanning duration (22 versus 56 seconds). The use of multidetector CT offers substantial improvements in the overall performance of CT angiography compared with single-detector CT [20].

In another landmark study comparing 4-channel MDCTA with DSA for the first time in 24 symptomatic PAOD patients, Rubin et al. (2001) reported a 100% concordance in revealing stenosis in segments shown on both MDCT angiography and conventional angiography [18]. In addition, MDCTA was able to depict 26 arterial segments that were not visualized with DSA distal to more occluded segments. A potential limitation of this study was that the assessment did not appear to have been performed in a blinded prospective manner, and inter-technique and inter-modality discrepancies were settled by consensus.

Martin et al. (2003) were among the first to determine the accuracy and reliability of MDCT angiography of the lower extremities in the evaluation of symptomatic atheroocclusive disease in a blinded manner prospectively [21]. The sensitivity and specificity for significant ($\geq$75%) stenosis was 87% and 98%, whereas for vessel occlusion it was 92% and 97%, respectively. Multidetector CTA again showed 110 more arterial segments than DSA; 90% were in the calves. The lowest agreement between the two techniques occurred in the calf vessel segments, likely resulting from the difficulty of accurately measuring the very small vessels and because of the inability of DSA to show several patent vessels seen on MDCT angiography [21]. The investigators did not achieve a complete concordance between CT and transcatheter angiography as reported by Rubin et al. [18], which could be explained by the fact that in this study both CT and DSA results were read in a blinded fashion. Another potential explanation is that MDCT studies were performed with a 5 mm collimation. The effective slice thickness in the study of Rubin et al. is twice as thin as that used in the study by Martin et al., allowing a better axial resolution with better z-axis coverage [18].

Ofer et al. (2003) evaluated 18 patients with suspected PAOD who were referred for elective digital subtraction angiography (DSA) with CT angiography (4-slice MDCT) from the level of the superior mesenteric artery to the pedal arteries in a single helical scan [22]. The 3.2 mm slices were reconstructed every 1.6 mm. An average total length of 1182 mm (range, 1081–1292 mm) was imaged in mean 48 seconds (range: 43–52 seconds) in a single helical acquisition. The study findings were graded according to six categories: 1, normal (0% stenosis); 2, mild (1–49% stenosis); 3, moderate (50–74% stenosis); 4, severe (75–99%

stenosis); 5, occluded; and 6, non-diagnostic. Grouping the six categories according to the threshold for treatment (categories 1 and 2 as one group and categories 3, 4, and 5 as the second group) resulted in an agreement of 92%. Although the authors reported an overall sensitivity and specificity of 91% and a specificity of 92% compared to DSA, the agreement for severe stenosis as well as occluded vessels was not reported [22].

Willmann et al (2003) in a landmark study compared the accuracy of 4-slice MDCTA with contrast-enhanced 3-D MR angiography for assessment of the aortoiliac in 46 consecutive patients (mean age: 68 years, 39 men) with DSA as the standard of reference [23]. The investigators using 1 mm nominal section thickness scanned the mean craniocaudal distance of 35 cm during one breath-hold. The excellent quality of CT angiograms obtained with a multidetector row CT scanner in this study is reflected in the sensitivity of 91% and specificity of 99% for the detection of hemodynamically significant arterial stenosis of aortoiliac arteries. There were no statistically significant differences in the diagnostic performance of MR angiography compared with that of MDCT angiography for the detection of significant arterial stenosis of the aortoiliac arteries (MRA has a sensitivity and specificity of 92% and 99%).

Ota et al (2004) also reported similar findings. A single-acquisition protocol with an automatic triggering system was performed that took an average of only 46 seconds for acquisition and approximately 15 minutes for the total examination [24]. The sensitivity, specificity, and accuracy of 4-slice MDCT angiography were all 99% respectively, in 24 patients with symptomatic lower extremity PAOD, compared to DSA of the aortoiliac and lower extremity arteries. In the non-calcified and mildly calcified segments, the sensitivity, specificity, and accuracy of MDCT angiography for the detection of more-than-mild stenosis were 100%, 100%, and 100%, respectively. The presence of dense calcifications and endoluminal stents are potential factors which may impair the quantification of the degree of PAOD. In these instances, cross-sectional viewing of the respective lesions may be beneficial [2]. In this study sufficient statistical diagnostic accuracy was not achieved using the axial images compared with the accuracy achieved using cross-sectional multiplanar reconstruction images and the axial images required more interobserver discussion to reach a final consensus. As a result, the authors emphasize the importance of careful observation of true cross-sectional images [24].

Despite careful 2-D imaging, severe calcifications of the peripheral arteries can limit accuracy and the ability to see within the lumen, similar to coronary CT angiography.

Catalano et al. (2004) also demonstrated that MDCT (4-slice) is highly accurate in the assessment of peripheral vascular disease in 50 patients with PAOD, independent of the grade of ischemia [25]. Arteries depicted at CT angiography and DSA were graded separately for degree of stenosis as 23 anatomic segments as follows: 1, normal patency;

2, moderate (≤50%) stenosis; 3, focal severe (>50%) stenosis; 4, multiple severe stenoses; and 5, occlusion. Three readers independently interpreted the images, Sensitivity, specificity, and accuracy, based on a consensus reading of MDCT angiograms, were 96%, 93%, and 94%, respectively. The level of interobserver agreement was high for the interpretation of both MDCT angiograms and DSA images. Among the vascular regions with the lowest level of interobserver agreement at interpretation of both DSA images and MDCT angiograms were the calf vessels, particularly the peroneal artery, because of differing interpretations of the vessel extent. For all readers, there was a tendency to overestimate the degree of stenosis, whereas instances of underestimation were few. Although a statistically significant difference ($p < 0.05$) between DSA and MDCT angiography was seen only in arteries graded 1 or 2, the erroneous interpretations did not result in any change in therapeutic approach. In fact, interobserver agreement was almost perfect even with regard to treatment recommendations [25].

Romano and coworkers (2004) compared intra-arterial DSA and four-channel MDCTA of the abdominal aorta and lower extremities prospectively in 42 consecutive untreated patients with PAOD (27 men, 15 women, age range 40–79 years) [26]. Overall sensitivity and specificity of MDCTA were 93% and 95%, respectively, with positive and negative predictive values of 90% and 97%. Independently from the examined region, 100% occlusions and normal arterial segments were correctly identified at MDCTA in all cases. The authors observed a slight decrease in MDCTA performance in the infrapopliteal arteries, particularly in sensitivity (85%) and positive predictive value (74%). However, even if the data pattern indicates a somewhat less accurate performance of MDCTA when analyzing infrapopliteal artery stenosis, the differences with the overall MDCTA performance and with the performance in the aortoiliac and femoropopliteal regions were found to be not statistically significant. It is important to point out that results analyzed on the basis of therapeutic approach when a consensus reading was obtained showed no statistical differences between the two imaging modalities [26].

In another prospective study by Portugaller et al. (2004), 50 patients (42 men, 8 women; age, 45–86 years; mean age, 68 ± 10 years) with peripheral arterial occlusive disease underwent multislice CTA and intra-arterial DSA within 7 days [27]. For detecting significant stenoses in all vessel regions, sensitivity and specificity ranged from 84% to 92% and from 74% to 78%, respectively, depending upon the post-processing technique employed.

In a recent study (2005), however, Edwards et al. have reported a much lower sensitivity than previously reported for sensitivity for treatable lesions (>50% stenosis), around 72–79% with a specificity of 93% [28]. The much lower sensitivity may be attributed to the utilization of volume-rendered software for this purpose rather than maximum intensity projection (MIP). Volumetric imaging combines the voxel processing of multiplanar reformation with the

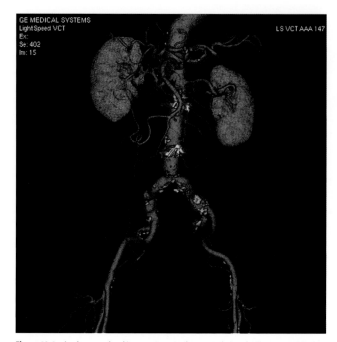

Figure 13.1. A volume-rendered image using a 64-detector LightSpeed VCT scanner (GE Medical Systems, Milwaukee Wisconsin). The calcifications are seen as white, the contrast-enhanced lumens of the aorta and vessels are red, and the kidneys are yellow.

techniques of tissue classification and surface shading with color codes to differentiate vascular from non-vascular structures (Figure 13.1). While any color schema can be applied, the most commonly employed create images in which contrast-enhanced blood (the lumen) is red, calcification is white, and other structures can be any other color. The degree of reliability with which these reformats adhere to the source data depends upon the choice of volume-rendering protocol (transfer function). However, as also reported by others, [18,21], 7% of segments that were visible with MDCTA in this study were not seen on DSA and were exclusively downstream to long-segment occlusions.

To the best of our knowledge there is only one study each that has evaluated the relative efficacy of 4-channel compared with 8-channel MDCTA and with 16-slice MDCTA, respectively [29,30]. In the study by Karcaaltincaba et al., both the 4- and 8-channel MDCT had scan coverage from iliac arteries to the level of the proximal femoral arteries [29]. For 4-channel MDCT, nominal slice thickness and beam pitch were 1.25 mm and 1.5, respectively, whereas for 8-channel MDCT they were 1.25 mm and 1.35 or 1.65, respectively. Compared with 4-channel MDCT, 8-channel MDCT aortoiliac angiography decreased contrast load (mean 45% decrease: 144 mL versus 83 mL of 300 mg iodine/mL contrast material) and decreased acquisition time (mean 51% shorter: 34.4 seconds versus 16.9 seconds) without a significant change in mean aortic enhancement (299 HU versus 300 HU, $p > 0.05$). As compared to 4-channel MDCT, aortoiliac CT angiography with 8-channel MDCT produces equivalent z-axis resolution with deceased contrast load and acquisition time without increased radiation exposure [29].

Wicky et al. (2004) performed a study to assess the level of vascular enhancement of gadolinium-enhanced aortoiliac computed tomographic (CT) angiography with a 16-detector row CT scanner and compared it with the results of previous similar studies that used four-detector row CT units [30]. Gadolinium-enhanced CT angiograms were obtained in 10 consecutive patients with contraindication to iodinated contrast medium with use of a 16-detector row CT scanner. In the region of interest, attenuation measurements (in HU) were obtained from the proximal abdominal aorta to the common femoral arteries during unenhanced, gadolinium-enhanced, and delayed acquisitions. The results were compared to those in the 15 consecutive patients who most recently had similar examinations performed on a four-detector row CT unit. Phantom studies with diluted gadolinium were conducted to compare attenuation between CT units. On four-detector row CT, throughout the scan length, mean enhancement values were 53.8 HU $\pm$ 5.3 and 15.0 HU $\pm$ 2.6 for gadolinium-enhanced and delayed series, respectively. For the 16-detector row CT unit, they were 76.1 HU $\pm$ 3.4 and 21.3 HU $\pm$ 1.3, respectively. As a result of a shorter scan time and a more optimal start time, the 16-detector row CT unit provided significantly greater and more consistent enhancement throughout the scan length compared with the four-detector row CTA. Both these studies demonstrate an overall better efficacy of 8–16-slice MDCTA compared to 4-slice scanners. We eagerly await more studies describing the diagnostic ability of identifying stenotic peripheral artery lesions. The potential of larger volumes of coverage with 40-and 64-detector-row MDCT will undoubtedly produce even greater accuracy, with lower contrast requirements and larger volumes of coverage per rotation. Due to lack of motion of the target vasculature, electron beam tomography (which improves temporal resolution) holds no distinct advantage in this application.

Other Applications

Assessment of Peripheral Arterial Bypass Grafts

Peripheral arterial bypass graft surgery is an established treatment for symptomatic PAOD when percutaneous interventional treatments have failed or are considered ineffective. However, around 30% of patients develop graft-related complications within the first 2 years after surgery [31]. Early identification of failing grafts by effective postoperative surveillance of peripheral arterial bypass grafts often averts impending graft failure and improves the secondary bypass graft patency rate [31].

Due to its non-invasive nature, as well as its rapid availability and access, low cost and high accuracy, duplex ultrasonography is considered to be a primary screening technique to detect of bypass graft patency as well com-

plications [32]. Apart from US, magnetic resonance (MR) angiography can also be used as a secondary technique in the assessment of peripheral arterial bypass grafts. However, the limited spatial resolution of the modality and the fact that vascular clips may simulate graft stenosis are potential limitations of MR angiography for graft assessment. Also there is a paucity of data regarding the use of MR angiography in the detection of graft-related arteriovenous fistulas, considering they are potential complications of peripheral bypass grafts [33].

Due to its high spatial resolution and lack of motion artifacts, CTA is a promising modality in the evaluation of graft patency (Figure 13.2). In a recent study, Willmann et al. investigated the technical feasibility of 4-slice MDCTA in the assessment of peripheral arterial bypass grafts and evaluated its accuracy and reliability in the detection of graft-related complications (graft stenosis, aneurysmal changes, and arteriovenous fistulas) in 65 consecutive patients with 85 peripheral arterial bypass grafts [34]. Each bypass graft was divided into three segments (proximal anastomosis, course of the graft body, and distal anastomosis), resulting in 255 segments. Image quality was rated as excellent in 250 (98%) and good in 252 (99%) of 255 bypass segments, respectively. When compared with duplex US and conventional DSA, sensitivity and specificity values of more than 95% were achieved by both readers with MDCT angiography for the diagnosis of arterial bypass graft-related complications (Kappa = 0.86–0.99). Opacification greater than 150 HU in 98% of the arterial segments of the peripheral arterial bypass graft was achieved in this study. The robustness and reliability of MDCT angiography are reflected by excellent interobserver agreement. The excellent accuracy of MDCTA in assessing bypass grafts patency as well complications, reported by Willmann et al. [34], suggest that it may be incorporated into a comprehensive graft assessment strategy as a secondary morphologic modality after functional assessment of the bypass graft with duplex US and that it may replace conventional angiography or DSA for this purpose.

Assessment of Arterial Injuries of Extremities

Direct contrast material-enhanced arteriography is the examination performed to assess arterial integrity in patients with extremity trauma. Arteriography depicts injuries that require therapeutic intervention, such as occlusions, arteriovenous fistulas, and pseudoaneurysms. Although generally considered safe, catheter-based arteriography may be associated with complications that result from the procedure itself. In the setting of peripheral vascular trauma, CTA has been reported to be highly accurate in assessing complicated or partial occlusions, arteriovenous fistulas, intimal flaps, and psuedoaneursyms [1,35]. Especially in the emergency room setting, the increased acquisition speed and a dedicated contrast injection pro-

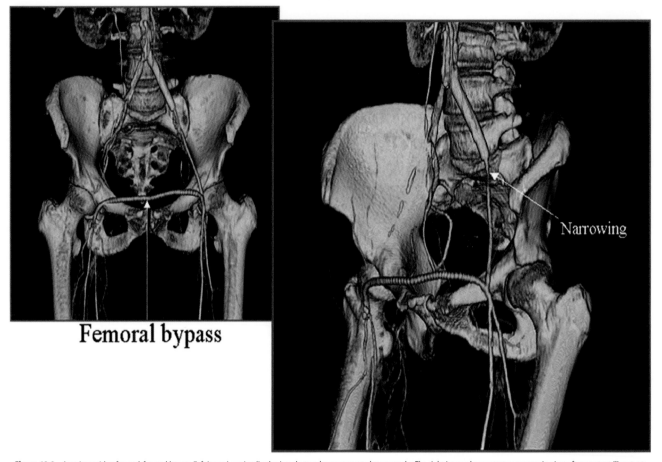

Figure 13.2. A patient with a femoral-femoral bypass (left image) as visualized using electron beam computed tomography. The right image demonstrates a narrowing just after a patent iliac stent.

tocol might add helpful information to the diagnostic workup of the traumatized patient.

Soto et al. compared helical CT arteriography with conventional angiography during a 19-month period in which 142 arterial segments in the proximal portions of the extremities of 139 patients were scanned for trauma. The sensitivity of CT arteriography was 95%, and the specificity was 99% for presence of arterial injuries as compared to conventional angiography [35]. In only 6 patients was additional conventional arteriography required for diagnosis because of technically inadequate or inconclusive CT examinations. However, a major limiting factor with MDCTA is that it is purely a diagnostic procedure, whereas catheter-based arteriography provides a means of therapy in patients with certain types of injuries. Most reports on endovascular therapy of arterial injuries have involved stent-graft repair of pseudoaneurysms or arteriovenous fistulas in the proximal arteries [36,37]. Therefore, catheter arteriography is still considered the first choice in patients with signs highly suggestive of pseudoaneurysm or fistula in proximal limb segments and at institutions in which endovascular intervention is an option [38].

MDCTA can also be used as a diagnostic tool in patients undergoing microsurgical reconstruction of the extremi-

ties [39]. When compared with traditional angiography, the acquisition time and examination costs were considerably lower. In a recent study, Bogdan et al. examined the utility of CT angiography for imaging of the upper extremity following trauma, as well as for patients with symptoms of vascular insufficiency [40]. Seventeen computed tomography angiograms were obtained in 14 patients over a 20-month period. All studies were obtained on an outpatient basis with contrast administered through a peripheral vein. All the studies demonstrated the pertinent anatomy and the intraoperative findings were as demonstrated in all cases. The average charge for CTA was $1140, compared to $3900 for traditional angiography. Greater experience with the technique is required before determining whether CTA should replace traditional and magnetic resonance angiography for preoperative imaging [39].

Detection of Deep Venous Thrombosis

Conventional venography is considered the gold standard technique for diagnosing deep venous thrombosis (DVT), allowing direct imaging of the inferior vena cava and deep veins of the calf, thigh, and pelvis. However, it is limited due to its invasive nature as well as being time-consuming and associated with post-procedure phlebitis. In addition, it does not adequately visualize the deep femoral veins, and is thus technically inadequate in 5–10% of the studies [41,42]. Sonography, owing to its high accuracy, non-invasiveness, speed, portability, and the fact that it does not require radiation or contrast material, has largely supplanted conventional venography in imaging the deep venous system of the thighs for thrombosis [43].

Peripheral venous CT may also be clinically valuable in demonstrating DVT especially the proximal extent into the iliac vein or inferior vena cava [8]. CT venography provides direct imaging of the inferior vena cava, pelvic, and lower extremity veins immediately after CT pulmonary angiography without injection of additional contrast material, adding only a few minutes to the examination. Indirect CT venography has been compared with US for the diagnosis of femoropopliteal DVT in several studies with sensitivity and specificity values for indirect CT venography in these studies ranging from 89% to 100% and 94% to 100%, respectively [41,44,45]. In Loud et al.'s study of 308 patients who had sonographic correlation, indirect CT venography was 97% sensitive and 100% specific for DVT in the thighs, and 4 patients had initially negative results from sonography and positive findings from CT venography, but repeated sonography helped to confirm the presence of DVT. More recently, Begemann et al. [42] obtained a sensitivity of 100% and a specificity of 96.6% in detecting DVT using MDCT venography in comparison with Doppler sonography.

Because DVT is the most important factor predisposing to pulmonary embolism (PE), a single examination capable of evaluating both the pulmonary arterial system and the pelvic and lower extremity venous system offers distinct advantages over other tests directed at either diagnosis alone [46]. Combined pulmonary angiography and venography of the extremities fills this role, and the results of one component can be used to guide therapy when the complementary component is not diagnostic, increasing the overall cost-effectiveness [46]. In recent years, studies have shown that indirect CT venography increases the diagnosis of thromboembolic disease by 15–38%, compared with the basic CT pulmonary angiographic examination [41,45]. In the largest study to date, 1590 consecutive patients underwent CT pulmonary angiography for suspected pulmonary embolism. In all these patients indirect CT venography was also performed from the iliac crest to the popliteal fossa [47]. Pulmonary embolism was detected in 243 (15%) of 1590 patients at CT pulmonary angiography, and DVT was detected in 148 (9%) patients at indirect CT venography. Among the 148 patients with DVT, pulmonary embolism was detected in 100 patients at CT pulmonary angiography. Thus, the addition of indirect CT venography to CT pulmonary angiography resulted in a 20% incremental increase in thromboembolic disease detection compared with that at CT pulmonary angiography alone (99% confidence interval: 17%, 23%).

Exposure to ionizing radiation is also greater with combined testing than with either alone, and this is particularly pertinent to radiosensitive tissues such as the ovaries and testes. Protocols using spaced sections rather than helical acquisition help reduce radiation doses but risk missing smaller venous thrombi. Although concern about exposure need not preclude clinically indicated examinations, physicians should be aware of the deleterious effects, particularly in younger patients, and remember that CT imaging contributes to the bulk of medical radiation exposure [46]. Rademaker et al., using a combined CT pulmonary angiographic and indirect CT venographic protocol, described patient gonadal doses on the order of 2.1–10.7 mSv, with variation between individuals and sex [48]. They found that the addition of indirect CT venography increases the gonadal radiation dose 500- to 2000-fold compared with CT pulmonary angiography alone. Fortunately, this increase in gonadal dose is well below the thresholds for deterministic radiation effects provided in the International Commission on Radiological Protection Publication 60, or ICRP-60, guidelines. In part because of these issues, the value of combining CT venography with CT pulmonary angiography is still debated, and in many institutions is not routinely included in the CT of pulmonary arteries protocol [47].

Scan Protocols

The scan parameters for a particular examination often require tailoring to the area of interest, the desired coverage, as well as the technical capabilities of the scanner [16]. The approach to image acquisition depends upon the detector configuration and the desired coverage [6]. The recently introduced faster scanners have had a profound effect on the angiographic study of the inflow and runoff vessels. Table 13.1 describes the scan parameters used in conjunction with 4-, 8- and 16-slice MDCT [9,10,49,50]. Compared to a 4-slice system, scan times are approximately

Table 13.1. Proposed scan parameters with 4, 8, and 16 slices for peripheral MDCTA

	4-slice MDCT	8-slice MDCT	16-slice MDCT
Collimation	2.5 mm	1.25 mm	0.75 mm
Slice thickness	3.0 mm	1.0–1.5 mm	1.0 mm
Reconstruction interval	1.5 mm	1 mm	0.8 mm
Gantry rotation	0.5 s	0.5 s	0.5 s
Table increment/360° gantry rotation	15 mm	16.75 mm	33 mm
Table feed	30 mm/s	27 mm/s	36 mm/s
Tube voltage	120 kV	100 mA	100 mA
Tube current	160 mA	100 mA	100 mA
Contrast concentration	300 mg/mL	350 mg/mL	350 mg/mL
Acquisition time	35–70 s	44–52 s	33–39 s
Number of slices	<1300	<1625	<2600

Adapted from Becker et al. [7], Jakobs et al. [9], Schoepf et al. [10], Fleischmann [49], Duddalwar [50].

3 times faster with 8-slice MDCT and 6 times faster with 16-slice MDCT scanners. The slice thickness usually depends upon the capabilities of the MDCT scanner [9]. A 4-slice MDCT usually allows for a complete assessment of 1200–1400 mm scan range within 40–50 seconds using 4 × 2.5 mm collimation. Usually, 16-slice MDCT covers this whole range with a collimation of 16 × 0.75 mm [9].

Electron beam tomography is performed using the continuous volume mode (Chapter 1), whereby the scanner simulates the MDCT, by taking continuous images of the volume of interest, without gating or pause. In this mode, the scanner can take 10 images per second, covering 1.5 mm to 6 mm per slice. Thus, large areas can be scanned with minimal contrast use. The most common protocols employed increase the image acquisition time from 100 ms per image to 200–300 ms per image, to improve tissue penetration and reduce image noise. Still, approximately 80 mL of contrast is all that is necessary to complete a runoff study.

Contrast Issues

An ideal CTA requires a combination of fine spatial resolution and perhaps most importantly "optimal intramural enhancement" synchronized with image acquisition [51]. However, it is dependent on a number of factors such as cardiac output, intravenous location, rate of injection, and pharmacokinetics of the contrast medium [50]. With faster acquisitions, contrast media delivery becomes more critical. In general, shorter acquisition times reduce the total amount of contrast media needed, but potentially require higher injection rates – or more precisely higher iodine administration. It is important to consider the following contrast issues while performing a peripheral examination.

Scanning Delay

In patients with CVD, the contrast transit time may be variable. Fleischmann et al. reported that the median transit time for contrast bolus from the aortopopliteal artery is 8 seconds (range 4–24 seconds) [52]. Thus, from a peripheral venous injection, the typical scan delays of 15 seconds for cardiac CT (Chapter 1) must now be further delayed by 8–10 seconds to allow the contrast to flow to the peripheral targets for imaging. The aortopopliteal transit time averages 10 seconds, representing an average contrast flow rate of 65 mm/s. There is significant variability among patients, however, with a minimum of 4 seconds (177 mm/s) and a maximum of 24 seconds (30 mm/s) – almost a 4-fold difference. It is important to note that there is no correlation between contrast flow rate and clinical stage of disease [7]. More likely, cardiac output and ejection fraction play a bigger role in the transit times for all contrast studies. As a result, the scan delay should not be estimated on the clin-

ical stage or degree of PAOD and contrast transit times are not predictable by any means other than direct measurement. Correct timing can be obtained by measuring the contrast time from a test bolus injection, or by automated bolus triggering [50]. In cases of peripheral vasculature the determination of delay time by a test bolus is generally considered more reliable than tracking the contrast media bolus [7,9]. The optimal delay time corresponds to the peak arrival time of a test bolus either in the abdominal artery or the popliteal artery or both if severe stenosis is suspected [7,9]. Several studies have proposed the use of a dual phase contrast injection protocol for a uniform vascular enhancement [7]. The dual measurement of the peak arrival time of the contrast media might compensate for significant differences concerning the arterial inflow in both legs [9].

Injection Flow Rates and Contrast Medium Volumes

The injection rate, the volume of the contrast, and the duration of injection all have interrelated effects on the course of arterial enhancement [49]. An optimum injection rate is important to achieve homogeneous opacification as well as good opacification of the smaller vessels. The contrast density level and synchronization of the contrast medium injection with image acquisition is critical [51]. This becomes especially important with the utilization of faster scanners (16–64 slices), as a higher injection rate is required to ensure sufficient filling of the peripheral arteries [9].

In his initial description of scanning of peripheral arteries with 4-MDCT, Rubin et al. used 180 mL of iodinated contrast medium injected at a rate of 3.5 mL/s, which results in a 51-second injection. Although the contrast injection is nearly 20 seconds less than the scan duration, the preliminary experience suggested that excellent arterial opacification is achieved throughout the scan volume [18]. This may be attributable to the substantial delay that tends to occur when blood travels from the aorta through the runoff vessels. Recent papers have reported that an injection rate of 3.5–4 mL/s with 300 mg iodine/mL will be able to provide sufficient enhancement of the peripheral vasculature [9,18,21,22].

The total amount of contrast media necessary depends on the scan duration [3]. With the feed of the CT table the scan follows the contrast bolus down to the periphery. Therefore, the duration of the contrast injection may be 5–10 seconds shorter than the actual scanning time [7,49]. A total volume of 120–160 mL of contrast media may be necessary to achieve sufficient enhancement of the entire vascular tree [7]. Faster scan times substantially reduce the total time needed for contrast material; however, the possibility to "outrun" the bolus at maximum table speed in patients with PAOD exists. As a result in these patients the table feed must not exceed 50 mm/s to run ahead of the contrast media bolus [7,49]. If the scanner can acquire data faster than that, then the scanning delay should be appropriately increased to allow the bolus to fill vessels distal to occluded segments. Recent CT technology with data acquisition of up to 16 slices per rotation enables scan duration to be reduced to less than 18 seconds. This can result in the potential reduction of contrast from approximate 150 mL in 4-slice MDCT systems to 80 mL in 16-slice CT scanners [53]. The 64-slice scanners now promise to cover this same territory in only 5–8 seconds, but "outrunning the contrast" will pose a significant risk if maximum speeds are used. Estimated contrast dose requirements drop to 50 mL for these newest scanners with great volume coverage.

The injection speed of the contrast can be reduced accordingly if higher contrast media is used [9]. Salute et al. have shown that the injection can be further reduced if a higher iodine concentration of 370–400 mg/mL is used [54]. Venditti et al. [55] reported that a higher iodine concentration provides greater vascular enhancement in MDCTA of the runoff vessels, allowing delivery of a greater amount of iodine. Thus contrast agents with elevated concentrations might become even more useful when even faster CT scanners with added detector rows become available in which the injection temporal window is further decreased [55].

Saline Chaser

The use of a saline chaser serves not only to reduce the amount of contrast medium needed but also prevents streaking artifacts. The saline chaser can be used by afterloading the contrast medium in a single barrel injector or more simply and accurately by using one of the double barrel injectors available [50]. In a recent study, Schoellnast et al. demonstrated that administration of a saline solution flush after the contrast material bolus in aortoiliac multi-slice CT angiography allows a further reduction of contrast material dose of approximately 17% without impairing the mean aortoiliac attenuation [56].

Post-processing

Image reconstruction is nearly as critical as the technique by which data are acquired in determining the diagnostic quality of the final product [16]. Various 3-D reformatting techniques are currently used in practice to aid in the visualization of peripheral vascular structures and their anatomic relationships. The most commonly used reformatting techniques include maximum intensity projection (MIP), multiplanar reformation (MPR), curved planar reformation (CPR), and volume rendering (VR). See Chapter 4 for more information regarding reconstruction techniques. Since all these techniques rely on contrast differences between the enhanced vascular lumen and surrounding structures, it is important that oral contrast not be given prior to the CT examination [3–6,57,58].

Maximum intensity projection is similar to conventional angiography in that it is a projection technique (Figures 13.3 and 13.4) [3]. The MIP algorithm, one of the most commonly used formats, has the capability to reveal the entire vascular tree in one image [50]. A ray is projected along the dataset in a user-selected direction and the

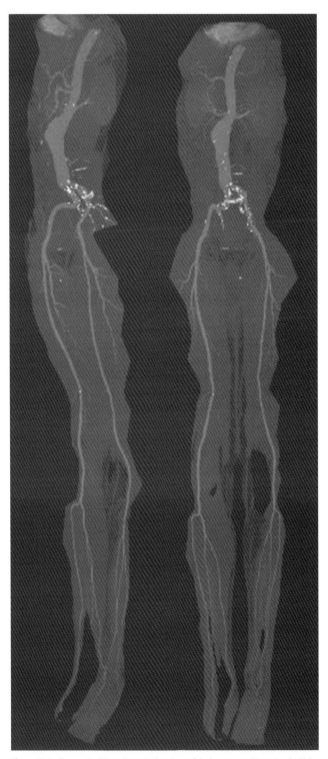

Figure 13.3. Two maximal intensity projection views of the lower extremities using the Light-Speed16, covering 1350 mm in 38 s, with a protocol of 16 × 1.25 mm slices. Larger slice thickness would allow for coverage at a much faster rate. Images courtesy Dr L. Tanenbaum, JFK, New Jersey.

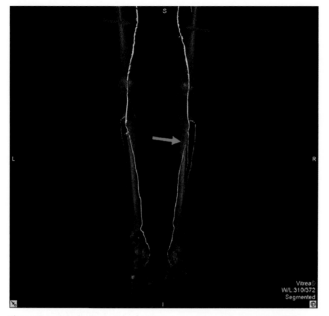

Figure 13.4. A maximal intensity image demonstrating dense calcifications in the mid-femoral arteries bilaterally (red arrows), making final clinical decision-making more difficult regarding the presence of high-grade disease of this region.

highest voxel value along the ray becomes the pixel value of the 2-D MIP image [50]. Usually only the density values of contrast or calcification are depicted, and regardless of where they are along the *x*-, *y*-, or *z*-axes, all such values will be reduced to a single plane [3]. However, the following issues need to be considered. Firstly, calcified plaques may cause misinterpretation of MIP images, especially at iliac, superficial femoral and popliteal levels (Figure 13.3). In such cases of heavy and circumferential calcifications, multiangle viewing of vessels with MIP display provides limited information. In the presence of extensive calcified plaques, especially in the distal small tibial arteries, it is difficult to produce MIP images with good diagnostic value. Underestimation or overestimation of arterial stenosis due to vessel wall calcifications on CT angiograms with MIP has been reported in several studies. Continuous calcification of the wall of an artery may cause a false diagnosis of patency, whereas the process of erasing these calcifications may result in a false diagnosis of high-grade stenosis or occlusion. When dense calcifications are present, the end product is of no, or questionable, diagnostic value [3,25]. Since the virtual rays used to generate MIP images are parallel, an MIP generated in an antero-posterior direction is identical to that generated in a posterior to anterior direction. Calcification of the anterior and posterior wall of the vessel along with the contrast-enhanced lumen in between are all depicted in a single plane. Volume rendering gives no information on lower-density tissues such as thrombus, and calcifications can make the VR or MIP image less diagnostic (Figure 13.4). With the MIP technique, the images are displayed with no surface shading or other devices to provide information

about the depth of the rendering, thus causing difficulty in assessing the 3-D relationships. The creation of MIP images usually involves removal of bony structures from the source images, and as a result is very time-intensive [16]. However, more powerful workstation applications allow for more rapid evaluation and processing, so this is no longer a significant limitation using any reconstruction technique. In spite of its limitations, MIP is considered to represent the best algorithm to display very fine details of PAOD [6,16] (Figure 13.5).

Multiplanar reformation (MPR) involves reconstruction of source data into sections in any arbitrarily defined plane, typically an oblique 2-D plane, and thus is potentially limited by vessel curvature and course as they are not confined to a single plane [3,16]. Similar to MPR, CPR is a single voxel thick tomogram, but it is capable of demonstrating an uninterrupted longitudinal cross-section because the display plane curves along the structure of interest (Figure 13.6) [5]. Curved planar reformations can be subsequently "straightened" to display relative lumen diameter over long segments and facilitate display of the relative density contributions of patent lumen, plaque, and calcification [3]. CPR along with MIP is the tool most widely used for image reconstruction in MDCTA [59]. A CPR enables visualization of both hard and soft plaques and is especially useful in cases of circumferential calcium, where it permits examination of the lumen adjacent to the calcium including regions of stenosis [6]. This technique provides the most accurate information on the vascular flow channel even in the presentation of atherosclerotic plaque (Figure 13.6) [59]. CPR techniques are currently favored for measurements of stenoses and aneurysms, but because the plane of both MPR and CPR is user defined, it is important to always provide an orthogonal plane to ensure a true center measurement is obtained [3]. However it is limited in the sense that CPR images are highly operator dependent because any inaccuracy in the selection of points that define a vessel may result in artifactual pseudostenoses [16]. Also, since CPR images are only one voxel thick, small or thin structures such as a dissection flap may not be included in a given CPR image, making it important to always generate at least two CPR images of a given structure in orthogonal planes. This task is simple and quick to perform once the points defining the plane have been selected (i.e., the orthogonal CPR image does not require a second set of points to be designated). According to Rubin and Fleischmann [6], it does not seem to provide as good an overview of the peripheral vasculature as does MIP.

Volume rendering represents the latest and most computer-intensive method for 3-D reconstruction (Figures 13.1, 13.7–13.10). VR is probably the most complex of the 3-D reconstruction techniques in widespread use. In general, the voxels within a dataset are assigned both a degree of opacity and a color as a function of their attenuation values. By changing this function, which is represented by a user-defined curve where either color or

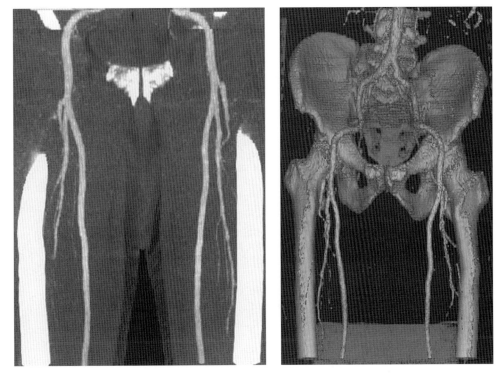

Figure 13.5. A maximal intensity projection image (left) and shaded surface display (right) demonstrating the same patient, who has essentially normal peripheral arteries bilaterally.

opacity is plotted against attenuation, structures of different attenuation can either be emphasized or de-emphasized (even to the point of invisibility) [16]. This technique renders the entire volume of data rather than just the surfaces and thus potentially provides more information than a surface model [50]. Volume rendering is a

technique that preserves all the density values found within a ray in the final 3-D image. For example, the VR image of a vessel will contain the different density values of the contrast, calcium, thrombus, vessel wall, muscle, and fat. There

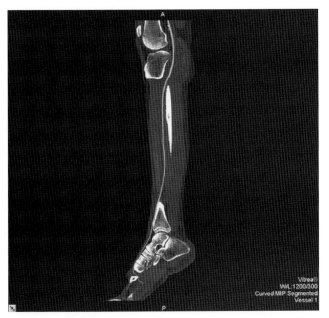

Figure 13.6. A curved maximal intensity projection of the popliteal and tibial artery using a 64-slice MDCT scanner (Toshiba).

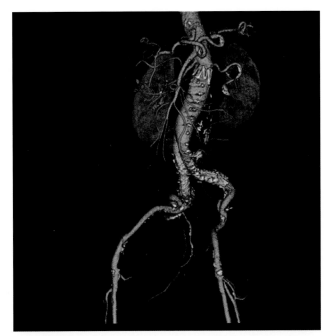

Figure 13.7. A volume-rendered image of an abdominal aorta and iliac arteries, including the kidneys. The white spots running down the aortic wall represent atherosclerotic plaques (calcified plaques). Volume rendering leaves the three-dimensional anatomy intact, so spatial relationships can be determined.

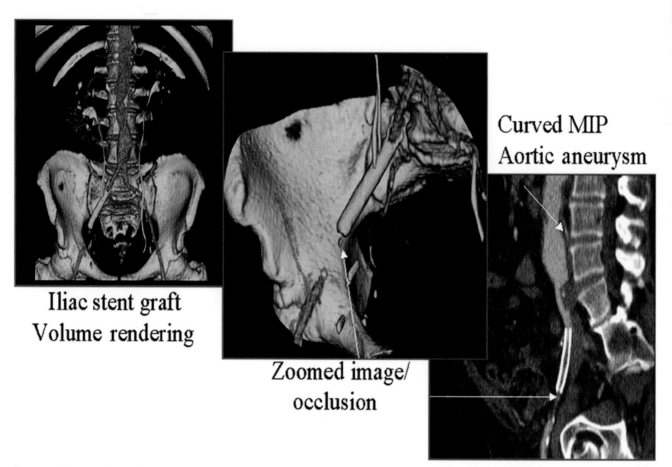

Curved MIP
Aortic aneurysm

Iliac stent graft
Volume rendering

Zoomed image/
occlusion

Figure 13.8. Patient with a history of right external iliac stent placement, now undergoing CT for follow-up. Subtotal occlusion of the stent can be seen, with no distal flow on volume rendering, and minimal contrast enhancement of a small lumen on MIP. Maximal intensity projection demonstrates smaller structures, so the residual lumen is visible using that technique. Imaging performed on EBCT.

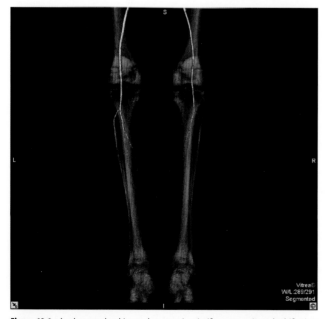

Figure 13.9. A volume-rendered image demonstrating significant tortuosity and calcifications (white structures running down the abdominal aorta). This image was performed with a 64-detector MDCT (LightSpeed VCT).

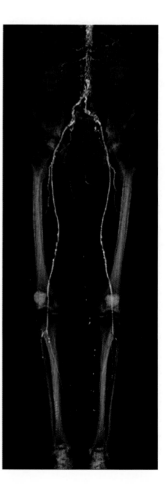

Figure 13.10. A volume-rendered image of the entire lower extremity, with bones left in the image. This allows for spatial relationships, a potential advantage when needing to know what vessel is diseased (i.e., popliteal versus femoral).

SSD } Shaded surface display
Discards all pixels <200 HU
VR } volume RENDERING
Pixels assigned a value.
MIP — { Maximal INTENSITY Projection
Relies on density differences
good for smaller vessels
+ LIMA

MPR → multiplanar Reformatting
i.e "curved surface reformation"
multiplanar reformatting

developed rapidly, substantial improvements must be made before physicians are freed from the confines of mandatory transverse section review [61].

Advantages and Limitations of MDCT Angiography

MDCTA has many advantages over traditional angiography. As compared to conventional angiography, CTA is able to demonstrate more anatomical details as well as having the capability to edit the overlying structures to provide unparalleled spatial details. It also allows 3-D visualization from any angle and in any direction, which cannot be achieved with projection techniques such as DSA [25]. Importantly, CT angiography eliminates the risk associated with arterial puncture as the contrast is delivered through a peripheral vein. Furthermore, extensive evidence exists regarding the reduced acquisition time, and MDCT angiography costs significantly less than DSA. In fact, CTA may effectively eliminate the required hospital stay following a conventional angiogram (approximately 6 hours) [40]. All these features make MDCTA not only an attractive imaging modality for elective assessment of peripheral vasculature, but also highly feasible for assessing arterial and venous trauma on an emergency basis [40]. The estimated time needed for MDCT peripheral angiography is 15 minutes for obtaining the dataset, and 10 minutes for post-processing, significantly faster than either invasive angiography or MR angiography.

Though MDCTA of peripheral arteries has great potential, it remains an emerging application with some limitations. As with all CTA examinations, radiation and iodinated contrast media are an issue [3]. Among imaging modalities that use ionizing radiation, CT produces one of the highest radiation doses per examination. Although CT accounts for only 5% of all radiographic imaging studies, the total radiation from CT imparted on the population accounts for 40–67% of all medical radiation [47]. Heuschmid et al. recently showed an effective dose of 6.70 mSv in male and 7.58 mSv in female patients [53]. The radiation exposure for a peripheral CTA examination is considered be around 4 times less than for DSA [18]. The relatively high dose of radiation in conventional angiography is predominately influenced by the large number of images acquired, with fluoroscopy accounting for less than 20% of the effective whole-body dose. Current scanners employ dose modulation tools, which alter the radiation dose depending on the type of body part and its size. Thus, a higher dose would be applied for aortoiliac vasculature of the abdomen and pelvis, but the dose is automatically reduced for the runoff of the legs [3]. Wintersperger et al. recently described a low-dose 16-slice MDCTA protocol for the abdominal vessels. Tube voltage was reduced from 120 to 100 kVp, thus allowing significant reduction in radiation

information. Rubin also considers this data "explosion" to be the greatest challenge of the new scanning technology [61]. As pointed out by Edwards et al., the challenge, however, for peripheral MDCTA is 2-fold: how is this large amount of information best analyzed, and how can it be presented to cardiologists, surgeons, and endovascular interventional radiologists in a standard angiographical format to assist treatment planning [28]. Current 3-D workstations substantially facilitate the analysis of large volumetric datasets. While their capabilities continue to exposure without reduction in signal-to-noise ratio and contrast-to-noise ratio [62].

Apart from the radiation doses, MDCT peripheral angiography is limited in some cases due to severe calcifications and time-consuming reconstruction procedures. While the reconstruction times have dramatically improved with newer workstations (it is literally possible to reconstruct an entire peripheral tree in seconds, while excluding venous structures and bones), severe vascular calcifications remain problematic (similar to coronary CTA) [53]. Stents most likely are not as big a limitation in the peripheral vessels as with the coronary vessels, as the often larger diameter stents have less problems with partial volume effects and blooming artifacts obscuring the lumen.

It is important to acknowledge that most of the data to date reflect performance on larger above-the-knee vessels. The ultimate clinical test of MDCTA for peripheral vascular disease will be its accuracy below the knee and, in particular, for small pedal vessels [3,21,24]. Heuschmid et al. evaluated 23 patients with peripheral arterial disease who underwent both multislice CTA (4-row) and intra-arterial DSA of the lower extremities [53]. Out of 442 segments proximal to the trifurcation, 386 were correctly assessed by multislice CTA (87.3%), and out of 126 segments distal to the trifurcation, 101 were rated correctly (80.2%). The smaller size of these vessels further complicates imaging with MDCT. Nonetheless, as a non-invasive modality, it has great promise, with 64-slice studies being able to cover the vascular territory in 10–15 seconds.

A past limitation included the lack of adequate post-processing software allowing for a fast and reliable display of peripheral arteries [7]. However, with recent developments, the solutions are now available. Using most current workstations, reconstructions (whether MIP, CMR, or volume rendering) can be done in seconds. The dose efficiency of CT detectors is increasing with added detector rows, and, most importantly, renewed awareness of radiation issues is taking hold in the medical community. On the data acquisition side, sophisticated means for reducing radiation dose are being implemented [10]. A very important step is the ongoing improvement in the performance of sophisticated software tools aimed at improving the visualization and characterization of vascular anatomy and pathology at multislice CT [10]. It is hoped that all these technological advancements will allow the minimally invasive MDCTA to play a major role in evaluating peripheral vasculature as it currently has in other vascular beds.

Some important features of MDCTA (4–16-slice scanners) are:

- A diagnostic examination can be obtained in 95% of cases.
- Sensitivity and specificity values of 95% for the detection of suprapopliteal stenoses.
- Sensitivity of 90% and specificity of 85–90% for grading infrapopliteal lesions.

- Diagnostic performance in critical limb ischemia and in diabetic patients with advanced disease could be reduced due to calcifications of the smaller vessels.
- Good interobserver correlations have been reported.
- Rate of false-negative examinations is very low (<2%).

Other Modalities

Sonography, which is used by some clinicians to depict the lower extremity arterial system, is relatively inexpensive and non-invasive and uses no ionizing radiation or contrast material (at present). Sonography has some major disadvantages: it remains a time-consuming and operator-dependent technique, with unsatisfactory results in the evaluation of lesions located in the calves or in the detection of lesions distal to high-grade stenosis [63,64]. Even in good hands, inconclusive duplex ultrasound examination is common due to frequent inability to visualize the abdominal or pelvic segments, calcified areas that cause acoustic shadowing, or slow flow downstream from occlusive disease [63,64]. Moneta et al. studied 150 patients and demonstrated that the sensitivity of sonography for depicting greater than 50% stenosis in the popliteal artery was only 67% [63]. In a recent meta-analysis, sonography was shown to have substantially lower sensitivity than MR for depicting peripheral vascular disease [64].

Magnetic resonance angiography (MRA) of the lower limbs has improved with the use of gadolinium-enhanced 3-D sequences together with improved patient tables, fast 3-D gradient-recalled echo acquisitions, as well as MR power injectors, dedicated surface coils, and state-of-the-art MR hardware and software [65]. Studies have demonstrated sensitivities and specificities of 81–97% and 60–96%, respectively [66,67]. There are many compelling advantages to the use of MR imaging, which in addition to the aforementioned benefits include less primary reconstructions owing to coronal acquisitions and no interference from high-signal-intensity non-arterial structures that are analogous to bone at CT angiography. Lack of ionizing radiation is a major advantage of MRA; as a result, patients with preexisting renal disease can undergo imaging without risk. It is these patients – especially those with diabetes – who often have concurrent peripheral vascular disease [65]. However, the typical patient undergoing MDCTA for peripheral vascular disease is relatively old, and MDCTA of the abdominal aorta and lower extremities has been shown to expose patients to a dose 3.9 times lower than that of DSA of the same area [2].

However, there are many reasons for CT angiography to be possibly a more attractive alternative to MR angiography. Currently, implanted pacemakers and defibrillators are known contraindications to MR imaging and may be common in patients with PAOD. Furthermore, patients with any of the following have strong contraindications: metallic valves, electronic infusion pumps, ferromagnetic intracranial clips or intra-ocular bodies, and epicardial electrodes. Claustrophobia is still a major problem with MR, affecting 2–10% of patients. Also therapeutically relevant mural calcifications are not depicted by MRA and the presence of endovascular metallic stents can result in significant artifacts [2]. Stents with EBT or MDCTA are not as problematic as with coronary CT, due to the larger diameters of stents often employed (Figure 13.9).

Compared to MRA, MDCTA has an increased volume coverage permitting acquisition of the aortoiliac arteries and the peripheral vessels of the lower extremity within one acquisition, combined with a high spatial resolution [18]. The limited spatial resolution of MR angiography is problematic, especially when evaluating vessels with small diameters. Rubin et al. achieved voxel dimensions of 0.7 × 0.7 × 1.25–3.2 mm to image the entirety of the lower extremity arterial system in 60–85 seconds with four-channel multidetector row CT. These voxel dimensions are 5 to 14 times smaller than those achieved with current MR angiographic techniques [66] and thus result in higher spatial resolution acquisition. Willmann et al. has demonstrated that voxel volumes are 9–19 times larger with MR angiography than with MDCT angiography and as a result may be an issue when assessing smaller vessel diameters or finer luminal abnormalities [23]. MR angiography has been shown to have lower specificity and diagnostic accuracy in the infrapopliteal region. Also, the possibility of localizing the arterial wall may be an advantage of MDCT angiography. Another potential advantage of MDCT angiography over MR angiography relates to the limited anteroposterior coverage of MR angiography, as a result of which additional vascular abnormalities, such as coexisting collateral pathways or extra-arterial findings, may be missed [23]. The short acquisition time also results in patient's preference for CT angiography for evaluating peripheral vasculature. According to the Willmann et al., the examination time (time from patient entry into the MR or CT suite until the source data are available for 3-D reconstruction), is significantly shorter for MDCT than for MR angiography (24 minutes versus 35 minutes; $p < 0.001$) [23]. In the same study, MDCT angiography was considered more comfortable than MR angiography and DSA [23]. There was no statistically significant difference in patient acceptance between MR angiography and DSA, although on average, patients rated MR angiography as more comfortable than DSA. However, time for generation of standardized 3-D reconstructions (including MIPs and volume-rendered images) was significantly more time-consuming for CT datasets than for MR datasets [23]. However, the workstations have progressed so quickly with CT, that currently it takes less than 1 minute to generate a complete MIP or volume-rendered dataset with EBT or MDCT angiography of the peripheral tree.

Another benefit of faster coverage with CT (especially compared to MR) is avoiding venous enhancement (contamination). Since the veins can fill just as brightly as the artery, and they run parallel, the artery is sometimes difficult to separate out from the venous distributions. The longer the acquisition, the more time the contrast-enhanced blood has to fill the veins, and cause this difficulty in imaging. The faster scanners, with more detectors, can completely avoid this, by scanning almost as fast as the contrast travels down the arterial circulation. MR, with significantly longer acquisition times, suffers greatly from this problem, and that is why many experts are moving to CT with peripheral imaging, in lieu of other methods. This is another reason why MR is thought to perform less well in the infrapopliteal arterial beds.

In general, the use of MR angiography or MDCT angiography in patients without contraindication to either modality may be influenced by several factors, including examination time, time for generation of 3-D reconstructions, time for image analysis, patient acceptance, and cost.

Cost-effectiveness

To date, little information is available on the cost-effectiveness of CT angiography compared with DSA for peripheral arterial disease and patents presenting with intermittent claudication. Visser et al. in a study used a decision model to compare the societal cost-effectiveness of CTA with that of gadolinium-enhanced MRA [68]. Cost-effectiveness was assessed in terms of the following parameters: the sensitivity for detection of significant stenoses, the proportion of cases requiring additional workup with DSA because of equivocal results, and the costs of MDCT angiography in the workup of patients with intermittent claudication. Main outcome measures were quality-adjusted life years (QALYs) and lifetime costs. The base evaluation used 60-year-old men with severe intermittent claudication and an assumed incremental cost-effectiveness threshold of $100,000 per QALY. The study revealed that a specific set of targets would allow a CTA workup to compete cost-effectively with an MRA workup for patients suffering from intermittent claudication caused by significant stenosis. According to the authors, DSA would always be more cost-effective than CTA if both angioplasty and bypass surgery were considered as treatment options. However, if they assumed that CTA involved no risks and had the diagnostic accuracy of DSA, then CTA would be more cost-effective than DSA. In conclusion, compared with currently used imaging examinations such as MR angiography, MDCT angiography has the potential to be cost-effective in the evaluation of patients with intermittent claudication [68].

Within the context of a randomized controlled trial, Adriaensen et al. compared confidence ratings and recommendations for additional imaging between patient groups for which CT or DSA was the initial test of choice [69]. Computed tomography angiography compared to DSA resulted in a lower confidence score (7.2 versus 8.2) and consequently more recommendations for additional imaging (35% versus 14%). However, it must be kept in mind that the confidence scores of both imaging tests are far above the threshold of 5.5. Diagnostic imaging tests recommended after initial CT angiography were duplex US, selective DSA, and/or DSA. Imaging tests recommended after initial DSA were duplex US, CT, MR imaging, and selective DSA. This demonstrates MDCTA has a place in the diagnostic imaging workup of patients prior to revascularization. Identification of patients in whom CT angiography can be expected to provide sufficient information should help with patient selection in the future. [69] However, further prospective studies are also warranted comparing MDCTA to MR angiography in terms of cost effectiveness, as this analysis may also guide physicians in choosing one or the other modality.

Future Directions

Katz and Hon [65] asked an important question following the initial study by Rubin et al. demonstrating the feasibility of 4-slice MDCTA in assessing the peripheral vasculature: "Where does multi-detector row helical CT angiography of the lower extremities fit into current imaging algorithms, particularly when compared with gadolinium-enhanced MR angiography and conventional angiography?" Conventional angiography is still exclusively performed as part of or prior to angioplasty, stent placement, and other arterial interventional procedures. However, considering the recent track record of CT angiography in replacing many conventional diagnostic angiographic procedures, it would not be surprising if CTA of the lower extremity arterial system began to replace conventional diagnostic angiography.

With the advent of 16–64-slice multidetector scanners, a further increase in the scanning speed without requiring additional output from the X-ray tube is possible. An eight-channel 500 ms scanner could be used to image the entire aortoiliac system with a 1.0 or 2.5 mm nominal section thickness in 23 or 9 seconds, respectively. The abdominal aorta and lower extremity runoff to the ankles could be imaged with a 2.5 mm nominal section thickness in 22 seconds. With a 16-channel system, the abdominal aorta and lower extremity runoff could be imaged in 11 seconds. The entire vascular system, from head to toe, of a 170 cm tall person could be imaged in 14 seconds with 2.5 mm nominal section thickness and a table feed rate of 120 mm/s [20]. However, larger series are needed to evaluate MDCTA performance in these updated scanners and ways to overcome the limitations such as increased processing time, lower accuracy in infrapopliteal vessels, as well as methods to reduce radiation and contrast dose. The image quality from 64-slice scanners is staggering, and the diagnostic potential is not yet realized (Figures 13.9 and 13.10). Emerging studies have provided strong evidence that MDCTA is not only highly accurate and reproducible, but also cost- and time-effective, and is very likely to replace conventional angiography for assessment of peripheral vasculature in most cases.

References

1. Lawler LP, Fishman EK. Multidetector row computed tomography of the aorta and peripheral arteries. Cardiol Clin 2003;21:607–629.
2. Catalano C, Napoli A, Fraioli F, Venditti F, Votta V, Passariello R. Multidetector-row CT angiography of the infrarenal aortic and lower extremities arterial disease. Eur Radiol 2003;13(Suppl 5):M88–M93.
3. Liddell RP, Lawler LP. Multidetector row CT angiography in the evaluation of the lower arterial system. Appl Radiol 2004;34–42.
4. Rubin GD. MDCT imaging of the aorta and peripheral vessels. Eur J Radiol 2003;45(Suppl 1):S42–S49.
5. Rubin GD. 3-D imaging with MDCT. Eur J Radiol 2003;45(Suppl 1): S37–S41.
6. Rubin GD, Fleischmann D. CT angiography of the lower extremities. Appl Radiol 2004;45–51.
7. Becker CR, Wintersperger B, Jakobs TF. Multi-detector-row CT angiography of peripheral arteries. Semin Ultrasound CT MR 2003; 24:268–279.
8. Reimer P, Landwehr P. Non-invasive vascular imaging of peripheral vessels. Eur Radiol 1998;8:858–872.
9. Jakobs TF, Wintersperger BJ, Becker CR. MDCT-imaging of peripheral arterial disease. Semin Ultrasound CT MR 2004;25:145–155.
10. Schoepf UJ, Becker CR, Hofmann LK, et al. Multislice CT angiography. Eur Radiol 2003;13:1946–1961.
11. Lawrence JA, Kim D, Kent KC, Stehling MK, Rosen MP, Raptopoulos V. Lower extremity spiral CT angiography versus catheter angiography. Radiology 1995;194:903–908.
12. Rieker O, Duber C, Schmiedt W, von Zitzewitz H, Schweden F, Thelen M. Prospective comparison of CT angiography of the legs with intraarterial digital subtraction angiography. AJR Am J Roentgenol 1996;166:269–276.
13. Raptopoulos V, Rosen MP, Kent KC, Kuestner LM, Sheiman RG, Pearlman JD. Sequential helical CT angiography of aortoiliac disease. AJR Am J Roentgenol 1996;166:1347–1354.
14. Beregi JP, Djabbari M, Desmoucelle F, Willoteaux S, Wattinne L, Louvegny S. Popliteal vascular disease: evaluation with spiral CT angiography. Radiology 1997;203:477–483.
15. Mesurolle B, Qanadli SD, El Hajjam M, Goeau-Brissonniere OA, Mignon F, Lacombe P. Occlusive arterial disease of abdominal aorta and lower extremities: comparison of helical CT angiography with transcatheter angiography. Clin Imaging 2004;28:252–260.
16. Chow LC, Rubin GD. CT angiography of the arterial system. Radiol Clin North Am 2002;40:729–749.
17. Prokop M. Multislice CT angiography. Eur J Radiol 2000;36:86–96.
18. Rubin GD, Schmidt AJ, Logan LJ, Sofilos MC. Multi-detector row CT angiography of lower extremity arterial inflow and runoff: initial experience. Radiology 2001;221:146–158.
19. Boll DT, Lewin JS, Duerk JL, Smith D, Subramanyan K, Merkle EM. Assessment of automatic vessel tracking techniques in preoperative planning of transluminal aortic stent graft implantation. J Comput Assist Tomogr 2004;28:278–285.
20. Rubin GD, Shiau MC, Leung AN, Kee ST, Logan LJ, Sofilos MC. Aorta and iliac arteries: single versus multiple detector-row helical CT angiography. Radiology 2000;215:670–676.
21. Martin ML, Tay KH, Flak B, et al. Multidetector CT angiography of the aortoiliac system and lower extremities: a prospective comparison with digital subtraction angiography. AJR Am J Roentgenol 2003;180:1085–1091.
22. Ofer A, Nitecki SS, Linn S, et al. Multidetector CT angiography of peripheral vascular disease: a prospective comparison with intra-arterial digital subtraction angiography. AJR Am J Roentgenol 2003;180:719–724.

23. Willmann JK, Wildermuth S, Pfammatter T, et al. Aortoiliac and renal arteries: prospective intraindividual comparison of contrast-enhanced three-dimensional MR angiography and multi-detector row CT angiography. Radiology 2003;226:798–811.

24. Ota H, Takase K, Igarashi K, et al. MDCT compared with digital subtraction angiography for assessment of lower extremity arterial occlusive disease: importance of reviewing cross-sectional images. AJR Am J Roentgenol 2004;182:201–209.

25. Catalano C, Fraioli F, Laghi A, et al. Infrarenal aortic and lower-extremity arterial disease: diagnostic performance of multi-detector row CT angiography. Radiology 2004;231:555–563.

26. Romano M, Mainenti PP, Imbriaco M, et al. Multidetector row CT angiography of the abdominal aorta and lower extremities in patients with peripheral arterial occlusive disease: diagnostic accuracy and interobserver agreement. Eur J Radiol 2004;50:303–308.

27. Portugaller HR, Schoellnast H, Hausegger KA, Tiesenhausen K, Amann W, Berghold A. Multislice spiral CT angiography in peripheral arterial occlusive disease: a valuable tool in detecting significant arterial lumen narrowing? Eur Radiol 2004;14:1681–1687.

28. Edwards AJ, Wells IP, Roobottom CA. Multidetector row CT angiography of the lower limb arteries: a prospective comparison of volume-rendered techniques and intra-arterial digital subtraction angiography. Clin Radiol 2005;60:85–95.

29. Karcaaltincaba M, Foley D. Four- and eight-channel aortoiliac CT angiography: a comparative study. Cardiovasc Intervent Radiol 2005;28(2):169–172.

30. Wicky S, Greenfield A, Fan CM, et al. Aortoiliac gadolinium-enhanced CT angiography: improved results with a 16-detector row scanner compared with a four-detector row scanner. J Vasc Interv Radiol 2004;15:947–954.

31. Idu MM, Buth J, Hop WC, Cuypers P, van de Pavoordt ED, Tordoir JM. Vein graft surveillance: is graft revision without angiography justified and what criteria should be used? J Vasc Surg 1998;27:399–411.

32. Mills JL, Harris EJ, Taylor LM Jr, Beckett WC, Porter JM. The importance of routine surveillance of distal bypass grafts with duplex scanning: a study of 379 reversed vein grafts. J Vasc Surg 1990;12:379–386.

33. Nielsen TG, Djurhuus C, Pedersen EM, Laustsen J, Hasenkam JM, Schroeder TV. Arteriovenous fistulas aggravate the hemodynamic effect of vein bypass stenoses: an in vitro study. J Vasc Surg 1996;24:1043–1049.

34. Willmann JK, Mayer D, Banyai M, et al. Evaluation of peripheral arterial bypass grafts with multi-detector row CT angiography: comparison with duplex US and digital subtraction angiography. Radiology 2003;229:465–474.

35. Soto JA, Munera F, Morales C, et al. Focal arterial injuries of the proximal extremities: helical CT arteriography as the initial method of diagnosis. Radiology 2001;218:188–194.

36. Patel AV, Marin ML, Veith FJ, Kerr A, Sanchez LA. Endovascular graft repair of penetrating subclavian artery injuries. J Endovasc Surg 1996;3:382–388.

37. Dorros G, Joseph G. Closure of a popliteal arteriovenous fistula using an autologous vein-covered Palmaz stent. J Endovasc Surg 1995;2:177–181.

38. Bettmann MA, Robbins A, Braun SD, Wetzner S, Dunnick NR, Finkelstein J. Contrast venography of the leg: diagnostic efficacy, tolerance, and complication rates with ionic and nonionic contrast media. Radiology 1987;165:113–116.

39. Klein MB, Karanas YL, Chow LC, Rubin GD, Chang J. Early experience with computed tomographic angiography in microsurgical reconstruction. Plast Reconstr Surg 2003;112:498–503.

40. Bogdan MA, Klein MB, Rubin GD, McAdams TR, Chang J. CT angiography in complex upper extremity reconstruction. J Hand Surg [Br.] 2004;29:465–469.

41. Cham MD, Yankelevitz DF, Shaham D, et al. Deep venous thrombosis: detection by using indirect CT venography. The Pulmonary

42. Begemann PG, Bonacker M, Kemper J, et al. Evaluation of the deep venous system in patients with suspected pulmonary embolism with multi-detector CT: a prospective study in comparison to Doppler sonography. J Comput Assist Tomogr 2003;27:399–409.

43. Lim KE, Hsu WC, Hsu YY, Chu PH, Ng CJ. Deep venous thrombosis: comparison of indirect multidetector CT venography and sonography of lower extremities in 26 patients. Clin Imaging 2004;28:439–444.

44. Loud PA, Katz DS, Klippenstein DL, Shah RD, Grossman ZD. Combined CT venography and pulmonary angiography in suspected thromboembolic disease: diagnostic accuracy for deep venous evaluation. AJR Am J Roentgenol 2000;174:61–65.

45. Loud PA, Katz DS, Bruce DA, Klippenstein DL, Grossman ZD. Deep venous thrombosis with suspected pulmonary embolism: detection with combined CT venography and pulmonary angiography. Radiology 2001;219:498–502.

46. Kanne JP, Lalani TA. Role of computed tomography and magnetic resonance imaging for deep venous thrombosis and pulmonary embolism. Circulation 2004;109:I15–I21.

47. Cham MD, Yankelevitz DF, Henschke CI. Thromboembolic disease detection at indirect CT venography versus CT pulmonary angiography. Radiology 2005;234:591–594.

48. Rademaker J, Griesshaber V, Hidajat N, Oestmann JW, Felix R. Combined CT pulmonary angiography and venography for diagnosis of pulmonary embolism and deep vein thrombosis: radiation dose. J Thorac Imaging 2001;16:297–299.

49. Fleischmann D. Present and future trends in multiple detector-row CT applications: CT angiography. Eur Radiol 2002;12(Suppl 2):S11–S15.

50. Duddalwar VA. Multislice CT angiography: a practical guide to CT angiography in vascular imaging and intervention. Br J Radiol 2004;77(Spec No 1):S27–S38.

51. Fleischmann D, Rubin GD, Bankier AA, Hittmair K. Improved uniformity of aortic enhancement with customized contrast medium injection protocols at CT angiography. Radiology 2000;214:363–371.

52. Fleischmann D. Aorto-popliteal bolus transit time in peripheral CT angiography: can fast acquisition outrun the bolus? Eur Radiol 2003;13:S268.

53. Heuschmid M, Krieger A, Beierlein W, et al. Assessment of peripheral arterial occlusive disease: comparison of multislice-CT angiography (MS-CTA) and intraarterial digital subtraction angiography (IA-DSA). Eur J Med Res 2003;8:389–396.

54. Salute L. Multi-slice computed tomography (MSCT) of the peripheral arteries. Clinical evaluation of a high contrast medium (400 mg/ml). Eur Radiol 2003;13:S268.

55. Venditti F. Contrast media administration in multi-detector-row spiral CT angiography (MDCTA) of peripheral arteries: optimization of contrast agent administration. Radiology 2003;229:542.

56. Schoellnast H, Tillich M, Deutschmann MJ, Deutschmann HA, Schaffler GJ, Portugaller HR. Aortoiliac enhancement during computed tomography angiography with reduced contrast material dose and saline solution flush: influence on magnitude and uniformity of the contrast column. Invest Radiol 2004;39:20–26.

57. Napoli A, Fleischmann D, Chan FP, et al. Computed tomography angiography: state-of-the-art imaging using multidetector-row technology. J Comput Assist Tomogr 2004;28(Suppl 1):S32–S45.

58. Chan FP, Rubin GD. MDCT angiography of pediatric vascular diseases of the abdomen, pelvis, and extremities. Pediatr Radiol 2005;35:40–53.

59. Fleischmann D. Future prospects in MDCT imaging. Eur Radiol 2003;13(Suppl 5):M127–M128.

60. Rieker O, Duber C, Neufang A, Pitton M, Schweden F, Thelen M. CT angiography versus intraarterial digital subtraction angiography for

assessment of aortoiliac occlusive disease. AJR Am J Roentgenol 1997;169:1133–1138.

61. Rubin GD. Data explosion: the challenge of multidetector-row CT. Eur J Radiol 2000;36:74–80.

62. Wintersperger BJ, Herzog P, Jakobs T, Reiser MF, Becker CR. Initial experience with the clinical use of a 16 detector row CT system. Crit Rev Comput Tomogr 2002;43:283–316.

63. Moneta GL, Yeager RA, Antonovic R, et al. Accuracy of lower extremity arterial duplex mapping. J Vasc Surg 1992;15:275–283.

64. Visser K, Hunink MG. Peripheral arterial disease: gadolinium-enhanced MR angiography versus color-guided duplex US – a meta-analysis. Radiology 2000;216:67–77.

65. Katz DS, Hon M. CT angiography of the lower extremities and aortoiliac system with a multi-detector row helical CT scanner: promise of new opportunities fulfilled. Radiology 2001;221:7–10.

66. Ruehm SG, Hany TF, Pfammatter T, Schneider E, Ladd M, Debatin JF. Pelvic and lower extremity arterial imaging: diagnostic performance of three-dimensional contrast-enhanced MR angiography. AJR Am J Roentgenol 2000;174:1127–1135.

67. Huber A, Heuck A, Baur A, et al. Dynamic contrast-enhanced MR angiography from the distal aorta to the ankle joint with a step-by-step technique. AJR Am J Roentgenol 2000;175:1291–1298.

68. Visser K, Kock MC, Kuntz KM, Donaldson MC, Gazelle GS, Hunink MG. Cost-effectiveness targets for multi-detector row CT angiography in the work-up of patients with intermittent claudication. Radiology 2003;227:647–656.

69. Adriaensen ME, Kock MC, Stijnen T, et al. Peripheral arterial disease: therapeutic confidence of CT versus digital subtraction angiography and effects on additional imaging recommendations. Radiology 2004;233:385–391.

14

Aortic, Renal, and Carotid CT Angiography

Matthew J. Budoff

Introduction

Volumetric datasets acquired with very thin slices (anywhere from 0.625 to 1.5 mm per image) will allow visualization of smaller structures with less partial volume averaging in the z-axis as well as superior 3-D and/or multiplanar imaging. Newer multidetector CT (MDCT) scanners have near isotropic voxels (similar z-axis to x-axis and y-axis imaging resolution), which results in improved multiplane reconstructions with higher resolution.

Computed tomographic angiography of other vascular beds is significantly easier to perform and interpret than coronary studies. There is no cardiac motion to contend with, so gating is most often not necessary. The exception is the ascending aorta, where pseudodissections have plagued earlier studies with single slice CT, due to motion artifacts [1]. Non-gated modes allow for very fast acquisition, and interpretation is significantly less complicated. Most of the large vessels of interest (carotid, renal, mesenteric) have significantly larger diameters than those of coronary arteries, as well as less tortuous courses. Renal and carotid arteries are usually straight structures, so reconstructions are significantly less complicated than coronary imaging. Also, due to the increased speed of newer systems (electron beam tomography and 16+ row multidetector computed tomography), venous enhancement is less common, so it is easier to see the arteries without superimposed contrast-filled structures. This is another reason why CT is most often superior to magnetic resonance imaging in these other vascular beds. Of course, the requirements of radiation (more significant for carotid imaging due to radiation-sensitive organs such as thyroid and orbits) and contrast (more significant for renal artery imaging due to the frequent coexistence of renal insufficiency and renal artery stenosis) make magnetic resonance more attractive for selective cases. In regard to the aorta, CT angiography can diagnose aneurysm, dissection, and wall abnormalities such as ulceration, calcification, or thrombus throughout the full length of the aorta as well as involvement of branch vessels.

Disease of the aorta or great vessels can present with a broad clinical spectrum of symptoms and signs. The accepted diagnostic gold standard, selective digital subtraction angiography, is now being challenged by state-of-the-art CT angiography (CTA) and MR angiography (MRA). Currently, in many centers, cross-sectional imaging modalities are being used as the first line of diagnosis to evaluate the cardiovascular system, and conventional angiography is reserved for therapeutic intervention.

Principles of Imaging

In aortic imaging, the volume coverage capabilities of MDCT come to full use without having to compromise on resolution of detail [2,3]. With the current configuration of 16-row (or greater) CT scanners, the entire abdominal aorta and the iliac arteries can be covered within seconds and with isotropic resolution (Chapter 1). Interrogation of the dataset can now be made in the anteroposterior (coronal) and lateral (sagittal) planes, which has been the convention with invasive angiography.

Larger collimation (more detectors) reduces contrast, as the imaging territory is covered in a shorter period of time. Another technique to minimize contrast is use of saline to flush the contrast through the system (Chapter 2). The saline chaser offers two significant benefits with CTA imaging. One is that the contrast is forced from the tubing and extremity veins into the central circulation, allowing for a reduction in the total dose of contrast. A second benefit is that the contrast sitting in the vein during imaging can cause partial volume (beam hardening) artifacts. Moving the contrast out of the venous system is important for cardiac imaging (where the scatter from the superior vena cava can cause artifacts in the right atrium and right coronary artery), carotid imaging (obscuring the proximal brachiocephalic artery or carotid base), and pulmonary imaging.

CT Technique

Understanding the principles of CTA techniques is essential to acquire diagnostic images consistently. This section reviews current CTA methods used in the evaluation of great vessels. The following broad approach is a guide to CT scan acquisition for various scanners.

1. Intravenous injection of 75–150 mL of a non-ionic contrast agent (300–370 mg I/mL), although decreasing with scanners with higher detectors.
2. Monophasic or biphasic injection rate: most commonly a monophasic injection at 4 mL/s (followed by a saline bolus).
3. Scan delay determined by test injection (10 mL at 4 mL/s) or by automated triggering (to achieve imaging to coincide with contrast arrival in the aortic root).
4. Pitch:
   - *For 4-row MDCT:* 4 × 2.50 mm detector configuration with 2.50 mm reconstruction thickness and pitch = 1.4 (table speed 14 mm/rotation, divided by 10 mm detector width), rotation speed 0.5 seconds, reconstructed at 1.00–1.25 mm interval for 3-D and MPR.
   - *For 8-row MDCT:* 8 × 1.25 mm detector configuration with 1.25–2.50 mm reconstruction thickness and pitch = 1.7 (table speed 16.8 mm/rotation divided by 10 mm detector width) during the arterial phase, reconstructed at 0.5–1.25 mm intervals for 3-D and MPR.
   - *For 16-detector MDCT:* 16 × 0.625 mm detector configuration with 1.25–2.50 mm reconstruction thickness and pitch = 1.7 (table speed 17.5 mm/ rotation divided by 10 mm detector width), reconstructed retrospectively with 0.3 mm interval for 3-D and MPR
   - *For 64-detector MDCT:* 64 × 0.625 mm detector configuration* with 1.25–2.50 mm reconstruction thickness and pitch = 1.375 (table speed 55 mm/ rotation divided by 40 mm detector width), reconstructed retrospectively with 0.3 mm interval for 3-D and MPR. (The 40 mm of detector width coverage per rotation used is currently available in the GE and Phillips systems. Siemens has 20 mm of collimation with the 64-MDCT scanner, with Toshiba allowing 32 mm of coverage per rotation (2005)).

Electron beam tomography (EBT) is performed by use of the continuous volume mode, whereby the scanner simulates the MDCT by taking continuous images of the volume of interest, without gating or pause. In this mode, the scanner can take 10 images per second, covering 1.5 mm to 6 mm per slice. Thus, large areas can be scanned with minimal contrast use. The most common protocols employed increase the image acquisition time from 100 ms per image to 200–300 ms per image, to improve tissue penetration and reduce image noise. Still, approximately 80 mL of contrast is all that is necessary to complete a thoracic and abdominal aortic study.

Aortic Imaging

The speed and ease of modern CTA make it the technique of choice for diagnosing chronic and acute aortic pathologic findings such as intramural hematoma, aneurysm, traumatic injuries, and dissection (Figure 14.1). With the current configuration of 16-row CT scanners, the entire abdominal aorta and the iliac arteries can be covered with isotropic resolution. Moreover, the high scan speed allows substantial reduction of the amount of contrast material used in earlier studies.

Aortic Dissection

The superior temporal resolution of EBT or MDCT significantly improves imaging of the aorta, because motion artifacts are eliminated in the ascending aorta. CT is often considered a superior method over other imaging methods for identification of aortic dissection (even invasive angiography in some cases), as the intimal flap is usually well delineated, even in branches of the aorta. The ability to visualize the great vessels into the transverse

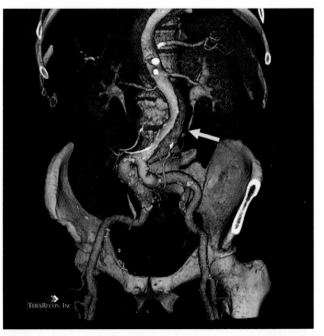

Figure 14.1. A volume-rendered image depicting an aortic dissection involving the abdominal aorta (arrow), starting below the renal arteries and ending prior to the iliac arteries. (Courtesy of TeraRecon, Inc.)

aorta, neck, and arms makes CT significantly more robust than transesophageal imaging and significantly better tolerated by patients. Because imaging protocols are less than 10 minutes (significantly shorter than MR or transesophageal echocardiography), even unstable patients can be evaluated and triaged quickly. With EBT, the flow mode also allows for assessing luminal flow in the true and false lumens.

Thoracic Imaging

CT is the primary means of imaging the lung, thoracic trauma (blunt and penetrating), aneurysms, and aortic dissections [4]. CT is playing an increasingly important role in the diagnosis and management of thoracic aortic pathology [5,6]. In the situation of an acute life-threatening event, CT can provide extensive information concerning the heart, aorta, and great vessels with a single scan protocol (Figure 14.2). In addition, during the same examination, the brain and spinal canal can be evaluated, if necessary. The entire global CT examination (head, cervical spine, chest, abdomen, and pelvis) can be completed on modern MDCT systems in less than 15 minutes [7].

Thoracic aortic imaging is the one area where gating to the cardiac cycle (similar to coronary CTA applications) is important [8]. The reduction in motion artifact provided by ECG gating is especially relevant to axial data from the ascending aorta. The evaluation of aneurysms of the ascending thoracic aorta and in the assessment of possible type A aortic dissection is improved with this methodology due to effective elimination of motion artifacts [9]. Moreover, the possibility of applying ECG-controlled X-ray tube dose modulation is an authentic step forward for reducing radiation exposure rates.

Comparison to Other Methods

Although MRI and transesophageal echocardiography can provide exquisite and unique information, the robust nature of CT often makes it the imaging modality of choice. Advantages are the ability to image the entire aorta and beyond, demonstration of surrounding structures and organs, quantitative measures of aneurysm size and location, and a rapid examination time. Limitations are the negative effects of iodinated contrast on renal function, the rare adverse reactions to iodinated contrast, and the inability to directly measure blood flow. A current MDCT protocol for CT angiography provides high-resolution arterial phase images from the thoracic inlet to the femoral arteries. This coverage incorporates the entire aorta, as well as the organs of the chest, abdomen, and pelvis. Beyond classifying dissections as involving the ascending (Stanford type A) or descending (type B), CT can demonstrate associated findings critical to patient care such as mediastinal hematoma, pericardial effusions, pseudoaneurysm formation, and active extravasation of contrast from the aorta. Quantitative measurement of aneurysm size, location and relation to branch vessels can be used for planning operative or intravascular repair and for monitoring postprocedure anatomy. The necessity for precise and quantitative measurements with CT has become more critical with the continued advancements in endovascular repair with stent-grafts [10,11].

Computed tomography angiography is less operator-dependent than transesophageal echocardiography, allows complete organ visualization, and is faster and more convenient for patients than magnetic resonance imaging and digital subtraction angiography. The latter issues are especially important with severely ill patients. In the setting of blunt and penetrating trauma, CT of the chest

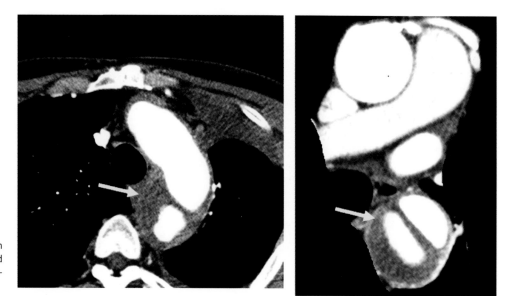

Figure 14.2. Thoracic aortic dissection extending into the transverse aorta (left) and descending thoracic aorta (right). The intramural thrombus is easily identified.

can be extremely useful in diagnosis and as an aid to surgical management [12]. Another major advantage over MR is that these examinations are performed in critically ill patients who may require mechanical ventilation, invasive monitoring, intravenous infusion pumps, and cardiac pacing.

Abdominal Aorta

Aortic aneurysm is associated with risk for sudden death due to aortic dissection or rupture and can occur associated with connective tissue disorders or acquired cardiovascular disease [13]. The ability to measure the diameter, wall thrombus, and calcification makes this an ideal modality for sequential following of patients, and to make an accurate assessment for surgical planning or medical therapy (Figure 14.3). The abdominal aorta is usually scanned before and following intravenous contrast enhancement, which enables detection of calcification of the arterial wall which will be partly obscured following contrast enhancement. It also provides a baseline for evaluating any vascular injury with hemorrhage or thrombus that will be seen on the post-contrast acquisition. Three-dimensional sagittal and coronal reconstructions are routinely performed (Figures 14.4 and 14.5).

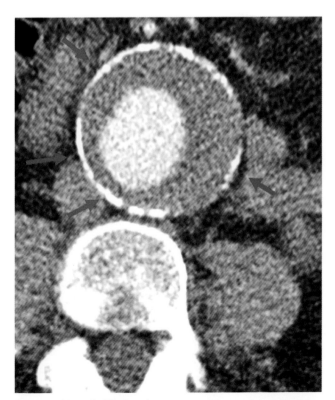

Figure 14.3. Aortic wall calcification and aneurysm on an axial image at the level of the abdominal aorta.

Common Indications for CTA of Abdominal Aorta

1. Detection and depiction of atherosclerotic occlusive disease or aneurysmal dilatation of the abdominal aorta and iliac arteries.
2. Preoperative assessment of aortoiliac aneurysms to determine whether open repair or stent grafting is indicated.
3. Follow-up for the size and progression or regression of abdominal aortic aneurysms.
4. Diagnose the presence and severity of complications following aortic stent-graft placement (leak, pseudoaneurysm, thrombus).
5. Detection and depiction of aortic dissection.
6. Detect the presence of aortic aneurysm rupture.

Accurate measurements of the aortic root diameter can be made easily and the extent of the aneurysm defined. Luminal thrombus is easily identified by differences in tissue density during contrast enhancement. The tomographic format of CT provides excellent definition of the relationship of aortic aneurysms to adjacent structures. Leakage of blood from the aneurysm or stent may be recognizable with contrast enhancement of surrounding tissues.

The two-dimensional images (axial data), maximal intensity projection, and multiplanar imaging allow accurate measurement of length, location, and diameter of aneurysms. The involvement of branch vessels (renals, mesenterics, iliacs, etc.) is also easily assessed with minimal contrast requirements. Computed tomography angiography has become the first-line modality for evaluation for planning stent-graft deployment (Figure 14.5) and post-procedural assessment (Figure 14.6). Cephalocaudal coverage from the celiac trunk to the proximal thighs provides a suitable study volume to detect aortic disease. Although the preoperative assessment requires a true early arterial phase to investigate all preoperative necessities (e.g. aortic neck diameters, angle and distance from the renal arteries), the postoperative study requires a biphasic scan protocol, allowing a more detailed inspection of the perigraft space to rule out possible endoleaks. High-resolution, thin slice protocols are preferable, especially for the post-processing task.

Several studies have demonstrated the accuracy of CT for the diagnosis of aortic diseases. Stueckle et al. compared conventional angiography to CTA in the diagnosis of morphologic changes in the abdominal aorta and its branches in 52 patients who underwent both MDCT and invasive angiography before surgical treatment [14]. All CT examinations were performed after administration of 100 mL contrast medium with a collimation of 4×1 mm and a pitch of 7. All aneurysms, occlusions, stenoses, and calcifications were diagnosed correctly by CTA in axial and multiplanar projections (sensitivity 1.0; specificity 1.0).

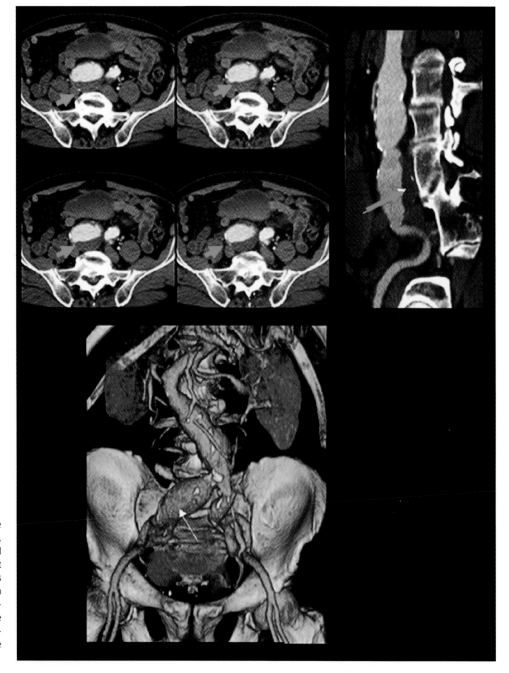

Figure 14.4. A representation of the two-dimensional axial images (top left), curved multiplanar reformat (top right) and volume-rendered images (bottom) of a patient with an abdominal aortic aneurysm. The iliacs and femoral bifurcations can be seen best in their true anatomic three-dimensional orientation with the volume-rendered image. The thrombus, however, is only visible on the two-dimensional images and curved MIP image (green arrows).

The degree of stenosis was overestimated in three cases when using axial projections. Three-dimensional volume-rendered CTA showed a sensitivity of 0.91 for aneurysms, 0.82 for stenoses, 0.75 for occlusions, and 0.77 for calcifications. The specificity was 1.0 in all cases. Multislice CT angiography seems to be similar to invasive angiography for abdominal vessels if multiplanar projections are used.

Nihan et al. described 25 patients (22 preoperative and 3 postoperative) who underwent EBT angiography prior to surgery, with results compared to surgical findings [15]. Among the 22 preoperatively evaluated patients, 17 patients had thoracic and/or abdominal aorta aneurysm with or without associated mural thrombus and calcified arteriosclerotic plaques, and 4 had dissection in the thoracic and abdominal aorta. The findings by CTA correlated with the surgical findings in all cases. In one preoperative patient, interventional angiography resulted in the misdiagnosis of occlusion in the proximal part of the abdominal aorta but EBA showed tortuosity and division anomaly of the abdominal aorta which could not be evaluated by interventional angiography because of technical limitations. There was one postoperative case of a patient with Marfan's syndrome who was found to have a pseudoaneurysm surrounding a graft in the ascending thoracic aorta with contrast extending from the pseudoaneurysmal space to the

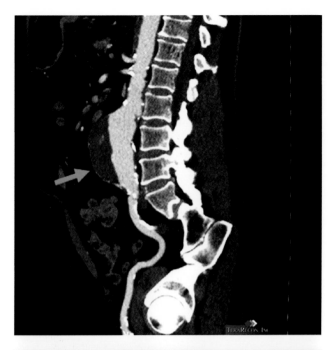

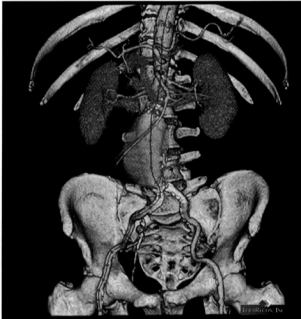

Comparison to Other Modalities

Like CT, MRA of the abdomen is always acquired as part of a routine lower extremity runoff procedure most commonly performed for symptoms of claudication.

With CT, the renals can be routinely evaluated during an abdominal aorta study. For MR, the evaluation of the renal arteries for characterizing potential renal artery stenosis in patients with hypertension must be done as a separate procedure, with different imaging protocols. This is also true for evaluation of a potential renal donor. In these patients, dedicated abdominal MRA acquisition is required with greater contrast enhancement, which is not feasible when the legs and feet must also be imaged at the same time. This is because there is a limit on the total volume of gadolinium, which is usually 60–75 mL for an adult. An abdominal MRA performed for the indications listed above is often scanned as part of the same procedure as a thoracic MRA, as it is for CT.

Conclusion

The simultaneous acquisition of multiple thin collimated slices in combination with enhanced gantry rotation speed

Figure 14.5. Abdominal aortic aneurysm with large intramural thrombus, seen on maximal intensity projection image (top, green arrow) and volume-rendered image (bottom, blue structure). (Courtesy of TeraRecon, Inc.)

right atrium. These findings were in addition to that found on conventional invasive angiography. These findings demonstrated that CTA is a highly accurate imaging method in all kinds of thoracic and abdominal aorta diseases in the preoperative and postoperative period with excellent 3-D images competitive in quality with interventional angiography. In some instances, CT angiography images give more information about the aortic diseases due to visualization of lumen, thrombus, and wall disease simultaneously, as compared to interventional angiography.

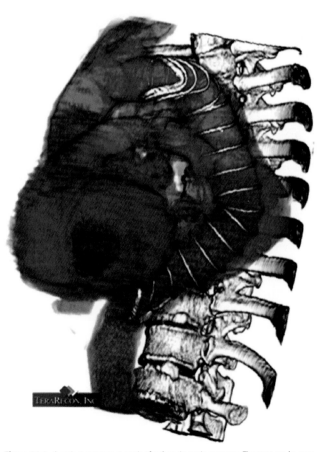

Figure 14.6. A patient status post repair of a thoracic aortic aneurysm. The stent can be seen, without scatter artifact or partial volume effect. (Courtesy of TeraRecon, Inc.)

offers thin slice coverage of extended volumes without any loss in spatial resolution. Using 4-detector-row CT scanners, the scan volume still has to be restricted and focused on dedicated abdominal vessel territories in order to provide high spatial resolution (1–2 mm), while 16-detector-row technology (or greater) now enables full abdominal coverage from the diaphragm to the groin without compromise of spatial resolution. This technique enables the evaluation of the whole arterial visceral vasculature (e.g. hepatic vessels, mesenteric vessels, renal arteries) and the aortic-iliac axis in a single data acquisition.

Renal and Mesenteric Arteries

CTA, combined with abdominal/parenchymal imaging, is a first-line diagnostic test in patients with suspected abdominal vascular emergencies, such as acute mesenteric ischemia, and an excellent tool to assess a wide variety of vascular abnormalities of the abdominal viscera. Important indications for directed renal artery imaging comprise the assessment of patients with suspected renal vascular hypertension to exclude hemodynamically significant renal artery stenosis as well as a complete preoperative assessment for renal transplant candidates. MDCT angiography of the renal arteries is performed with a high-resolution protocol (thickness of 1–1.25 mm or less). Achieving adequate coverage to encompass the entire kidneys and the origins of accessory renal arteries is easily accomplished in a scan of less than 10 seconds duration, or as part of the aortic evaluation (described above). With adequate selection of acquisition parameters (thin collimation) high spatial-resolution volumetric datasets for subsequent 2-D and 3-D reformation can be acquired (Figure 14.7). Whereas fast acquisitions allow a reduction of total contrast volume in the setting of CTA, this is not the case when CTA is combined with a second-phase abdominal MDCT acquisition for parenchymal (e.g. hepatic) imaging. Renal CTA is an accurate and reliable test for visualizing vascular anatomy and renal artery stenosis, and therefore a viable alternative to MRA in the assessment of patients with renovascular hypertension and in potential living related renal donors.

Methods

Routine clinical practice follows the rule of thumb that the injection duration should match the acquisition time. Biphasic injection protocols, with an initially high injection rate followed by a slower continuing injection phase, ensure optimal opacification of the renal arteries (Chapter 2). Note that high-concentration contrast material requires only moderate injection flow rates (maximum of 4.5 mL/s) to achieve high iodine administration rates [16].

By using a half-second MDCT scanner and a 1 mm nominal section thickness, Willmann et al. [17] obtained

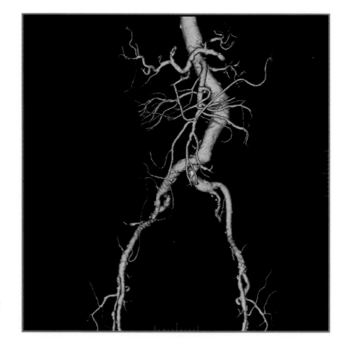

Figure 14.7. A volume-rendered image of the abdominal aorta and vessels (including exquisite detail of the mesenteric and iliac arteries) using 64-detector MDCTA.

excellent quality CT angiograms (92% and 99% sensitivity and specificity, respectively) for the detection of hemodynamically significant arterial stenosis of aortoiliac and renal arteries. When compared to MR angiography, there is no statistically significant difference between 3-D MR angiography and MDCT angiography in the detection of hemodynamically significant arterial stenosis of the aortoiliac and renal arteries. This study also demonstrated that patient acceptance of the CT study is higher than either invasive angiography or MR angiography.

Tepe et al. used 3-D EBT angiography to evaluate renal artery lesions, as well as vascular variants that it is crucial to detect before surgery [18]. Forty patients underwent EBT (GE-Imatron, C 150 ultrafast CT scanner, San Francisco, CA) of the renal arteries. The study demonstrated that both maximal intensity projection (MIP) and volume-rendered images were excellent in demonstrating stenosis of the renal arteries. Accessory and main renal arteries were easily depicted, and stenosis shown with high accuracy. In this study, among 40 renal angiography patients, 21 had stenosis of the renal arteries with different percentages. A total of 12 accessory renal arteries (5 left, 7 right) were detected. CT, with its non-invasive volume rendering (VR) and MIP techniques, is easy to apply and is functional and accurate for neoplasms, renal vascular anatomy, and renal artery stenosis.

While most vascular beds have demonstrated an advantage of MIP imaging over VR for accurate stenosis detection (especially coronary artery imaging), renal vasculature seems more amenable to quantitation with VR. One study specifically compared overall image quality and vascular delineation on MIP and VR images. The authors found that all main and accessory renal arteries depicted at invasive angiography were also demonstrated on MIP and VR images [19]. VR performed slightly better than MIP for quantification of stenoses greater than 50% (VR: $r^2 = 0.84$, $p < 0.001$; MIP: $r^2 = 0.38$, $p = 0.001$) and significantly better for severe stenoses (VR: $r^2 = 0.83$, $p < 0.001$; MIP: $r^2 = 0.21$, $p = 0.1$). For detection of stenosis, VR yielded a substantial improvement in positive predictive value (VR: 95% and 90%; MIP: 86% and 68% for stenoses greater than 50% and 70%, respectively). Image quality obtained with VR was not significantly better than that with MIP; however, vascular delineation on VR images was significantly better (Figure 14.8). The VR technique of renal MR angiography enabled more accurate detection and quantification of renal artery stenosis than did MIP, with significantly improved vascular delineation.

Another study evaluated findings in 50 main and 11 accessory renal arteries [20]. All arteries depicted on conventional angiograms were visualized on MIP and VR images. Receiver operating characteristic (ROC) analysis for MIP and VR images demonstrated excellent discrimination for the diagnosis of stenosis of at least 50% (area under the ROC curve, 0.96–0.99). While in this study, sensitivity was not significantly different for VR and MIP (89% versus 94%, $p > 0.1$), specificity was greater with VR (99% versus 87%, $p = 0.008$ to 0.08). Stenosis of at least 50% was overestimated with CT angiography in four accessory renal arteries, but three accessory renal arteries not depicted at conventional angiography were depicted at CT angiography. In the evaluation of renal artery stenosis, CT angiography with VR is faster and more accurate than CT angiography with MIP. Accessory arteries not depicted

with conventional angiography were depicted with both CT angiographic algorithms.

Computed tomography angiography is a highly reliable technique for detection of renal artery stenosis as well as for morphologic assessment (Figure 14.8). In patients with renal insufficiency, magnetic resonance angiography or color-coded duplex ultrasound should remain the initial examination performed, depending on local expertise and availability.

Mesenteric Vasculature

MDCT angiography has become a valuable minimally invasive tool for the visualization of normal vascular anatomy and its variants as well as for pathologic conditions affecting the mesenteric vessels (Figures 14.9 to 14.11) [17,21,22]. Indications for MDCT angiography include not only acute and chronic ischemia, aneurysm, and dissection but preoperative vascular assessment for patients undergoing liver lesion embolization as well as in the setting of liver transplantation [23,24]. Protocols for typical aortic imaging (described above) are used to image the mesenteric vasculature. The reconstructed images allow for easy evaluation of all abdominal vasculature. Volume rendering is most often used, predominantly due to the complex anatomy, making MIP imaging more difficult (Figure 14.11). Since the arteries are highly tortuous, leaving the 2-D plane often (and traveling both caudally and cranially at different times), these vessels pose the most challenge with axial interpretations. With coronary imaging, the arteries run cranial to caudal, without significant exception. Thus,

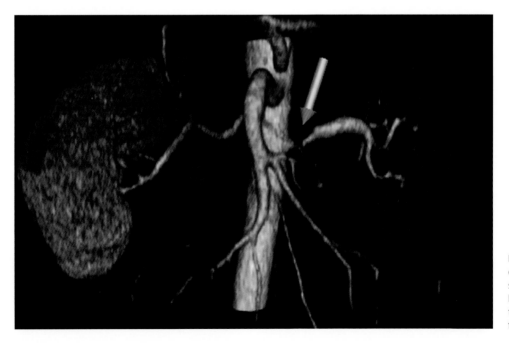

Figure 14.8. A volume-rendered EBT study of the renal arteries, depicting a high-grade stenosis of the left renal artery (arrow). The left kidney also opacifies less (darker color) than the right kidney, suggesting decreased blood flow and significance of the visualized stenosis.

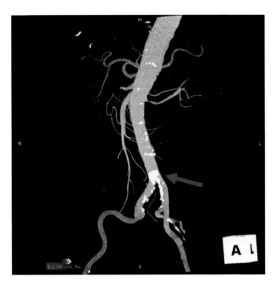

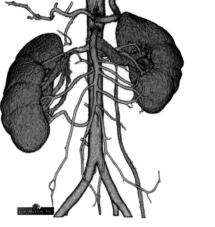

Figure 14.9. Maximal intensity projection of the abdominal aorta, demonstrating severe calcifications at the iliac bifurcation (arrow, left image). The right image demonstrates a normal arterial bed in another patient, displayed using volume rendering. (Courtesy of TeraRecon, Inc.)

interpreting with MIP or axial imaging is fairly straight-forward, as the operator needs to systematically go from the most cranial images to the most caudal to follow the respective arteries. With mesenteric imaging, the arteries commonly turn both cranially and caudally, and volume rendering makes visualization of the entire dataset with one reconstruction possible. No studies of the diagnostic potential of the different reconstruction methods have been reported.

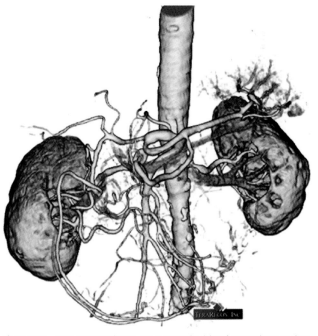

Figure 14.11. Three-dimensional image demonstrating the ability of computed tomography to visualize the abdominal arteries, including the gastric arteries in this case. Reconstruction performed on Aquarius Workstation, TeraRecon, San Mateo, CA. (Courtesy of TeraRecon, Inc.)

Carotid Artery CT Angiography

Ischemic cerebrovascular events are often due to athero-sclerotic narrowing of the carotid bifurcation (Figure 14.12) [25]. Invasive angiography is the current reference standard for the evaluation of obstructive carotid artery disease. Computed tomography angiography is a robust technique in assessing carotid artery stenosis, allowing excellent visualization of the lumen of the carotid artery using intravenous contrast (Figure 14.13). Subsequent refinement of magnetic resonance imaging, ultrasound,

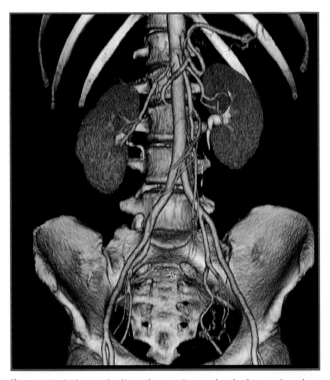

Figure 14.10. A volume-rendered image demonstrating normal renal and mesenteric arteries, as well as aorta and iliac arteries bilaterally. Large volumes of coverage (spanning multiple vascular beds) can be imaged with a single scan.

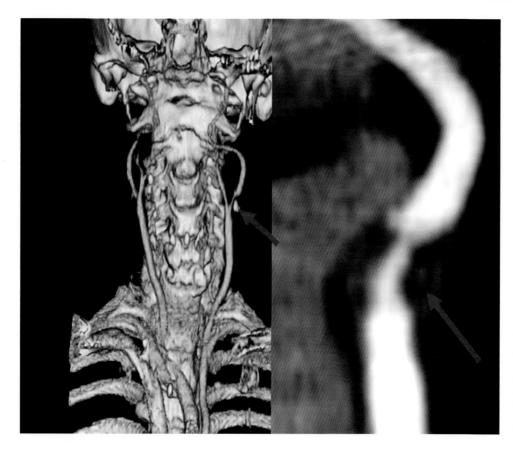

Figure 14.12. Two patients with carotid stenosis at the bifurcation. The left image is a volume-rendered image, with a high-grade stenosis at the proximal portion of the internal carotid, with a dense calcification also seen. The right image demonstrates a maximal intensity projection image of the same region, with a tight stenosis and thrombus present.

and CT techniques has led to changes in clinical practice whereby many centers have now abandoned conventional X-ray angiography in place of safer imaging modalities [26]. Computed tomography angiography offers details of the entire relevant neurovascular axis by excluding significant carotid disease and intracranial disease [27].

Coupling non-contrast-enhanced cranial CT imaging with CT perfusion imaging and CTA of the entire cerebrovascular axis is both safe and feasible [28]. Current practice is to use CTA to facilitate patient triage and provide specific information to rule out large vessel stenosis in patients with transient ischemic attacks, suspected stroke, or in

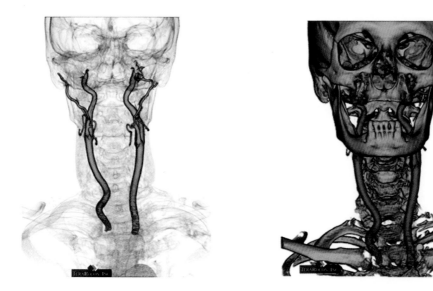

Figure 14.13. Three-dimensional images of normal carotid arteries bilaterally. (Courtesy of TeraRecon, Inc.)

patients with carotid bruits. Furthermore, clarification of equivocal results of carotid ultrasound or MRA is also a common indication. This chapter will address the clinical applications of CT angiography of the carotid and vertebral arteries.

Since treatment has demonstrated a large reduction in strokes by performing carotid endarterectomy [26,29] in symptomatic patients with a stenosis of more than 70%, accurate assessment of carotid disease is important. Furthermore, endarterectomy in patients with a symptomatic moderate carotid stenosis of 50–69% produced a moderate reduction in the risk of stroke [30]. Randoux et al. prospectively compared gadolinium-enhanced magnetic resonance (MR) angiography and computed tomographic (CT) angiography with invasive angiography for use in detecting atheromatous stenosis and plaque morphology at the carotid bifurcation in 22 patients [31]. There was significant correlation between CTA, enhanced MRA, and invasive angiography. Severe internal carotid artery (ICA) stenoses were detected with high sensitivity and specificity: 100% and 100%, respectively, with CT angiography; 93% and 100%, respectively, with enhanced MRA. Luminal surface irregularities and ulcerations were most frequently seen at CTA. Most studies suggest that CT angiography is the best modality for analyzing plaque morphology because it allows visualization of the atheromatous plaque. Detection of ulcerated plaques may prove to be important, since it has been suggested that the presence of plaque ulceration is a risk factor for embolism [32]. However, the inability of invasive angiography to depict plaque ulceration is well documented [33,34], partly because of the limited number of views that are typically obtained. In the case in which CT angiography depicted an ulceration that was not depicted at gadolinium-enhanced MR angiography, this could be due to a lack of spatial resolution at gadolinium-enhanced MR angiography.

CT angiography and gadolinium-enhanced MR angiography have both proved reliable and fast techniques to evaluate the degree of ICA stenosis [34]. CT angiography has some substantial benefits, including its accuracy and lack of invasiveness [35], and improved spatial and temporal resolution as compared with MR angiography.

Methods for Carotid CT Angiography

Carotid CT angiographic images are obtained with patients placed in the supine position with the head tilted back as far as possible to avoid inclusion of dental hardware. Spiral data can be acquired with a 0.5 to 1.5 mm collimation starting at the seventh cervical vertebra and proceeding as far cephalad as possible. Some centers suggest starting at the CT parameters including a field of view (FOV) of 15 × 15 cm and a section thickness of 1 mm. With a power injector, 80–140 mL of non-ionic contrast medium is injected at a rate of 2.5 mL/s into an antecubital vein. Administration of each bolus was followed immediately by a 20 mL saline

flush. The acquisition is initiated after the start of the administration of contrast medium, the time of which was determined by a test of circulation time.

EBT scanning for carotid stenosis utilizes the 50 to 100 ms exposure times per slice, using the continuous volume mode and a 10-second breath-hold. The angle of the jaw is angled up, to get the jawbone (and possible associated metal fillings) out of the axial images that include the carotid bifurcation. A total of 60–80 mL of contrast is utilized, injected at a rate of 3 mL/s.

In general, good image quality is essential. A CT angiographic image of good quality is easily obtained if the patient does not move during the study. Given the faster scan times with increased detector systems, this is even easier. A breath-hold acquisition is not necessary. Compared with invasive angiography and CTA, a major limitation of gadolinium-enhanced MR angiography is spatial resolution. By using automatic triggering with detection of the contrast material bolus, it is fairly straightforward to selectively obtain an arterial phase image. Previous studies [36] have shown that a combination of optimal tracking volume placement and adjustment of tracking volume size ensures optimal sensitivity to the contrast material bolus. By choosing a 5 × 20 mm tracker volume placed in the aortic arch, bolus arrival was always detected. Careful timing is very important, with arterial enhancement critical. It is vital to make sure that there is no venous filling when images are obtained. Obtaining images too early will lead to non-enhanced images, and obtaining images late allows for venous enhancement. Large jugular veins filled with contrast in close proximity to the carotid arteries can make the interpretation of carotid arteries more difficult.

Transverse source images are reconstructed in 1 mm increments by using a small FOV (15 cm). These parameters allowed a spatial resolution of 1.0 × 0.3 × 0.3 mm. Total coverage is approximately 18 cm. The images are then analyzed with axial images and maximal intensity projection or curved multiplanar reconstruction. Total postprocessing time is approximately 5 minutes per carotid artery. Precision of length and degree of stenosis is reported to depend more on measurement technique than on acquisition parameters [37]. The accuracy of stenosis measurement depends on the scanning plane, which ideally should be perpendicular to the carotid artery used to obtain magnified transverse oblique images. Most authors consider maximal intensity projection or curved multiplanar reconstructions the most accurate techniques for measurements. Volume rendering is considered the least accurate technique for measurement.

Comparison to MR

Gadolinium-enhanced MR angiography is an appropriate technique for evaluating ICA stenosis [38–40]. Clinically relevant stenosis and occlusions of the ICA were correctly detected with good sensitivity and specificity and good interobserver agreement. Most studies [39,40] with gadolinium-enhanced MR angiography demonstrate overestimation of the degree of stenosis [41]. Artifacts due to excessive section thickness, necessary with current MR systems, cause a partial volume effect [42,43]. The signal loss can also be explained by the presence of hemodynamic modifications. The decreased flow caused by stenosis leads to a reduced concentration of contrast agent in the distal arterial lumen, which may also explain why overestimation of stenosis with gadolinium-enhanced MR angiography can occur [44], especially for evaluating the degree of stenosis in small-vessel lumens.

Plaques that are more prone to disruption, fracture, or fissuring may be associated with a higher risk of embolization, occlusion, and consequent ischemic neurologic events [45]. Plaque irregularities are more frequent at CT angiography than at invasive angiography or contrast-enhanced MR angiography.

In general, studies demonstrate that MR angiography sometimes performs inferiorly to CT angiography, mainly due to lower spatial resolution. MR has been postulated to demonstrate inflammation, and MRI-derived measurements of fibrous-cap and lipid-core thickness have the potential for identifying vulnerable carotid plaques in vivo, although this application is still very experimental [46]. CT does not have the same potential for demonstrating flow or inflammation.

Invasive angiography has long been considered the standard for evaluation of carotid stenosis but has well-known risks and limitations. Invasive angiography allows only a limited number of views, which can lead to an underestimation of the degree of stenosis by as much as 40% [47] when compared with histologic correlation. Invasive angiography is also a relatively expensive technique that uses numerous resources. Finally and perhaps most importantly, there is a small but definite risk of major complications secondary to the procedure itself. The Asymptomatic Carotid Atherosclerosis Study Committee reported a 1.2% risk of persisting neurologic deficit or death following invasive angiography, while the surgical risk was 1.5%. The risks associated with CT angiography are markedly lower with similar or lower radiation exposures and no catheter-induced risks.

Almost all authors consider that calcified plaque is a limitation of CT angiography. This can be minimized when multiplanar volume reconstruction is used, although circumferential calcified plaques will still cause problems. Carotid arteries tend to calcify less than either coronary or peripheral arteries (perhaps due to the fact that carotid arteries are more elastic and less muscular), so dense circumferential calcifications occur less frequently in this vascular bed.

CTA has been shown to have a pooled sensitivity of 95% and specificity of 98% for the detection of >70% stenoses, even if only older scanners are used. Differentiation between lipid, fibrous, and calcified plaques may be possible, especially with e-Speed EBT scanning. Carotid CTA has come of age and can be used to quantify stenoses more precisely than ultrasound, to detect tandem stenoses and for the workup of acute stroke patients. The e-Speed EBT scanner has the additional advantage of a very low radiation profile, allowing for minimal risk to the patient, and maximum visualization of the arteries in question.

Imaging the Vertebral Artery

Although conventional intra-arterial angiography remains the gold standard method for imaging the vertebral artery, non-invasive modalities such as ultrasound, multislice computed tomographic angiography and magnetic resonance angiography are constantly improving and are playing an increasingly important role in diagnosing vertebral artery pathology in clinical practice. Normal anatomy, normal variants, and a number of pathologic entities such as vertebral atherosclerosis, arterial dissection, arteriovenous fistula, subclavian steal syndrome, and vertebrobasilar dolichoectasia can be seen.

Summary

During the past decade, we have been witness to a tremendous development in the field of CT imaging. CTA has gained remarkably by improvements in scan time and image quality, replacing diagnostic angiography in many cases of peripheral, carotid, and renal angiography. These vascular beds do not suffer from motion artifacts, so imaging with CT is ideal. CTA is less expensive, less invasive, and allows simultaneous visualization of large anatomic areas from multiple angles using 3-D display. Nevertheless, along with exciting advances, MDCT also carries some emerging and important issues such as increased patient radiation exposure and continued exposure to iodinated contrast.

References

1. Rooholamini SA, Stanford W: Ultrafast computed tomography in the diagnosis of aortic aneurysms and dissections. In: Stanford W, Rumberger J (eds) Ultrafast computed tomography in cardiac imaging: principles and practice. Mount Kisco, NY: Futura Publishing, 1992: 287–310.
2. Katz DS, Hon M. CT angiography of the lower extremities and aortoiliac system with a multi-detector row helical CT scanner: promise of new opportunities fulfilled. Radiology 2001;221:7–10.
3. Kim JK, Park SY, Kim HJ, et al. Living donor kidneys: usefulness of multi-detector row CT for comprehensive evaluation. Radiology 2003;229:869–876.
4. Fishman JE. Imaging of blunt aortic and great vessel trauma. J Thorac Imaging 2000;15(2):97–103.
5. Kouchoukos NT, Dougenis D. Surgery of the thoracic aorta. N Engl J Med 1997;336(26):1876–1888.
6. Rubin GD. Helical CT angiography of the thoracic aorta. J Thorac Imaging 1997;12(2):128–149.

7. Rubin GD, Shiau MC, Leung AN, Kee ST, Logan LJ, Sofilos MC. Aorta and iliac arteries: single versus multiple detector-row helical CT angiography. Radiology 2000;215(3):670–676.

8. Gotway MB, Dawn SK. Thoracic aorta imaging with multislice CT. Radiol Clin North Am 2003;41:521–543.

9. Roos JE, Willmann JK, Weishaupt D, et al. Thoracic aorta: motion artifact reduction with retrospective and prospective electrocardiography assisted multi-detector row CT. Radiology 2002;222:271–277.

10. Galla JD, Ergin MA, Lansman SL, et al. Identification of risk factors in patients undergoing thoracoabdominal aneurysm repair. J Cardiac Surg 1997;12:292–299.

11. Semba CP, Kato N, Kee ST, et al. Acute rupture of the descending thoracic aorta: repair with use of endovascular stent-grafts. J Vascular Intervent Rad 1997;8(3):337–342.

12. Zinck SE, Primack SL. Radiographic and CT findings in blunt chest trauma. J Thorac Imaging 2000;15(2):87–96.

13. Lu B, Dai RP, Jing BL, et al. Electron beam tomography with three-dimensional reconstruction in the diagnosis of aortic diseases. J Cardiovasc Surg 2000;41:659–668.

14. Stueckle CA, Haegele KF, Jendreck M, et al. Multislice computed tomography angiography of the abdominal arteries: comparison between computed tomography angiography and digital subtraction angiography findings in 52 cases. Australas Radiol 2004;48(2):142–147.

15. Nihan E, Levent A, Sekup A. Assessment of aortic diseases with electron beam tomographic angiography. EBT Symposium 2003;11–15.

16. Fleischmann D. Multiple detector-row CT angiography of the renal and mesenteric vessels. Eur J Radiol 2003;45(Suppl 1):S79–S87.

17. Willmann JK, Wildermuth S, Pfammatter T, et al. Aortoiliac and renal arteries: prospective intraindividual comparison of contrast-enhanced three-dimensional MR angiography and multi-detector row CT angiography. Radiology 2003;226:798–811.

18. Tepe SM, Memisoglu E, Kural AR. Three-dimensional noninvasive contrast-enhanced electron beam tomography angiography of the kidneys: adjunctive use in medical and surgical management. Clin Imaging 2004;28(1):52–58.

19. Mallouhi A, Schocke M, Judmaier W, et al. 3D MR angiography of renal arteries: comparison of volume rendering and maximum intensity projection algorithms. Radiology. 2002;223(2):509–516.

20. Johnson PT, Halpern EJ, Kuszyk BS, et al. Renal artery stenosis: CT angiography – comparison of real-time volume-rendering and maximum intensity projection algorithms. Radiology 1999 May; 211(2):337–343.

21. Laghi A, Iannaccone R, Catalano C, et al. Multislice spiral computed tomography angiography of mesenteric arteries. Lancet 2001;358: 638–639.

22. Lawler LP, Fishman EK. Celiomesenteric anomaly demonstration by multidetector CT and volume rendering. J Comput Assist Tomogr 2001;25:802–804.

23. Erbay N, Raptopoulos V, Pomfret EA, et al. Living donor liver transplantation in adults: vascular variants important in surgical planning for donors and recipients. Am J Roentgenol 2003;181:109–114.

24. Byun JH, Kim TK, Lee SS, et al. Evaluation of the hepatic artery in potential donors for living donor liver transplantation by computed tomography angiography using multidetector-row computed tomography: comparison of volume rendering and maximum intensity projection techniques. J Comput Assist Tomogr 2003;27: 125–131.

25. Kannel WB. Current status of the epidemiology of brain infarction associated with occlusive arterial disease. Stroke 1971;2:295–318.

26. North American Symptomatic Carotid Endarterectomy Trial Collaborators. Beneficial effect of carotid endarterectomy in symptomatic patients with high-grade carotid stenosis. N Engl J Med 1991; 325:445–453.

27. Smith WS, Roberts HC, Chuang NA, et al. Safety and feasibility of a CT protocol for acute stroke: combined CT, CT angiography, and CT perfusion imaging in 53 consecutive patients. Am J Neuroradiol 2003;24:688–690.

28. Na DG, Ryoo JW, Lee KH, et al. Multiphasic perfusion computed tomography in hyperacute ischemic stroke: comparison with diffusion and perfusion magnetic resonance imaging. J Comput Assist Tomogr 2003;27:194–206.

29. Collaborative Group. MRC European Carotid Surgery Trial: interim results for symptomatic patients with severe (70–99%) or with mild (0–29%) carotid stenosis – European Carotid Surgery Trialists. Lancet 1991;337:1235–1243.

30. Barnett HJ, Taylor DW, Eliasziw M, et al. Benefit of carotid endarterectomy in patients with symptomatic moderate or severe stenosis: North American Symptomatic Carotid Endarterectomy Trial Collaborators. N Engl J Med 1998;339:1415–1425.

31. Randoux B, Marro B, Koskas F, et al. Carotid artery stenosis: prospective comparison of CT, three-dimensional gadolinium-enhanced MR, and conventional angiography. Radiology. 2001;220(1):179–185.

32. Hatsukami TS, Ferguson MS, Beach KW, et al. Carotid plaque morphology and clinical events. Stroke 1997;28:95–100.

33. Comerota AJ, Katz ML, White JV, Grosh JD. The preoperative diagnosis of the ulcerated carotid atheroma. J Vasc Surg 1990;11:505–510.

34. Runge VM, Kirsch JE, Lee C. Contrast-enhanced MR angiography. J Magn Reson Imaging 1993;3:233–239.

35. Marro B, Zouaoui A, Koskas F, et al. Computerized tomographic angiography scan following carotid endarterectomy. Ann Vasc Surg 1998;12:451–456.

36. Castillo M, Wilson JD. CT angiography of the common carotid artery bifurcation: comparison between two techniques and conventional angiography. Neuroradiology 1994;36:602–604.

37. Cinat M, Lane CT, Pham H, Lee A, Wilson SE, Gordon I. Helical CT angiography in the preoperative evaluation of carotid artery stenosis. J Vasc Surg 1998;28:290–300.

38. Leclerc X, Martinat P, Godefroy O, et al. Contrast-enhanced three-dimensional fast imaging with steady-state precession (FISP) MR angiography of supraaortic vessels: preliminary results. Am J Neuroradiol 1998;19:1405–1413.

39. Slosman F, Stolpen AH, Lexa FJ, et al. Extracranial atherosclerotic carotid artery disease: evaluation of non-breath-hold three-dimensional gadolinium-enhanced MR angiography. Am J Roentgenol 1998;170:489–495.

40. Scarabino T, Carriero A, Magarelli N, et al. MR angiography in carotid stenosis: a comparison of three techniques. Eur J Radiol 1998;28:117–125.

41. Cronqvist M, Stahlberg F, Larsson EM, Lonntoft M, Holtas S. Evaluation of time-of-flight and phase-contrast MRA sequences at 1.0 T for diagnosis of carotid artery disease. I. A phantom and volunteer study. Acta Radiol 1996;37:267–277.

42. Remonda L, Heid O, Schroth G. Carotid artery stenosis, occlusion, and pseudo-occlusion: first-pass, gadolinium-enhanced, three-dimensional MR angiography – preliminary study. Radiology 1998; 208:95–102.

43. Levy RA, Prince MR. Arterial-phase three-dimensional contrast-enhanced MR angiography of the carotid arteries. Am J Roentgenol 1996;167:211–215.

44. Evans AJ, Richardson DB, Tien R, et al. Poststenotic signal loss in MR angiography: effects of echo time, flow compensation, and fractional echo. Am J Neuroradiol 1993;14:721–729.

45. Eliasziw M, Streifler JY, Fox AJ, Hachinski VC, Ferguson GG, Barnett HJ. Significance of plaque ulceration in symptomatic patients with high-grade carotid stenosis: North American Symptomatic Carotid Endarterectomy Trial. Stroke 1994;25:304–308.

46. Fayad ZA, Sirol M, Nikolaou K, Choudhury RP, Fuster V. Magnetic resonance imaging and computed tomography in assessment of atherosclerotic plaque. Curr Atheroscler Rep 2004;6(3):232–242.

47. Ho VB, Foo TK. Optimization of gadolinium-enhanced magnetic resonance angiography using an automated bolus-detection algorithm. Invest Radiol 1998;33:515–523.

15

Cardiovascular Magnetic Resonance Imaging: Overview of Clinical Applications

Jerold S. Shinbane, Patrick M. Colletti, and Gerald M. Pohost

Introduction

Although magnetic resonance imaging technology has been available for decades, detailed visualization of cardiac anatomy had remained challenging due to cardiac motion. Technologic advances in cardiovascular magnetic resonance (CMR) imaging now allow this modality to comprehensively visualize cardiovascular structures and function. CMR and cardiovascular CT are complementary technologies, each with unique strengths and limitations. An understanding of these techniques allows selection of the study most appropriate for a particular clinical or research issue. The strengths of CMR include evaluation of tissue characteristics, myocardial perfusion, ventricular function, myocardial metabolism, viability, shunts, valvular function, and peripheral vasculature without the need for potentially nephrotoxic contrast media or X-ray irradiation. The paramagnetic element gadolinium, when attached to a chelating agent like DTPA, provides a means for contrast enhancement, allowing assessment of perfusion and delayed enhancement to detect acutely infarcted myocardium and myocardial scar. Paramagnetic contrast agents are safe and have greatly expanded the applications of CMR. CMR spectroscopy provides noninvasive assessment of myocardial metabolism, allowing a mechanistic understanding of myocardial function when using ^{31}P to depict the high-energy phosphates, phosphocreatine and ATP, and inorganic phosphate to evaluate intracellular pH.

The strengths of cardiovascular CT technologies currently include a greater ability to characterize coronary vasculature, shorter study times, and the ability to image patients with pacemakers, defibrillators, and other devices incompatible or difficult to use within a CMR system. Additionally, CT allows quantitation of coronary artery calcium for risk stratification. Both CT and CMR technologies are advancing rapidly, and therefore future applications may reflect changes in these above strengths and limitations.

There are some contraindications to CMR. These largely consist of implanted devices including pacemakers,

implantable cardiac defibrillators, and certain other devices that have been felt to be absolute contraindications to magnetic resonance imaging [1–3], although recent publications have suggested that under the right circumstances patients with implanted pacemakers may be safely scanned using CMR approaches [4,5]. Most prosthetic heart valves and annuloplasty rings can be safely scanned [6], but specific details of compatibility need to be assessed individually prior to patient study. All patients require a complete history for any prosthetic materials or metal depositions which may be relative contraindications for magnetic resonance imaging. Due to acoustic noise associated with scanning, ear protection should be provided [7]. Claustrophobia, although a problem for some patients, results in failed examinations in only a small minority of patients (<2%) [8,9]. Larger bore magnets, open magnets, and visual devices allowing patients to see out of the magnet may make this even less of an issue in the future.

Similar to CT technology, cardiac gating has been a major advance in CMR imaging [10]. Electrocardiographic (ECG) triggering, though, can be challenging, as the magnetic field can interfere with sensing of the QRS complex. Attention to skin preparation, lead placement, and ECG vector can improve the ability to perform ECG gating [11,12].

A variety of novel contrast agents are being assessed in CMR [13,14], but the main agent in current clinical use is gadolinium-DTPA [15]. As opposed to iodinated contrast agents used in CT, which enhance vascular structures by increasing CT Hounsfield units, gadolinium is a paramagnetic agent which alters the magnetic properties of water in close proximity to the contrast agent. Additionally, techniques such as black blood imaging and bright blood imaging allow for differentiation of vasculature without the injection of a contrast agent (Figure 15.1). CMR sequences and technology are rapidly evolving with 3-D real-time acquisition and increased field strengths to 3 Tesla with attendant increased signal-to-noise ratio [16,17]. The effects and safety of field strengths greater than 3 Tesla require further investigation [18].

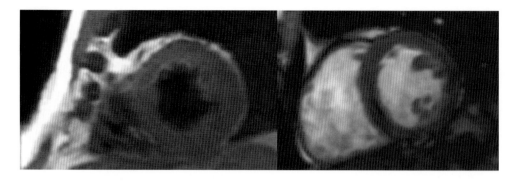

Figure 15.1. Black blood image (left panel) and bright blood image (right panel) demonstrating left ventricular cavity. (Images courtesy of Toshiba Medical Systems.)

Coronary Artery Visualization

CMR techniques are useful for the diagnosis of proximal coronary artery disease (Figure 15.2) [19,20]. Additionally, CMR can assess patency and stenoses of coronary artery bypass grafts [21]. Advances in technique have improved the ability to visualize coronary arteries with respiratory gating [22,23], but issues of cardiac, coronary artery, and respiratory motion, as well as problems with assessment of small caliber vessels, still remain. Anomalous coronary arteries can be diagnosed with CMR [19,24,25]. In addition to definition of anatomy of anomalous coronary artery origin, CMR can also assess functional significance through perfusion imaging. CT has historically assessed coronary arteries more optimally [19], but advances in technology are improving this technique [19,26–29]. The assessment of multiple components including coronary anatomy, ventricular function, rest perfusion, adenosine perfusion, and delayed enhancement provides comprehensive evaluation with increased accuracy [20].

Since myocardial infarction can occur due to plaque rupture and thrombosis in coronary arteries without obstructive disease, there is a need to attempt to characterize plaques potentially at higher risk for rupture [30,31]. CMR can assess tissue characteristics of vessel wall and atheromas, with assessment of fibrous tissue, fat, and calcified lesion components, but further investigation is required to identify characteristics of vulnerable plaques [32,33]. CMR can assess for vascular remodeling with changes in wall thickness and lumen size [34]. Noncalcified plaque detection and quantification between CMR and CT have been comparable, but CMR provides greater information on tissue characteristics [35].

Assessment of Cardiac Substrates

CMR can characterize cardiac structures and function by reproducibly assessing right and left ventricular volumes, ejection fraction, wall thickness and wall motion [36–44]. The ability to comprehensively assess ejection fraction, wall motion, perfusion, and viability is a great strength of CMR in the characterization of myocardial substrates associated with coronary artery disease as well as other cardiovascular disease processes.

Rest and stress first pass imaging as well as delayed enhancement imaging with CMR are important for characterization of ischemia, myocardial infarction, and ischemic cardiomyopathy (Figures 15.3–15.7). The first pass study after gadolinium injection can assess

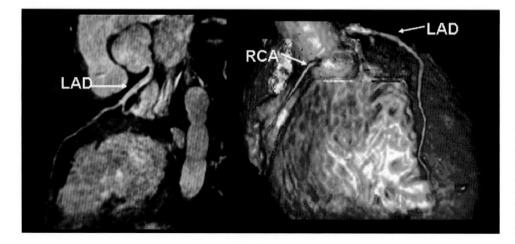

Figure 15.2. CMR coronary arteriogram demonstrating 2-D image of a left anterior descending coronary artery and a 3-D volume-rendered image demonstrating visualization of a right coronary artery and left anterior descending coronary artery. LAD = left anterior descending coronary artery, RCA = right coronary artery. (Images courtesy of Toshiba Medical Systems.)

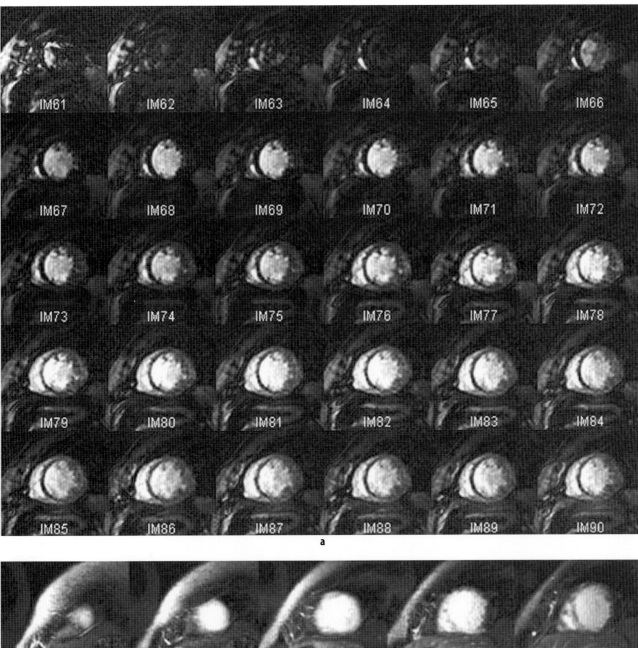

a

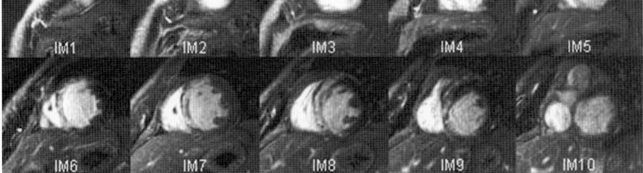

b

Figure 15.3. a First pass myocardial perfusion study with serial short axis images demonstrating a perfusion deficit in the anterior wall and septum. **b** Delayed enhancement study with serial short axis images demonstrating non-viability of the anterior wall and entire septum.

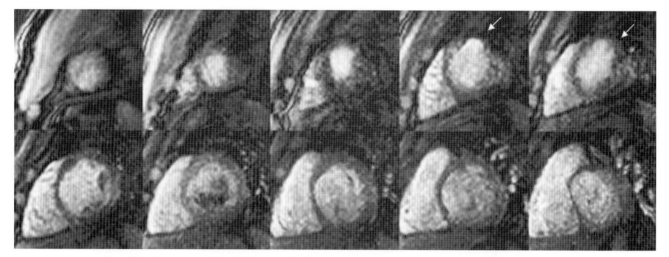

Figure 15.4. First pass myocardial perfusion imaging study with serial short axis images demonstrating a perfusion deficit in the anterior wall.

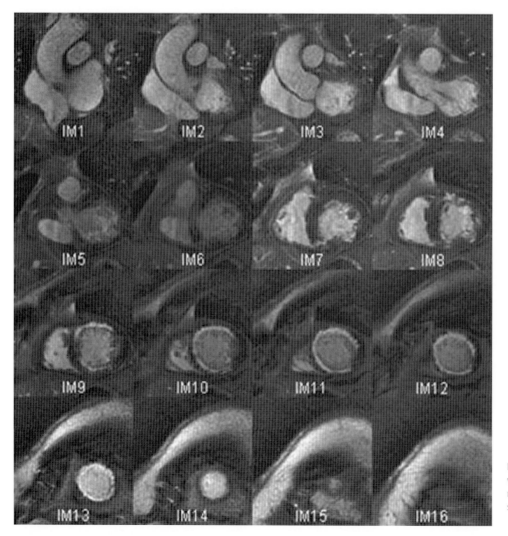

Figure 15.5. Delayed enhancement study with serial short axis images demonstrating non-viability of the anterior, septal, and inferior subendocardium.

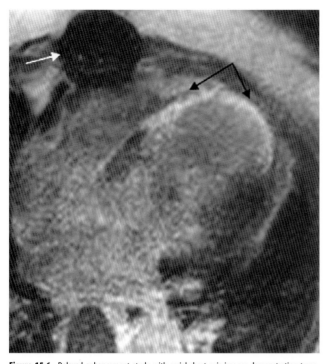

Figure 15.6. Delayed enhancement study with serial short axis images demonstrating transmural non-viability of the apical septum with wall thinning. Note the magnetic susceptibility artifact associated with sternal wires (white arrow).

myocardial perfusion [45]. With delayed enhancement images, usually obtained 10 minutes after injection, gadolinium has cleared from normal myocardium, but causes enhancement of non-viable, fibrosed tissue. Additionally, stress techniques such as dobutamine, persantine, and adenosine can be used to assess for evidence of ischemia [20,46,47]. Dobutamine CMR can be used to assess for ischemia and demonstrated a higher diagnostic accuracy than dobutamine echocardiography [48]. Additionally, dobutamine CMR is helpful in the assessment of patients with poor echo windows [49]. Dobutamine CMR can also assess for functional improvement after revascularization of ischemic cardiomyopathy [50]. The use of

CMR assessment of response to percutaneous coronary intervention with first pass imaging evaluated in the baseline state and with dipyridamole has been reported [47].

In ischemic cardiomyopathy, gadolinium delayed enhancement images can assess for areas of viability prior to potential revascularization. Specifically, in patient with ischemic cardiomyopathy, delayed hyperenhancement correlates with lack of viability defined by thallium single photon emission CT [51]. Soon after acute myocardial infarction, gadolinium delayed enhancement CMR images assessment of infarct size correlates with other clinical indices of infarct size [52]. The degree of wall thickening correlates with degree of myocardial non-enhancement on delayed images after recent myocardial infarction and predicts improvement in wall thickening as assessed by study at a later time [53].

A multimodal approach including assessment of coronary vasculature, cardiac function, rest and stress perfusion, and delayed enhancement, can be used for comprehensive assessment of cardiac substrates associated with coronary artery disease with a high accuracy [20]. In addition, gadolinium enhancement can be a useful tool in the assessment of fibrosis associated with dilated non-ischemic cardiomyopathy [54]. The presence and degree of gadolinium enhancement can predict remodeling response to beta blockers in both ischemic and non-ischemic cardiomyopathy [54].

CMR has proven useful in the diagnosis, characterization, and follow-up of patients with hypertrophic cardiomyopathy, with assessment for regional wall thickness, indexed ventricular mass, ejection fraction, and hemodynamic data including gradients (Figures 15.8 and 15.9) [55–57]. The presence, extent, and pattern of gadolinium delayed enhancement may potentially provide additional prognostic information [58,59]. Preoperative and follow-up studies may be useful in patients undergoing surgical myocardial resection or coronary artery septal embolization [57,60].

Myocardial tissue characteristics and gadolinium enhancement may also be useful in the assessment of inflammatory and infiltrative processes. Tissue character-

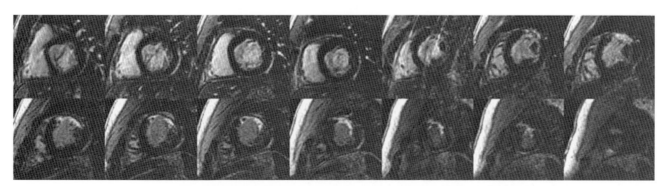

Figure 15.7. Delayed enhancement study with serial short axis images demonstrating non-viability of the anterior wall.

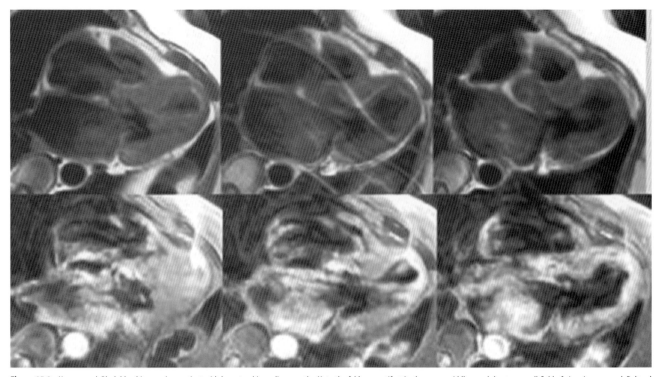

Figure 15.8. Upper panel: Black blood images in a patient with hypertrophic cardiomyopathy. Note the fold over artifact in the upper middle panel due to a small field of view. Lower panel: Delayed enhancement image demonstrating delayed gadolinium myocardial enhancement.

istics seen on CMR may help to differentiate amyloid from hypertrophic cardiomyopathy [61]. Gadolinium enhanced CMR can identify inflammation and fibrosis associated with cardiac sarcoidosis [62]. Additionally, changes associated with treatment of cardiac sarcoidosis with steroids have been reported [63]. Gadolinium enhancement associated with the inflammatory process in Chagas disease has also been reported [64].

A frontier in CMR is the assessment and understanding of microvascular coronary artery disease. Phosphorus-31 nuclear magnetic resonance spectroscopy has provided a window into the assessment of myocardial metabolism through assessment of myocardial high-energy phosphates. This tool has allowed insight into mechanisms of chest pain in the absence of obstructive coronary artery disease [65–68]. Studies have demonstrated direct evidence

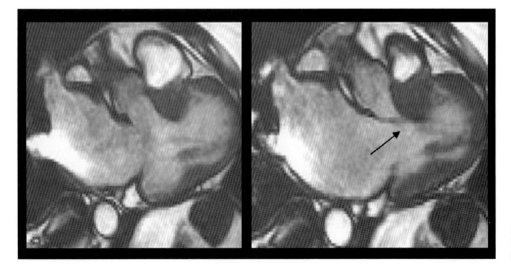

Figure 15.9. CMR images demonstrating hypertrophic cardiomyopathy with systolic anterior motion of the mitral valve (arrow).

of metabolic abnormalities consistent with ischemia in women with chest pain without obstructive coronary artery disease, and proven essential in forwarding the understanding of microvascular coronary artery disease. A stress-induced reduction in myocardial phosphocreatine–adenosine triphosphate ratio in women with chest pain without evidence of obstructive coronary artery disease has been shown to be predictive of greater rates of angina, as well as use of cardiac catheterization, and healthcare resources [67].

Congenital Heart Disease

The ability of CMR to provide comprehensive assessment of cardiovascular structure and function, as well as extracardiac thoracic structure, makes it useful in the diagnosis, facilitation of surgical or other procedural intervention, and follow-up of patients with congenital heart disease. Assessment of congenital heart disease was one of the first clinical applications of CMR [69–71]. CMR can comprehensively assess simple and complex congenital heart disease in the native state or after surgical treatment (Figures 15.10 and 15.11) [72–87].

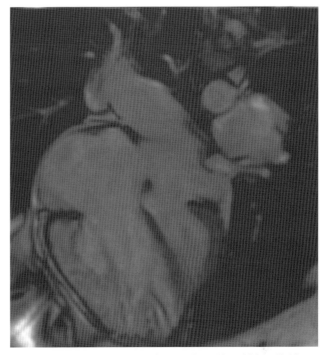

Figure 15.10. CMR image demonstrating a large secundum atrial septal defect, with right ventricular enlargement and hypertrophy and right atrial enlargement.

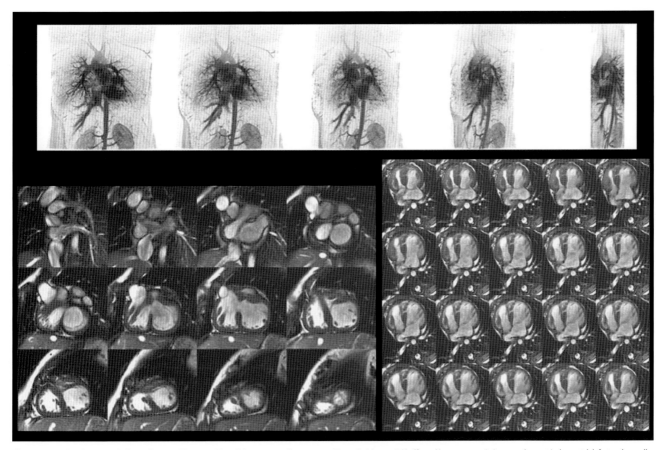

Figure 15.11. Complex congenital heart disease with transposition of the great vessels, status post Mustard with an atrial baffle and large non-restrictive muscular ventricular septal defect and a smaller muscular ventricular septal defect.

Assessment of ventricular function is extremely important in patients with congenital heart disease, with worse prognosis with ventricular dysfunction late after surgical repair of such anomalies as tetralogy of Fallot [88]. Baseline as well a dobutamine stress CMR can assess ventricular function and has been used to assess right ventricular dysfunction in patients with chronic right ventricular pressure overload secondary to congenital heart disease [82]. Additionally, cardiac shunts can be accurately assessed over the spectrum of pulmonary to systemic shunt ratios [77].

CMR is useful in pre-procedure planning for surgical approaches to congenital heart disease [83]. Studies can also provide information important to the pre-procedural planning of interventional cardiology procedures, such as atrial septal defect closure, with ability to assess such factors as defect size and rim characteristics [86]. Post-surgical imaging is important for the follow-up of surgically treated congenital heart disease, with reports demonstrating the utility of post-surgical follow-up for tetralogy

of Fallot [75,79], Mustard's operation for transposition of the great vessels [73,74], and follow-up of arterial switch for transposition of the great vessels [87].

In addition to congenital aortic lesions such as coarctation of the aorta, CMR can diagnose acquired vascular heart disease including aneurysm, dissection, and wall abnormalities such as penetrating ulcers, calcification or thrombus with ability to assess all aortic segments (Figures 15.12 and 15.13) [89]. CMR can characterize valves (Figures 15.14 and 15.15) and can assess for such abnormalities as significant aortic valve stenosis, with measurement of pressure gradients, velocity-time integral and valve dimensions which correlate well with echocardiogram [90].

Imaging approaches that are faster and more operator-independent should increase the utility of CMR for the assessment of congenital heart disease [84]. Real-time cardiac catheterization guided by magnetic resonance in compatible laboratory settings is being investigated for use in the assessment of congenital heart disease [91].

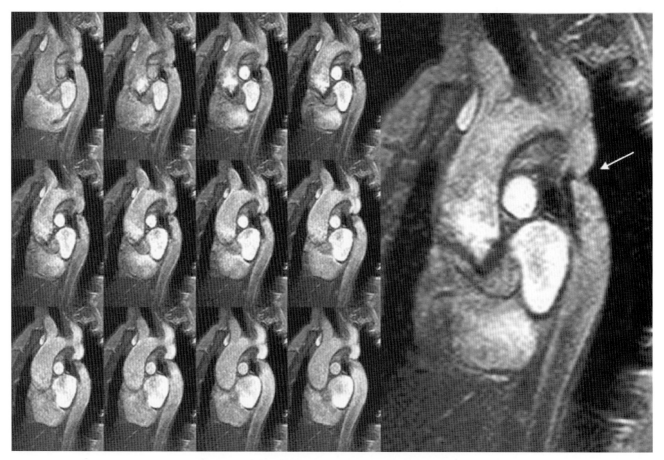

Figure 15.12. Serial sagittal slices demonstrating coarctation of the aorta (arrow).

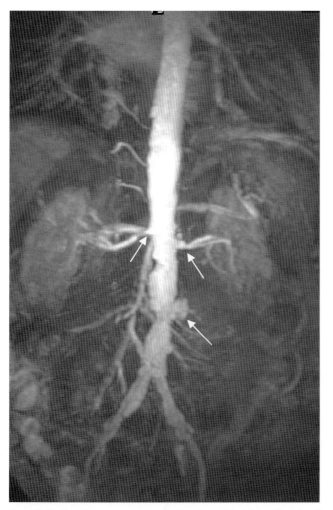

Figure 15.13. Magnetic resonance aortogram demonstrating multifocal plaques, bilateral renal artery stenosis (upper arrows), and a saccular aneurysm of infrarenal aorta (lower arrow).

Cardiac Masses

Assessment with CMR is useful in the diagnosis and characterization of cardiac masses due to the ability to comprehensively assess tissue characteristics of a mass, as well as relation of a mass to surrounding cardiac and thoracic structures (Figures 15.16–15.19). In regard to assessment of cardiac thrombi, CMR can visualize thrombi in both the atria and ventricles [92,93]. Although transesophageal echocardiography is the current method of choice for assessment of left atrial thrombi, CMR has been compared to transesophageal echocardiography in patients with non-rheumatic atrial fibrillation, showing high concordance with transesophageal echocardiography [92].

Benign tumors, primary malignant tumors, and metastatic malignant tumors have been identified with CMR, including fibromas, lipomas, myxomas, mesotheliomas, sarcomas, lymphomas, melanomas, and metastatic carcinomas [94–105]. The location of a mass, tissue characteristics of the mass, and presence or absence of pericardial involvement or pleural effusion are important

clues to assessment for potential benign or malignant etiology when findings are compared to actual histologic examination [106].

Cardiac Electrophysiology Applications

Due to the comprehensive nature of CMR, it has been shown to be useful in cardiac electrophysiology in the assessment for structural and functional abnormalities associated with electrophysiologically related disease processes. The major limitation to assessment of patients with electrophysiologically relevant issues is the preexistence of devices including pacemakers and implantable cardiac defibrillators. Issues reported have included pacemaker malfunction and lead heating [1–3]. As mentioned previously, some studies question whether scanning of patients with pacemakers using 1.5 Tesla systems is an absolute contraindication [4,5].

Diagnosis and characterization of ischemic and non-ischemic dilated cardiomyopathy is essential to risk stratification of patients for the primary prevention of sudden cardiac death. Due to multiple trials which have demonstrated benefit of placement of an implantable cardiac defibrillator based on severity of cardiac systolic dysfunction, the quantitative assessment of function in dilated ischemic and non-ischemic cardiomyopathy has become an important issue [107,108]. As previously detailed, CMR can characterize cardiac structure and function by reproducibly assessing ventricular volumes, ejection fraction, wall thickness, and wall motion [36–44].

Other applications relate to the assessment of electrophysiologically relevant disease processes involving the right ventricle. CMR can provide reproducible assessment of right ventricular size and function [43]. Arrhythmogenic right ventricular dysplasia is associated with ventricular arrhythmias and sudden cardiac death [109,110]. The diagnosis is challenging to make and involves multiple possible diagnostic factors, including clinical symptoms, family history, ECG findings, results of electrophysiology study, and structural/functional abnormalities of the right ventricle. Abnormalities associated with right ventricular dysplasia can be missed with many imaging modalities. CMR has become the diagnostic modality most commonly used to assess for arrhythmogenic right ventricular dysplasia, as CMR can differentiate tissue characteristics between fat and myocardium, as well as providing assessment of right ventricular size, shape, and function.

The initial focus of CMR identification of arrhythmogenic right ventricular dysplasia related to characterization of intramyocardial fat, but intramyocardial fat may also be present in normal subjects [111]. Initially, there was overdiagnosis of arrhythmogenic right ventricular dysplasia, partially due to focus on fat involvement and thinning of the right ventricle [112]. More recent focus has been on right ventricular size, shape, and function [113]. As CMR is contraindicated in patients with implantable cardiac

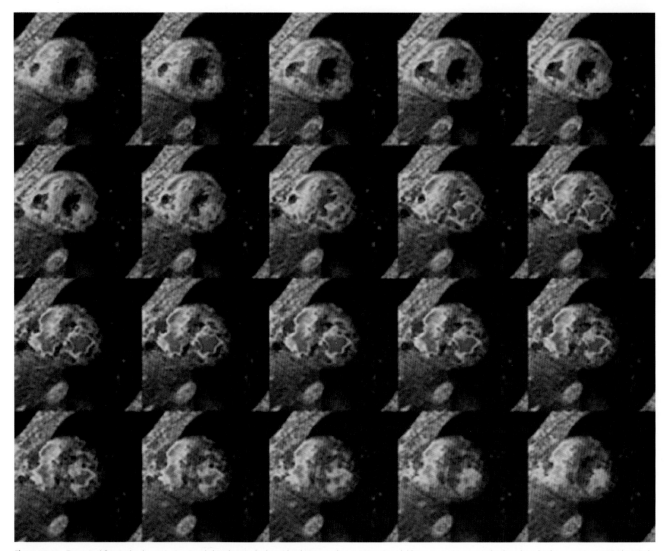

Figure 15.14.   Transmitral flow in the short axis view 2 cm below the mitral valve with velocity encoding at 200 cm/s, with blue representing ventricular diastole and red representing ventricular systole.

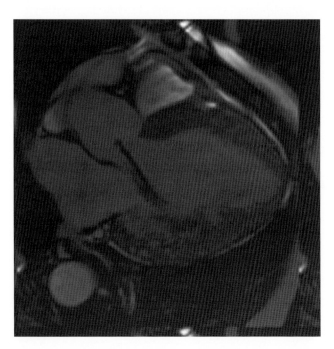

Figure 15.15.   Mild aortic regurgitation with an eccentric jet.

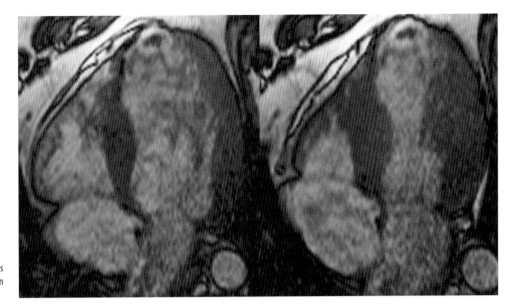

Figure 15.16. Diastolic and systolic images demonstrating an apical myocardial infarction with aneurysm and thrombus.

defibrillators, comprehensive diagnosis needs to be performed in patients suspected of having this diagnosis prior to device placement. Arrhythmogenic right ventricular dysplasia may mimic Brugada syndrome; therefore MRI can be useful as part of the workup for Brugada syndrome assessing for structural abnormalities associated with arrhythmogenic right ventricular dysplasia [114]. Study with CMR for assessment of structural changes associated with Brugada syndrome has only demonstrated subtle anatomic findings in comparison to normal volunteers [115].

Assessment of atrial anatomy is important to the understanding and treatment of supraventricular arrhythmias. Issues related to left atrial anatomy are particularly impor-

tant for cather ablation for atrial fibrillation. Techniques for atrial fibrillation ablation are in evolution, and involve either segmental catheter ablation of the pulmonary veins or circumferential electrical isolation of the pulmonary veins [116–118]. CMR can characterize the left atrium, as well as location, shape, complexity, and individual variation of pulmonary veins, facilitating preoperative planning for atrial fibrillation ablation procedures [119–122]. Similar to cardiovascular CT, the superimposition of real-time catheter positions and electrical recordings on 3-D CMR images obtained pre-procedure may prove to be useful in the performance of ablation procedures [123–125]. Animal models are being used to assess

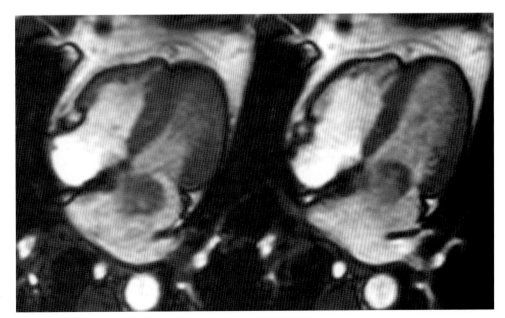

Figure 15.17. Image demonstrating a large left atrial myxoma.

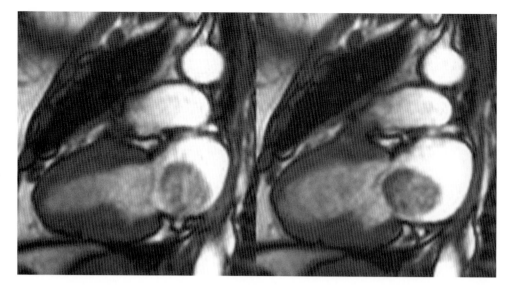

Figure 15.18. Large left atrial myxoma which obstructs the mitral valve during atrial systole.

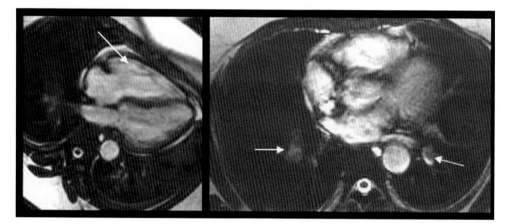

Figure 15.19. Left panel: Four-chamber view demonstrating right ventricular enlargement (arrows). Right panel: Localizer image demonstrating multiple pulmonary emboli (arrow).

real-time mapping, potentially with the ability to visualize radiofrequency catheter ablation lesions [125,126].

Similar to cardiovascular CT, CMR has been used to diagnose and provide surveillance for pulmonary vein stenosis, a potential complication of atrial fibrillation ablation [127–130]. In addition to providing roadmaps for ablation, pre-procedure studies can serve as templates to assess for changes in pulmonary vein anatomy on post-procedure studies. As the time course of pulmonary vein stenosis has not been fully defined, CMR may become a useful tool for the long-term follow-up for possible pulmonary vein stenosis [131].

Summary

Cardiovascular magnetic resonance imaging provides a multifaceted and comprehensive assessment for the diagnosis and treatment of cardiovascular disease, including cardiovascular structures, function, tissue characterization, myocardial perfusion, and metabolism. Applications

include the assessment of coronary artery disease, pathologic myocardial substrates, congenital heart disease, thoracic vasculature, valvular function, masses, and electrophysiologically relevant substrates. Advances in technology will continue to lead to novel clinical and research applications.

References

1. Lauck G, von Smekal A, Wolke S, et al. Effects of nuclear magnetic resonance imaging on cardiac pacemakers. Pacing Clin Electrophysiol 1995;18:1549–1555.
2. Achenbach S, Moshage W, Diem B, Bieberle T, Schibgilla V, Bachmann K. Effects of magnetic resonance imaging on cardiac pacemakers and electrodes. Am Heart J 1997;134:467–473.
3. Vahlhaus C, Sommer T, Lewalter T, et al. Interference with cardiac pacemakers by magnetic resonance imaging: are there irreversible changes at 0.5 Tesla? Pacing Clin Electrophysiol 2001;24:489–495.
4. Gimbel JR, Johnson D, Levine PA, Wilkoff BL. Safe performance of magnetic resonance imaging on five patients with permanent cardiac pacemakers. Pacing Clin Electrophysiol 1996;19:913–919.

5. Martin ET, Coman JA, Shellock FG, Pulling CC, Fair R, Jenkins K. Magnetic resonance imaging and cardiac pacemaker safety at 1.5-Tesla. J Am Coll Cardiol 2004;43:1315–1324.

6. Shellock FG. Prosthetic heart valves and annuloplasty rings: assessment of magnetic field interactions, heating, and artifacts at 1.5 Tesla. J Cardiovasc Magn Reson 2001;3:317–324.

7. Counter SA, Olofsson A, Grahn HF, Borg E. MRI acoustic noise: sound pressure and frequency analysis. J Magn Reson Imaging 1997;7:606–611.

8. Francis JM, Pennell DJ. Treatment of claustrophobia for cardiovascular magnetic resonance: use and effectiveness of mild sedation. J Cardiovasc Magn Reson 2000;2:139–141.

9. Sarji SA, Abdullah BJ, Kumar G, Tan AH, Narayanan P. Failed magnetic resonance imaging examinations due to claustrophobia. Australas Radiol 1998;42:293–295.

10. Lanzer P, Botvinick EH, Schiller NB, et al. Cardiac imaging using gated magnetic resonance. Radiology 1984;150:121–127.

11. Chia JM, Fischer SE, Wickline SA, Lorenz CH. Performance of QRS detection for cardiac magnetic resonance imaging with a novel vectorcardiographic triggering method. J Magn Reson Imaging 2000;12:678–688.

12. Dimick RN, Hedlund LW, Herfkens RJ, Fram EK, Utz J. Optimizing electrocardiograph electrode placement for cardiac-gated magnetic resonance imaging. Invest Radiol 1987;22:17–22.

13. Storey P, Danias PG, Post M, et al. Preliminary evaluation of EVP 1001-1: a new cardiac-specific magnetic resonance contrast agent with kinetics suitable for steady-state imaging of the ischemic heart. Invest Radiol 2003;38:642–652.

14. Flacke S, Fischer S, Scott MJ, et al. Novel MRI contrast agent for molecular imaging of fibrin: implications for detecting vulnerable plaques. Circulation 2001;104:1280–1285.

15. Carr DH, Brown J, Bydder GM, et al. Gadolinium-DTPA as a contrast agent in MRI: initial clinical experience in 20 patients. AJR Am J Roentgenol 1984;143:215–224.

16. Nayak KS, Cunningham CH, Santos JM, Pauly JM. Real-time cardiac MRI at 3 tesla. Magn Reson Med 2004;51:655–660.

17. McGee KP, Debbins JP, Boskamp EB, Blawat L, Angelos L, King KF. Cardiac magnetic resonance parallel imaging at 3.0 Tesla: technical feasibility and advantages. J Magn Reson Imaging 2004;19:291–729.

18. Kangarlu A, Burgess RE, Zhu H, et al. Cognitive, cardiac, and physiological safety studies in ultra high field magnetic resonance imaging. Magn Reson Imaging 1999;17:1407–1416.

19. Budoff MJ, Achenbach S, Duerinckx A. Clinical utility of computed tomography and magnetic resonance techniques for noninvasive coronary angiography. J Am Coll Cardiol 2003;42:1867–1878.

20. Plein S, Greenwood JP, Ridgway JP, Cranny G, Ball SG, Sivananthan MU. Assessment of non-ST-segment elevation acute coronary syndromes with cardiac magnetic resonance imaging. J Am Coll Cardiol 2004;44:2173–2181.

21. Bunce NH, Lorenz CH, John AS, Lesser JR, Mohiaddin RH, Pennell DJ. Coronary artery bypass graft patency: assessment with true ast imaging with steady-state precession versus gadolinium-enhanced MR angiography. Radiology 2003;227:440–446.

22. Achenbach S, Kessler W, Moshage WE, et al. Visualization of the coronary arteries in three-dimensional reconstructions using respiratory gated magnetic resonance imaging. Coron Artery Dis 1997;8:441–448.

23. Kessler W, Laub G, Achenbach S, Ropers D, Moshage W, Daniel WG. Coronary arteries: MR angiography with fast contrast-enhanced three-dimensional breath-hold imaging – initial experience. Radiology 1999;210:566–572.

24. Post JC, van Rossum AC, Bronzwaer JG, et al. Magnetic resonance angiography of anomalous coronary arteries. A new gold standard for delineating the proximal course? Circulation 1995;92:3163–3171.

25. Bunce NH, Rahman SL, Keegan J, Gatehouse PD, Lorenz CH, Pennell DJ. Anomalous coronary arteries: anatomic and functional assessment by coronary and perfusion cardiovascular magnetic resonance in three sisters. J Cardiovasc Magn Reson 2001;3:361–369.

26. Achenbach S, Ropers D, Regenfus M, et al. Noninvasive coronary angiography by magnetic resonance imaging, electron-beam computed tomography, and multislice computed tomography. Am J Cardiol 2001;88:70E–73E.

27. Regenfus M, Ropers D, Achenbach S, et al. Noninvasive detection of coronary artery stenosis using contrast-enhanced three-dimensional breath-hold magnetic resonance coronary angiography. J Am Coll Cardiol 2000;36:44–50.

28. Regenfus M, Ropers D, Achenbach S, et al. Comparison of contrast-enhanced breath-hold and free-breathing respiratory-gated imaging in three-dimensional magnetic resonance coronary angiography. Am J Cardiol 2002;90:725–730.

29. Ropers D, Regenfus M, Stilianakis N, et al. A direct comparison of noninvasive coronary angiography by electron beam tomography and navigator-echo-based magnetic resonance imaging for the detection of restenosis following coronary angioplasty. Invest Radiol 2002;37:386–392.

30. Naghavi M, Libby P, Falk E, et al. From vulnerable plaque to vulnerable patient: a call for new definitions and risk assessment strategies: Part I. Circulation 2003;108:1664–1672.

31. Naghavi M, Libby P, Falk E, et al. From vulnerable plaque to vulnerable patient: a call for new definitions and risk assessment strategies: Part II. Circulation 2003;108:1772–1778.

32. Nikolaou K, Becker CR, Muders M, et al. Multidetector-row computed tomography and magnetic resonance imaging of atherosclerotic lesions in human ex vivo coronary arteries. Atherosclerosis 2004;174:243–252.

33. Fayad ZA, Fuster V, Nikolaou K, Becker C. Computed tomography and magnetic resonance imaging for noninvasive coronary angiography and plaque imaging: current and potential future concepts. Circulation 2002;106:2026–2034.

34. Kim WY, Stuber M, Bornert P, Kissinger KV, Manning WJ, Botnar RM. Three-dimensional black-blood cardiac magnetic resonance coronary vessel wall imaging detects positive arterial remodeling in patients with nonsignificant coronary artery disease. Circulation 2002;106:296–299.

35. Viles-Gonzalez JF, Poon M, Sanz J, et al. In vivo 16-slice, multidetector-row computed tomography for the assessment of experimental atherosclerosis: comparison with magnetic resonance imaging and histopathology. Circulation 2004;110:1467–1472.

36. Cranney GB, Lotan CS, Dean L, Baxley W, Bouchard A, Pohost GM. Left ventricular volume measurement using cardiac axis nuclear magnetic resonance imaging. Validation by calibrated ventricular angiography. Circulation 1990;82:154–163.

37. Rumberger JA, Behrenbeck T, Bell MR, et al. Determination of ventricular ejection fraction: a comparison of available imaging methods. The Cardiovascular Imaging Working Group. Mayo Clin Proc 1997;72:860–870.

38. Scharhag J, Schneider G, Urhausen A, Rochette V, Kramann B, Kindermann W. Athlete's heart: right and left ventricular mass and function in male endurance athletes and untrained individuals determined by magnetic resonance imaging. J Am Coll Cardiol 2002;40:1856–1863.

39. Rominger MB, Bachmann GF, Pabst W, Rau WS. Right ventricular volumes and ejection fraction with fast cine MR imaging in breath-hold technique: applicability, normal values from 52 volunteers, and evaluation of 325 adult cardiac patients. J Magn Reson Imaging 1999;10:908–918.

40. Kaji S, Yang PC, Kerr AB, et al. Rapid evaluation of left ventricular volume and mass without breath-holding using real-time interactive cardiac magnetic resonance imaging system. J Am Coll Cardiol 2001;38:527–533.

41. Plein S, Smith WH, Ridgway JP, et al. Measurements of left ventricular dimensions using real-time acquisition in cardiac magnetic resonance imaging: comparison with conventional gradient echo imaging. Magma 2001;13:101–108.

42. Ioannidis JP, Trikalinos TA, Danias PG. Electrocardiogram-gated single-photon emission computed tomography versus cardiac magnetic resonance imaging for the assessment of left ventricular volumes and ejection fraction: a meta-analysis. J Am Coll Cardiol 2002;39:2059–2068.

43. Grothues F, Moon JC, Bellenger NG, Smith GS, Klein HU, Pennell DJ. Interstudy reproducibility of right ventricular volumes, function, and mass with cardiovascular magnetic resonance. Am Heart J 2004;147:218–223.

44. Lethimonnier F, Furber A, Balzer P, et al. Global left ventricular cardiac function: comparison between magnetic resonance imaging, radionuclide angiography, and contrast angiography. Invest Radiol 1999;34:199–203.

45. Manning WJ, Atkinson DJ, Grossman W, Paulin S, Edelman RR. First-pass nuclear magnetic resonance imaging studies using gadolinium-DTPA in patients with coronary artery disease. J Am Coll Cardiol 1991;18:959–965.

46. Kuijpers D, Janssen CH, van Dijkman PR, Oudkerk M. Dobutamine stress MRI. Part I. Safety and feasibility of dobutamine cardiovascular magnetic resonance in patients suspected of myocardial ischemia. Eur Radiol 2004;14:1823–1828.

47. Al-Saadi N, Nagel E, Gross M, et al. Improvement of myocardial perfusion reserve early after coronary intervention: assessment with cardiac magnetic resonance imaging. J Am Coll Cardiol 2000;36:1557–1564.

48. Nagel E, Lehmkuhl HB, Bocksch W, et al. Noninvasive diagnosis of ischemia-induced wall motion abnormalities with the use of high-dose dobutamine stress MRI: comparison with dobutamine stress echocardiography. Circulation 1999;99:763–770.

49. Hundley WG, Morgan TM, Neagle CM, Hamilton CA, Rerkpattanapipat P, Link KM. Magnetic resonance imaging determination of cardiac prognosis. Circulation 2002;106:2328–2333.

50. Samady H, Choi CJ, Ragosta M, Powers ER, Beller GA, Kramer CM. Electromechanical mapping identifies improvement in function and retention of contractile reserve after revascularization in ischemic cardiomyopathy. Circulation 2004;110:2410–2416.

51. Ansari M, Araoz PA, Gerard SK, et al. Comparison of late enhancement cardiovascular magnetic resonance and thallium SPECT in patients with coronary disease and left ventricular dysfunction. J Cardiovasc Magn Reson 2004;6:549–556.

52. Ingkanisorn WP, Rhoads KL, Aletras AH, Kellman P, Arai AE. Gadolinium delayed enhancement cardiovascular magnetic resonance correlates with clinical measures of myocardial infarction. J Am Coll Cardiol 2004;43:2253–2259.

53. Ichikawa Y, Sakuma H, Suzawa N, et al. Late gadolinium-enhanced magnetic resonance imaging in acute and chronic myocardial infarction: improved prediction of regional myocardial contraction in the chronic state by measuring thickness of nonenhanced myocardium. J Am Coll Cardiol 2005;45:901–909.

54. Bello D, Shah DJ, Farah GM, et al. Gadolinium cardiovascular magnetic resonance predicts reversible myocardial dysfunction and remodeling in patients with heart failure undergoing beta-blocker therapy. Circulation 2003;108:1945–1953.

55. Dong SJ, MacGregor JH, Crawley AP, et al. Left ventricular wall thickness and regional systolic function in patients with hypertrophic cardiomyopathy. A three-dimensional tagged magnetic resonance imaging study. Circulation 1994;90:1200–1209.

56. Devlin AM, Moore NR, Ostman-Smith I. A comparison of MRI and echocardiography in hypertrophic cardiomyopathy. Br J Radiol 1999;72:258–264.

57. Schulz-Menger J, Strohm O, Waigand J, Uhlich F, Dietz R, Friedrich MG. The value of magnetic resonance imaging of the left ventricular outflow tract in patients with hypertrophic obstructive cardiomyopathy after septal artery embolization. Circulation 2000;101:1764–1766.

58. Moon JC, McKenna WJ, McCrohon JA, Elliott PM, Smith GC, Pennell DJ. Toward clinical risk assessment in hypertrophic cardiomyopathy with gadolinium cardiovascular magnetic resonance. J Am Coll Cardiol 2003;41:1561–1567.

59. Teraoka K, Hirano M, Ookubo H, et al. Delayed contrast enhancement of MRI in hypertrophic cardiomyopathy. Magn Reson Imaging 2004;22:155–161.

60. White RD, Obuchowski NA, Gunawardena S, et al. Left ventricular outflow tract obstruction in hypertrophic cardiomyopathy: presurgical and postsurgical evaluation by computed tomography magnetic resonance imaging. Am J Card Imaging 1996;10:1–13.

61. Fattori R, Rocchi G, Celletti F, Bertaccini P, Rapezzi C, Gavelli G. Contribution of magnetic resonance imaging in the differential diagnosis of cardiac amyloidosis and symmetric hypertrophic cardiomyopathy. Am Heart J 1998;136:824–830.

62. Nemeth MA, Muthupillai R, Wilson JM, Awasthi M, Flamm SD. Cardiac sarcoidosis detected by delayed-hyperenhancement magnetic resonance imaging. Tex Heart Inst J 2004;31:99–102.

63. Shimada T, Shimada K, Sakane T, et al. Diagnosis of cardiac sarcoidosis and evaluation of the effects of steroid therapy by gadolinium-DTPA-enhanced magnetic resonance imaging. Am J Med 2001;110:520–527.

64. Bocchi EA, Kalil R, Bacal F, et al. Magnetic resonance imaging in chronic Chagas' disease: correlation with endomyocardial biopsy findings and gallium-67 cardiac uptake. Echocardiography 1998;15:279–288.

65. Buchthal SD, den Hollander JA, Merz CN, et al. Abnormal myocardial phosphorus-31 nuclear magnetic resonance spectroscopy in women with chest pain but normal coronary angiograms. N Engl J Med 2000;342:829–835.

66. Butterworth EJ, Evanochko WT, Pohost GM. The 31P-NMR stress test: an approach for detecting myocardial ischemia. Ann Biomed Eng 2000;28:930–933.

67. Johnson BD, Shaw LJ, Buchthal SD, et al. Prognosis in women with myocardial ischemia in the absence of obstructive coronary disease: results from the National Institutes of Health-National Heart, Lung, and Blood Institute-Sponsored Women's Ischemia Syndrome Evaluation (WISE). Circulation 2004;109:2993–2999.

68. Pohost GM, Forder JR. From the atomic nucleus to man: nuclear magnetic resonance spectroscopy, the next horizon in diagnostic cardiology. J Am Coll Cardiol 2003;42:1594–1595.

69. Goldman MR, Pohost GM. Nuclear magnetic resonance imaging. The potential for cardiac evaluation of the pediatric patient. Cardiol Clin 1983;1:521–525.

70. Fletcher BD, Jacobstein MD, Nelson AD, Riemenschneider TA, Alfidi RJ. Gated magnetic resonance imaging of congenital cardiac malformations. Radiology 1984;150:137–140.

71. Boxer RA, Singh S, LaCorte MA, Goldman M, Stein HL. Cardiac magnetic resonance imaging in children with congenital heart disease. J Pediatr 1986;109:460–464.

72. Nishimura T, Fujii T. Double-chambered right ventricle demonstrated by magnetic resonance imaging before cardiac catheterization – case report. Angiology 1988;39:259–262.

73. Rees S, Somerville J, Warnes C, et al. Comparison of magnetic resonance imaging with echocardiography and radionuclide angiography in assessing cardiac function and anatomy following Mustard's operation for transposition of the great arteries. Am J Cardiol 1988;61:1316–1322.

74. Theissen P, Kaemmerer H, Sechtem U, et al. Magnetic resonance imaging of cardiac function and morphology in patients with transposition of the great arteries following Mustard procedure. Thorac Cardiovasc Surg 1991;39(Suppl 3):221–224.

75. Greenberg SB, Faerber EN, Balsara RK. Tetralogy of Fallot: diagnostic imaging after palliative and corrective surgery. J Thorac Imaging 1995;10:26–35.

76. Watanabe H, Hayashi JI, Sugawara M, Yagi N. Complete unilateral anomalous connection of the left pulmonary veins to the coronary sinus with unroofed coronary sinus syndrome: a case report. Thorac Cardiovasc Surg 1999;47:193–195.

77. Arheden H, Holmqvist C, Thilen U, et al. Left-to-right cardiac shunts: comparison of measurements obtained with MR velocity mapping and with radionuclide angiography. Radiology 1999;211: 453–458.

78. Hahm JK, Park YW, Lee JK, et al. Magnetic resonance imaging of unroofed coronary sinus: three cases. Pediatr Cardiol 2000;21: 382–387.

79. Helbing WA, de Roos A. Clinical applications of cardiac magnetic resonance imaging after repair of tetralogy of Fallot. Pediatr Cardiol 2000;21:70–79.

80. Ferrari VA, Scott CH, Holland GA, Axel L, Sutton MS. Ultrafast three-dimensional contrast-enhanced magnetic resonance angiography and imaging in the diagnosis of partial anomalous pulmonary venous drainage. J Am Coll Cardiol 2001;37:1120–1128.

81. Geva T, Greil GF, Marshall AC, Landzberg M, Powell AJ. Gadolinium-enhanced 3-dimensional magnetic resonance angiography of pulmonary blood supply in patients with complex pulmonary stenosis or atresia: comparison with x-ray angiography. Circulation 2002;106:473–478.

82. Tulevski II, van der Wall EE, Groenink M, et al. Usefulness of magnetic resonance imaging dobutamine stress in asymptomatic and minimally symptomatic patients with decreased cardiac reserve from congenital heart disease (complete and corrected transposition of the great arteries and subpulmonic obstruction). Am J Cardiol 2002;89:1077–1081.

83. Haramati LB, Glickstein JS, Issenberg HJ, Haramati N, Crooke GA. MR imaging and CT of vascular anomalies and connections in patients with congenital heart disease: significance in surgical planning. Radiographics 2002;22:337–347; discussion 348–349.

84. Razavi RS, Hill DL, Muthurangu V, et al. Three-dimensional magnetic resonance imaging of congenital cardiac anomalies. Cardiol Young 2003;13:461–465.

85. Sorensen TS, Korperich H, Greil GF, et al. Operator-independent isotropic three-dimensional magnetic resonance imaging for morphology in congenital heart disease: a validation study. Circulation 2004;110:163–169.

86. Durongpisitkul K, Tang NL, Soongswang J, Laohaprasitiporn D, Nanal A. Predictors of successful transcatheter closure of atrial septal defect by cardiac magnetic resonance imaging. Pediatr Cardiol 2004;25:124–130.

87. Taylor AM, Dymarkowski S, Hamaekers P, et al. MR coronary angiography and late-enhancement myocardial MR in children who underwent arterial switch surgery for transposition of great arteries. Radiology 2005;234(2):542–547.

88. Ghai A, Silversides C, Harris L, Webb GD, Siu SC, Therrien J. Left ventricular dysfunction is a risk factor for sudden cardiac death in adults late after repair of tetralogy of Fallot. J Am Coll Cardiol 2002;40:1675–1680.

89. Hartnell GG. Imaging of aortic aneurysms and dissection: CT and MRI. J Thorac Imaging 2001;16:35–46.

90. Caruthers SD, Lin SJ, Brown P, et al. Practical value of cardiac magnetic resonance imaging for clinical quantification of aortic valve stenosis: comparison with echocardiography. Circulation 2003;108: 2236–2243.

91. Razavi R, Hill DL, Keevil SF, et al. Cardiac catheterisation guided by MRI in children and adults with congenital heart disease. Lancet 2003;362:1877–1882.

92. Ohyama H, Hosomi N, Takahashi T, et al. Comparison of magnetic resonance imaging and transesophageal echocardiography in detection of thrombus in the left atrial appendage. Stroke 2003;34: 2436–2439.

93. Barkhausen J, Hunold P, Eggebrecht H, et al. Detection and characterization of intracardiac thrombi on MR imaging. AJR Am J Roentgenol 2002;179:1539–1544.

94. Brechtel K, Reddy GP, Higgins CB. Cardiac fibroma in an infant: magnetic resonance imaging characteristics. J Cardiovasc Magn Reson 1999;1:159–161.

95. Burri H, Bloch A, Hauser H. Characterization of an unusual right atrial mass by echocardiography, magnetic resonance imaging, computed tomography, and angiography. Echocardiography 1999; 16:393–396.

96. Kamiya H, Ohno M, Iwata H, et al. Cardiac lipoma in the interventricular septum: evaluation by computed tomography and magnetic resonance imaging. Am Heart J 1990;119:1215–1217.

97. Salanitri JC, Pereles FS. Cardiac lipoma and lipomatous hypertrophy of the interatrial septum: cardiac magnetic resonance imaging findings. J Comput Assist Tomogr 2004;28:852–856.

98. Matsuoka H, Hamada M, Honda T, et al. Morphologic and histologic characterization of cardiac myxomas by magnetic resonance imaging. Angiology 1996;47:693–688.

99. Watanabe AT, Teitelbaum GP, Henderson RW, Bradley WG Jr. Magnetic resonance imaging of cardiac sarcomas. J Thorac Imaging 1989;4:90–92.

100. Inoko M, Iga K, Kyo K, et al. Primary cardiac angiosarcoma detected by magnetic resonance imaging but not by computed tomography. Intern Med 2001;40:391–395.

101. Tahara T, Takase B, Yamagishi T, et al. A case report on primary cardiac non-Hodgkin's lymphoma: an approach by magnetic resonance and thallium-201 imaging. J Cardiovasc Magn Reson 1999;1:163–167.

102. Schrem SS, Colvin SB, Weinreb JC, Glassman E, Kronzon I. Metastatic cardiac liposarcoma: diagnosis by transesophageal echocardiography and magnetic resonance imaging. J Am Soc Echocardiogr 1990;3:149–153.

103. Mousseaux E, Meunier P, Azancott S, Dubayle P, Gaux JC. Cardiac metastatic melanoma investigated by magnetic resonance imaging. Magn Reson Imaging 1998;16:91–95.

104. Testempassi E, Takeuchi H, Fukuda Y, Harada J, Tada S. Cardiac metastasis of colon adenocarcinoma diagnosed by magnetic resonance imaging. Acta Cardiol 1994;49:191–196.

105. Kaminaga T, Takeshita T, Kimura I. Role of magnetic resonance imaging for evaluation of tumors in the cardiac region. Eur Radiol 2003;13(Suppl 4):L1–10.

106. Hoffmann U, Globits S, Schima W, et al. Usefulness of magnetic resonance imaging of cardiac and paracardiac masses. Am J Cardiol 2003;92:890–895.

107. Moss AJ, Zareba W, Hall WJ, et al. Prophylactic implantation of a defibrillator in patients with myocardial infarction and reduced ejection fraction. N Engl J Med 2002;346:877–883.

108. Bardy GH, Lee KL, Mark DB, et al. Amiodarone or an implantable cardioverter-defibrillator for congestive heart failure. N Engl J Med 2005;352:225–237.

109. Corrado D, Thiene G, Nava A, Rossi L, Pennelli N. Sudden death in young competitive athletes: clinicopathologic correlations in 22 cases. Am J Med 1990;89:588–596.

110. Tabib A, Loire R, Chalabreysse L, et al. Circumstances of death and gross and microscopic observations in a series of 200 cases of sudden death associated with arrhythmogenic right ventricular cardiomyopathy and/or dysplasia. Circulation 2003;108:3000–3005.

111. di Cesare E. MRI assessment of right ventricular dysplasia. Eur Radiol 2003;13:1387–1393.

112. Bomma C, Rutberg J, Tandri H, et al. Misdiagnosis of arrhythmogenic right ventricular dysplasia/cardiomyopathy. J Cardiovasc Electrophysiol 2004;15:300–306.

113. Bluemke DA, Krupinski EA, Ovitt T, et al. MR Imaging of arrhythmogenic right ventricular cardiomyopathy: morphologic findings and interobserver reliability. Cardiology 2003;99:153–162.

114. Wilde AA, Antzelevitch C, Borggrefe M, et al. Proposed diagnostic criteria for the Brugada syndrome: consensus report. Circulation 2002;106:2514–2519.

115. Papavassiliu T, Wolpert C, Fluchter S, et al. Magnetic resonance imaging findings in patients with Brugada syndrome. J Cardiovasc Electrophysiol 2004;15:1133–1138.

116. Nakagawa H, Aoyama H, Beckman KJ, et al. Relation between pulmonary vein firing and extent of left atrial-pulmonary vein connection in patients with atrial fibrillation. Circulation 2004;109: 1523–1529.

117. Pappone C, Rosanio S, Oreto G, et al. Circumferential radiofrequency ablation of pulmonary vein ostia: A new anatomic approach for curing atrial fibrillation. Circulation 2000;102:2619–2628.

118. Oral H, Knight BP, Ozaydin M, et al. Segmental ostial ablation to isolate the pulmonary veins during atrial fibrillation: feasibility and mechanistic insights. Circulation 2002;106:1256–1262.

119. Hauser TH, McClennen S, Katsimaglis G, Josephson ME, Manning WJ, Yeon SB. Assessment of left atrial volume by contrast enhanced magnetic resonance angiography. J Cardiovasc Magn Reson 2004;6: 491–497.

120. Lickfett L, Kato R, Tandri H, et al. Characterization of a new pulmonary vein variant using magnetic resonance angiography: incidence, imaging, and interventional implications of the "right top pulmonary vein". J Cardiovasc Electrophysiol 2004;15:538–543.

121. Kato R, Lickfett L, Meininger G, et al. Pulmonary vein anatomy in patients undergoing catheter ablation of atrial fibrillation: lessons learned by use of magnetic resonance imaging. Circulation 2003; 107:2004–2010.

122. Mansour M, Holmvang G, Sosnovik D, et al. Assessment of pulmonary vein anatomic variability by magnetic resonance imaging: implications for catheter ablation techniques for atrial fibrillation. J Cardiovasc Electrophysiol 2004;15:387–393.

123. Dickfeld T, Calkins H, Zviman M, et al. Anatomic stereotactic catheter ablation on three-dimensional magnetic resonance images in real time. Circulation 2003;108:2407–2413.

124. Dickfeld T, Calkins H, Zviman M, et al. Stereotactic magnetic resonance guidance for anatomically targeted ablations of the fossa ovalis and the left atrium. J Interv Card Electrophysiol 2004;11: 105–115.

125. Reddy VY, Malchano ZJ, Holmvang G, et al. Integration of cardiac magnetic resonance imaging with three-dimensional electroanatomic mapping to guide left ventricular catheter manipulation. Feasibility in a porcine model of healed myocardial infarction. J Am Coll Cardiol 2004;44:2202–2213.

126. Lardo AC, McVeigh ER, Jumrussirikul P, et al. Visualization and temporal/spatial characterization of cardiac radiofrequency ablation lesions using magnetic resonance imaging. Circulation 2000; 102:698–705.

127. Robbins IM, Colvin EV, Doyle TP, et al. Pulmonary vein stenosis after catheter ablation of atrial fibrillation. Circulation 1998;98: 1769–1775.

128. Taylor GW, Kay GN, Zheng X, Bishop S, Ideker RE. Pathological effects of extensive radiofrequency energy applications in the pulmonary veins in dogs. Circulation 2000;101:1736–1742.

129. Yang M, Akbari H, Reddy GP, Higgins CB. Identification of pulmonary vein stenosis after radiofrequency ablation for atrial fibrillation using MRI. J Comput Assist Tomogr 2001;25:34–35.

130. Dill T, Neumann T, Ekinci O, et al. Pulmonary vein diameter reduction after radiofrequency catheter ablation for paroxysmal atrial fibrillation evaluated by contrast-enhanced three-dimensional magnetic resonance imaging. Circulation 2003;107:845–850.

131. Arentz T, Jander N, von Rosenthal J, et al. Incidence of pulmonary vein stenosis 2 years after radiofrequency catheter ablation of refractory atrial fibrillation. Eur Heart J 2003;24:963–969.

16

Congenital Heart Disease and Computed Tomography

Jamil AboulHosn and Ronald J. Oudiz

Introduction

Congenital heart disease (CHD) of moderate to severe complexity afflicts nearly 2% of all live births [1]. In the Western world these cases are often recognized at or shortly after birth because of the vigilant auscultation for murmurs and observation for cyanosis. Advances in the field of fetal echocardiography and videoscopic surgery have made intrauterine diagnosis and treatment possible in some cases [2]. The surgical and medical management of these cases has advanced at a dizzying pace in the past fifty years, allowing many patients with complex CHD to survive to adulthood where previously childhood or infant mortality was the norm. In contrast to the systematic attention and care provided in the developed world, the picture remains grim for a child born with complex CHD in the developing world. Less than 1% of children with CHD are appropriately identified and treated [3–4]. Repaired, palliated, or untreated, many patients with congenital heart disease survive into adulthood. These patients often have complex cardiac anatomy and present a real challenge to the clinician.

The suspicion of congenital heart disease begins with the history and physical examination and confirmation is sought by various imaging modalities, hemodynamic assessment, and electrocardiographic patterns. Patients who have had previous surgery often require frequent imaging to determine the adequacy of operative repair or palliation. Echocardiography and cardiac catheterization have been the primary modalities used to serve this purpose [5]. Cardiac catheterization, widely viewed as the gold standard, is invasive and complications, although uncommon, can be serious [6]. Echocardiography has been the non-invasive workhorse in this field [7–8]. However, the quality of the studies is highly dependent on body habitus and echocardiographic windows. Moreover, the extracardiac but intrathoracic vasculature and anatomy is not well imaged [8]. This is no small limitation given the frequency of associated intra- and extracardiac anomalies in patients with congenital heart disease. It is upon this backdrop that magnetic resonance imaging (MRI) and computed tomography (CT) are carving a niche as key imaging tools in CHD.

MRI has been utilized more extensively in the CHD field than CT for a number of reasons [9]. First, MRI does not deliver any radiation. In contrast, one CT study will deliver nearly 1000 millirads to the skin of the back [10]. This may seem negligible in most adults when compared to the 10,000 millirads a patient is exposed to with invasive catheterization and angiography. However, no amount of radiation is considered safe. Moreover, the evaluation of most congenital cases begins in infancy and childhood when radiation is most likely to cause lasting damage and produce malignancies. Considering that the average radiation dose from one year of television viewing is 1 millirad, the 1000 millirads from one CT seems excessive if another means of diagnosis is readily available. That has led to the near exclusion of CT in favor of MRI in the pediatric population. Not so in the adult population where advances in image acquisition, speed, and clarity have propelled CT to the forefront of non-invasive imaging. Moreover, electrocardiographic gating of studies at multiple points in systole and diastole allows the evaluation of dynamic processes such as ventricular wall motion [11]. The provision of such functional information had been the domain of MRI until recently and this had steered many CHD specialists in the direction of MRI. MRI does have the ability to very accurately determine plasma velocity and valvar areas whereas CT requires the accompaniment of echocardiography [12–13]. However, the static anatomy of small vessels (especially coronaries) is far more accurately imaged by CT in a fraction of the time needed for MRI [14]. Both modalities can be rendered into three-dimensional images that are useful in clarifying the often complex anatomic relationships in patients with CHD. In truth, both modalities have strengths and weaknesses. However, the previously lopsided playing field is being evened out by advances in CT image quality, decreases in radiation dose, and the provision of accurate functional information. Furthermore, MRI most often requires significant sedation in children, not necessary with the very fast study times with CT. Currently, CT is being used extensively at many centers for the evaluation of adult patients with CHD.

This chapter will provide an overview of CHD, with or without previous surgery, that is compatible with survival into adulthood. For the sake of organizing a large and heterogeneous panoply of conditions a simple anatomic classification of CHD will be used [15]. This includes four major categories that can occur in isolation or combination. These are:

1. defects (communications, shunts)
2. obstructions (stenosis, atresia)
3. transpositions
4. dysplasias.

The evolution and indications for various surgical techniques will also be addressed in a succinct manner. CT is widely used for planning and assessing the results of operative interventions [16]. The goal of this chapter is to summarize and clarify the current role and future potential of cardiac CT in the evaluation of patients with CHD.

Defects

Atrial Septal Defects

Atrial septal defects (ASD) are the most common defect in adults with congenital heart disease, accounting for 40% of lesions in adults older than 40 years [17]. The development of the atrial septum begins with outgrowth of the septum primum from the roof of the atria to the endocardial cushion. Thereafter, the mid-portion of this septum dissolves, creating the ostium primum. This is followed by outgrowth of the septum secundum from the roof of the atrium. Hence, at birth there are two curtains of atrial septum, the septum primum inferior and leftward to the septum secundum. Failure of the septum primum to fuse with the endocardial cushions leads to the development of a primum ASD. Failure of the septum secundum to grow in and cover the ostium primum leads to development of a secundum ASD. The various types of atrial septal defects and their locations are displayed in Figure 16.1.

The septum secundum ASDs are the most common type. They are usually of little clinical consequence in the first two decades of life. However, if these defects are not repaired they often lead to right heart volume overload, moderate pulmonary hypertension, and atrial tachyarrhythmias. This is especially true in patients with large defects and a left to right shunt ratio of >1.5 : 1. Moreover, these defects can occasionally be a portal through which systemic venous thromboemboli may cross to the systemic arterial circulation, leading to arterial embolic complications such as stroke. Hence, closure of such defects is preferred.

The treatment of patients with ostium secundum ASD has evolved rapidly in the past 10 years. Surgical closure

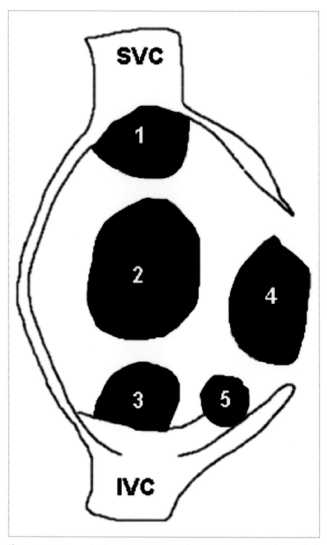

Figure 16.1. Anatomy of various atrial septal defects. The right atrial free wall has been excised. 1, Superior sinus venosus type (frequency 15%); 2, secundum type (60%); 3, inferior sinus venosus type (<5%); 4, primum type (20%); 5, coronary sinus type (<1%).

had been the preferred treatment because operative outcomes are excellent. However, surgical closure carries a 5.4% 1-year major complication rate [18]. Transcatheter closure of ostium secundum ASDs was first attempted by King and Mills in 1976 [19]. Since that time, numerous devices and approaches have been designed to improve both efficacy and safety [20]. Recent studies have demonstrated the efficacy, safety, and lower cost of such devices as compared to conventional surgical techniques [18,21–23]. The body of evidence is especially compelling for the Amplatzer® septal occluder. The widespread acceptance of percutaneous closure techniques is rapidly occurring. However, procedural success is highly dependent on the pre-procedural assessment of patients. Defect sizing and determination of adequate rims are essential for selecting appropriate patients for transcatheter closure. Transthoracic and transesophageal echocardiography have traditionally been used for this assessment. However, echocardiography often underestimates the defect size

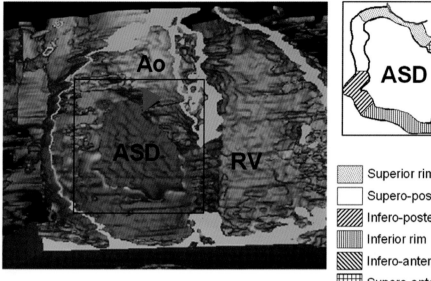

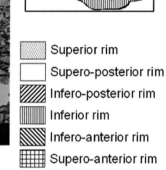

Superior rim

Supero-posterior rim

Infero-posterior rim

Inferior rim

Infero-anterior rim

Supero-anterior rim

Figure 16.2. Three-dimensional surface-rendered reconstruction of a secundum atrial septal defect (ASD) as seen from a right anterior oblique and slightly caudal projection. The rims appear adequate except for a partial absence of the superior rim. This defect measured 34 mm at its largest diameter. Ao = aorta; RV = right ventricle.

[24]. Cardiac CT provides excellent quality images of the atrial septum that can be reconstructed to provide a three-dimensional view of these often non-geometric defects (Figure 16.2). Moreover, assessment of atrial septal rims is feasible. These properties make CT an ideal non-invasive method for determining ASD size, shape, and candidacy for percutaneous closure. Post-percutaneous device closure tomography clearly demonstrates the position of the device, absence of thrombus, and any potential impingement of nearby structures (Figure 16.3). Superior sinus venosus atrial septal defects are often accompanied by partial anomalous pulmonary venous return, usually from the right upper and middle lung lobes (Figure 16.4). Such defects cannot be closed percutaneously. Operative intervention is often necessary because the shunted volume is invariably large and leads to right ventricular enlargement, pulmonary arterial hypertension, and tachyarrhythmias. Cardiac CT with angiography clearly demonstrates anomalous pulmonary venous drainage as shown in Figure 16.4. Occasionally, the presence of an ASD is accompanied by other unsuspected pertinent anatomic findings. CT with angiography may demonstrate other associated abnormalities that may not have been suspected by echocardiography (Figure 16.5). Accurate determination of shunt fractions is also feasible. The arterial time–concentration curve produced after intravenous injection of an indicator (iodine) demonstrates a recirculation hump on the downslope of the curve with left to right shunts (Figure 16.5) or early appearance and hump on the upslope of the curve with right to left shunts. The area under the curve is indicative of the shunted volume [25].

Ventricular Septal Defects

Ventricular septal defects (VSD) are the most common shunting lesions in infants. The majority of these are small muscular defects that close with time. The interventricular septum can be divided into four main regions (Figure 16.6):

1. The inlet septum is formed by the endocardial cushions and separates the tricuspid and mitral valvar annuli. Defects in this region are known as inlet septal defects and are commonly associated with primum ASD and atrioventricular septal defect. Cleft, straddling, or overriding atrioventricular valves are often associated with such defects. Patients with trisomy 13 are more likely than the general

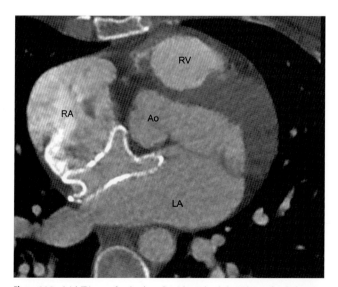

Figure 16.3. Axial CT image of an Amplatzer® atrial septal occluder 24 hours after deployment. The device is not impinging on important nearby structures such as the anterior mitral leaflet or the right upper pulmonary vein. RA = right atrium, LA = left atrium, Ao = aortic root, RV = right ventricular outflow tract.

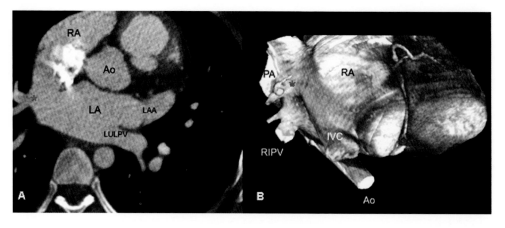

Figure 16.4. A Axial CT image of a sinus venosus ASD with anomalous right upper pulmonary vein draining into the SVC/RA junction (*). **B** 3-D volume-rendered reconstruction of the same case as viewed from a right lateral and caudal projection. Right atrium = RA, left atrium = LA, LULPV = left upper lobe pulmonary vein, RIPV = right inferior pulmonary vein, Ao = aorta, LAA = left atrial appendage, PA = pulmonary artery, IVC = inferior vena cava.

population to develop endocardial cushion defects with associated VSD. These defects generally do not close spontaneously and often lead to or are associated with pulmonary hypertension. They are best seen in a four-chamber axial cut at the level of the tricuspid and mitral annuli. They are uncommon in the general population.

2. The outlet septum is formed by tissue extending from the crista supraventricularis to the pulmonary valve. Defects in this region are known as supracristal or subarterial VSDs (Figure 16.7A). These defects are uncommon but may be located directly below an aortic sinus of Valsalva. The absence of a portion of this septum below the aortic valve weakens the underpinnings of the sinuses and may lead to aortic regurgitation and aneurysm formation. Sakakibara and Konno [26] described the development of aneurysms of the sinuses of Valsalva which may rupture into an adjoining chamber or obstruct subpulmonary outflow (Figure 16.7B).

3. The membranous septum is a small fibrous area inferior to the aortic valve. Membranous and perimembranous defects occur below the aortic valve (Figure 16.6). This portion of the septum is often thin and not well visualized by cardiac CT. Intact membranous ventricular septum may be mistaken for a defect. Therefore careful inspection for the presence or absence of associated features such as right ventricular hypertrophy or pulmonary artery enlargement may suggest or make suspect the presence of a defect. These are the most common type of VSD in the adult. Fifty percent of these will close spontaneously, usually in childhood. Some are large and unrestrictive. Unrepaired these may result in systemic levels of pulmonary hypertension and the Eisenmenger complex (Figure 16.8). These patients invariably have right ventricular hypertrophy and may suffer from biventricular dysfunction. Restrictive defects generally do not result in systemic levels of pulmonary hypertension. The clinical significance is largely dependent

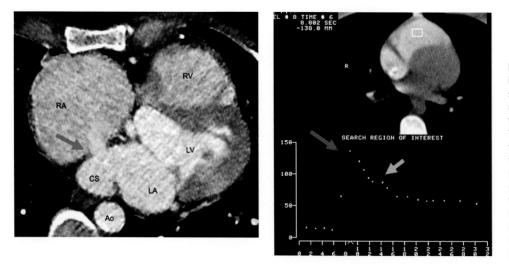

Figure 16.5. Small secundum ASD measuring 9.5 mm in diameter with small left to right shunting. The image on the left shows a coronary sinus (CS) that is unroofed and drains into the left atrium. The right atrium (RA) is dilated. The image on the right is the corresponding flow study, demonstrating a peak of contrast in the right ventricle at 8 seconds (red arrow, normal RV filling) and then a smaller, second peak at 14 seconds (the shunting of contrast from the left side, corresponding to enhancement of the LV). The area under the second curve (blue arrow) represents the amount of left to right shunt. LA = left atrium, Ao = aorta, LV = left ventricle, RV = right ventricle.

anism noted for subarterial defects. Surgical closure is generally recommended if the shunt fraction is >1.5 or if there is evidence of left-sided enlargement or failure. Repaired patients and those with small defects generally have an excellent outcome. Percutaneous closure of membranous and perimembranous defects is increasingly being used with a success rate that is comparable to surgical repair.

4. Muscular VSDs often close spontaneously during childhood. They may be single or multiple. They are often difficult to visualize surgically but are well seen on echocardiography or cardiac CT. These may be a result of trauma or myocardial infarction (Figure 16.9).

The management of VSDs is dependent on their size and shunt fraction. The goal is to prevent pulmonary hypertension, preserve ventricular function, and prevent bacterial endocarditis. Small muscular VSDs often close spontaneously in childhood and warrant infrequent follow-up. In larger VSDs closure is required. Surgical closure with pericardial patching had been the only means by which these defects were closed. Nitinol (nickel and titanium alloy) percutaneous VSD closure devices have been developed for both muscular and perimembranous defects. Large unrepaired VSDs will result in irreversible pulmonary hypertension (Eisenmenger complex) with reversal of shunt direction. The presence of Eisenmenger complex has been a contraindication for closure because of the high incidence of pulmonary ventricular failure in the face of suprasystemic pulmonary vascular resistance. A small but growing body of evidence suggests that this contraindication may not be absolute. The development of a variety of agents that decrease pulmonary vascular resistance (nitric oxide, endothelin blockers, prostacyclins) may prevent right ventricular failure after defect closure. Pulmonary artery banding with subsequent worsening of hypoxemia may result in reversal of pulmonary vascular changes permitting defect closure at a later time [27]. The hallmarks of CT findings in patients with the Eisenmenger complex resulting from VSD are:

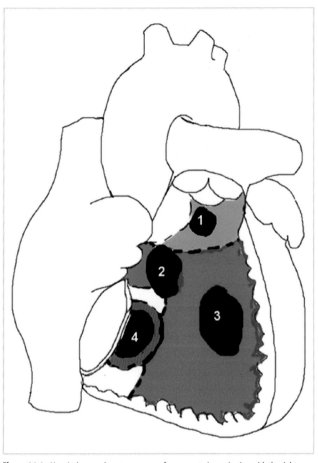

Figure 16.6. Ventricular septal anatomy as seen from an anterior projection with the right ventricular free wall removed. Outlet septum (purple), inlet septum (green), membranous septum (blue), and muscular septum (red). Ventricular septal defects: 1, subarterial defect; 2, perimembranous defect; 3, muscular defect; 4, inlet defect.

on size and location. The shunt fraction is highly dependent on defect size and when significant may lead to left ventricular volume overload and potential failure. Aortic regurgitation occurs in 20% of patients via the same mech-

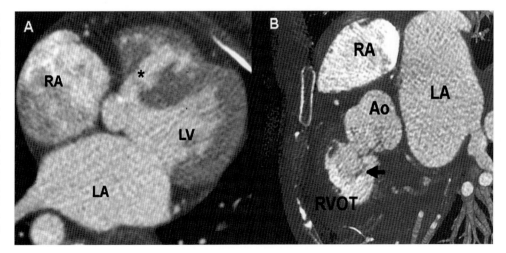

Figure 16.7. A Axial CT angiogram image of a patient with a small subarterial VSD (*). Note the hypertrophied right ventricular outflow tract. This patient had developed a "two chambered right ventricle" as a result of right ventricular outflow tract (RVOT) muscular hypertrophy encouraged by the impact of turbulent, high-velocity flow across the VSD. Note this patient also has a right-sided aortic arch. **B** Volume-rendered CT angiogram of a 35-year-old man who had been diagnosed with a small subarterial VSD at 13 years of age. The arrow points to a sinus of Valsalva aneurysm protruding into the RVOT and causing mild stenosis (25 mmHg gradient on catheterization). The aneurysm had ruptured and this patient had continuous flow from the aorta (Ao) to the RVOT. RA = right atrium, LA = left atrium, LV = left ventricle.

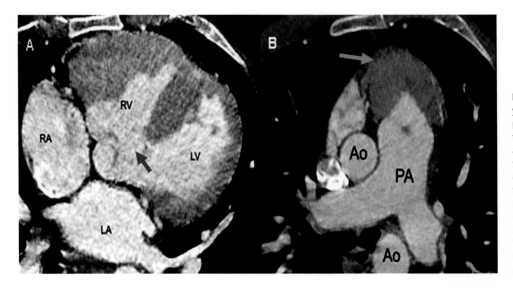

Figure 16.8. **A** Axial CT angiogram of a 36-year-old cyanotic man with a large (18 mm) perimembranous VSD (arrow). His right ventricular (RV) muscle mass is increased (148 g) and the RV has a moderately depressed ejection fraction (39%). The left ventricular (LV) ejection fraction is mildly reduced (47%). By the indicator dilution method his shunt is reversed with Qp:Qs of 0.5. **B** Axial image at the level of the pulmonary valve. Note the severe hypertrophy of the RV outflow tract (arrow). The pulmonary artery (PA) is very dilated, indicating severe pulmonary hypertension. RA = right atrium, LA = left atrium, and Ao = aorta.

1. dilated main pulmonary artery
2. right ventricular hypertrophy
3. dilated, uncalcified, and tortuous coronary arteries
4. absence of aortic atherosclerosis or calcium
5. pulmonary neovascularization
6. in situ thromboses and calcification within the pulmonary arterial tree.

In contrast to the existing and rapidly expanding understanding of calcification in the systemic circulation, there is a paucity of knowledge regarding this process in the pulmonary arterial circulation. William Osler in 1892 [28] observed a sclerotic process in the main pulmonary trunk in "... all conditions which for a long time increase the tension in the lesser circulation." Calcium deposits have been noted on chest radiography in the pulmonary arterial tree of patients with congenital heart disease and the Eisenmenger syndrome [29]. The literature is sparse and often contradictory. Perloff and Child reviewed the computed tomographic characteristics of patient with primary

pulmonary hypertension (PPH) or the Eisenmenger complex and noted that mild to extensive mural calcific deposits occurred in 26% of patients with the Eisenmenger complex and 23% of patients with PPH [30]. However, these deposits were not quantified and no histologic correlations were sought. Moderate to massive thromboses were identified in 29% of patients with the Eisenmenger complex and were absent in patients with PPH. Such massive thromboses in patients with cyanotic congenital heart disease are associated with aneurysmal dilation of the pulmonary trunk and a poor prognosis. It is unclear if calcium deposits help or hinder such processes, but it does appear that calcium deposits are decreased in aneurysmal pulmonary vessels. Extensive mural calcification may limit dilation, possibly by damping intraluminal pulse pressure, but this hypothesis needs further investigation. The available literature on pulmonary arterial calcification suggests a relationship between pulmonary pressures, disease process, presence of thrombus, and vessel size/morphology. However, these relationships are not clearly understood. Computed tomography (CT) accurately and

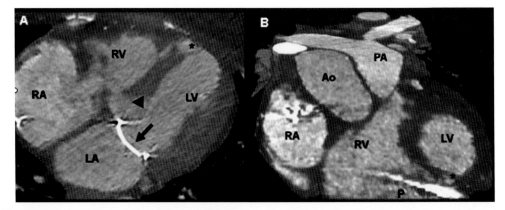

Figure 16.9. **A** Axial CT angiogram of a 57-year-old woman with an apical muscular VSD (*) from a myocardial infarct. Note the thinned infarcted left ventricular apex. The arrow points to a prosthetic mitral valve. The patient did not have a membranous VSD. However, this axial image does give the false impression that a defect is present in the membranous septum (black arrowhead). Echocardiography can be used to confirm or refute the presence of a membranous VSD in such cases. **B** Volumerendered reconstruction of the same patient as viewed from an anteroposterior projection. The small muscular VSD (*) is located near the tip of pacing lead (P). RA = right atrium, LA = left atrium, LV = left ventricle, RV = right ventricle, and PA = pulmonary artery.

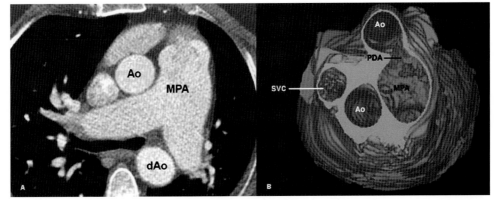

Figure 16.10. **A** Axial CT angiogram of a 57-year-old patient with PDA and Eisenmenger complex. This slice is below the level of the PDA. Note the dilated main pulmonary artery (MPA) as compared to the ascending aorta (Ao). Note the increased contrast density in the descending aorta (dAo) as compared to the Ao as a result of right to left shunting from the large PDA. **B** Three-dimensional surface reconstruction of the same CT angiogram as viewed from an anteroposterior cranial projection. The MPA and aortic arch have been unroofed to reveal a large PDA. SVB = superior vena cava.

non-invasively provides valuable information about the amount, location, and characteristics of calcium deposits [31,32]. Moreover, CT with angiography facilitates accurate determinations of vessel shape, dimensions, and the presence of any thrombotic material. Hence, CT is an excellent tool for analyzing the dilemma of pulmonary calcification.

Patent Ductus Arteriosus

The ductus arteriosus is a communication between the distal aortic arch and the proximal left pulmonary artery that is vital in fetal life for shunting of the mother's oxygenated blood to the systemic fetal circulation. In patients with pulmonary atresia or hypoplastic left heart syndrome, the patency of the ductus arteriosus is essential for survival. Urgent surgical intervention is needed to prevent this communication from constricting and closing within 7–10 days after birth. Failure of the ductus to close results in patent ductus arteriosus (PDA). The clinical significance of a PDA, as in the case of VSD, is dependent on the defect size and hence the shunt fraction. Small defects with a negligible shunt volume are clinically well tolerated but do carry a moderate risk of endarteritis. Endarteritis in patients with PDA most commonly involves the pulmonary artery segment most battered by the PDA jet. Larger PDAs carry a higher risk of endarteritis as well as a higher potential for causing irreversible pulmonary hypertension (Eisenmenger syndrome) (Figure 16.10). The shunt direction and fraction can be calculated using the indicator dilution method (see above) with regions of interest placed at the left atrium and descending aorta. As with ASD and VSD, when irreversible pulmonary hypertension is absent, surgical closure had been the treatment of choice for moderate to large PDAs, until the advent of percutaneous closure devices. These devices consist of coil embolization and nitinol-based devices. Correct sizing of such devices is imperative to successful defect closure. Cardiac CT provides clear images of such defects that facilitate pre-procedural sizing as well as post-procedural evaluation of coil or device placement.

Aorto-pulmonary window is a rare lesion that is clinically difficult to differentiate from PDA. A large communication is usually present between the ascending aorta and the main pulmonary artery. The absence of arterial wall tissue at this level can be seen on CT. Moreover, these patients develop irreversible pulmonary hypertension if the aorto-pulmonary window is not repaired before adulthood. Indicator dilution curves with the regions of interest placed on the left atrium and descending aorta accurately determine the left to right shunt fraction. The shunted volume is determined in part (as in PDA) by the size of the defect, which is usually large. Associated lesions are frequent and can be identified by cardiac CT. They include ASD, VSD, tetralogy of Fallot (TOF), subaortic stenosis, and PDA. Anomalous coronary anatomy is often present and should be evaluated.

Obstructions

In the realm of CHD, the general category of "obstructions" refers to a collection of heterogeneous lesions with one aspect in common, they obstruct anterograde blood flow. The systematic approach to obstructions is fundamentally important. CT angiography (CTA) can be effectively used to evaluate various obstructions by following the path of the contrast across axial slices in a systematic manner. In most cases the contrast injection is via the right or left antecubital veins. In our clinical experience, when CHD is present or suspected, injection of contrast through the left arm is preferable in order to determine if a left superior vena cava (SVC) is present. The subclavian vein, innominate vein, and superior vena cava should be clearly delineated. In patients with low cardiac output or obstruction to anterograde blood flow at the valvar or arterial level, the contrast flow within the innominate vein, SVC, and right atrium becomes very sluggish. The contrast tends to swirl and layer, often giving the impression that a thrombus is present (Figure 16.11).

Obstruction at the right atrial level is rare but may result from atrial tumors, persistence of the right venous valve

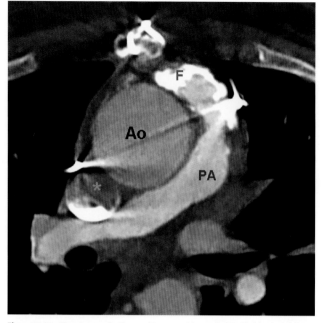

Figure 16.11. CT angiogram of a 46-year-old woman with a repaired double inlet single left ventricle. The patient had a modified Fontan operation with placement of a valved aortic homograft from the right atrial appendage to the main pulmonary artery (PA). The Fontan conduit was complicated by stenosis necessitating percutaneous placement of an endovascular stent (F), which appears bright on CTA. This stent lumen had become narrowed and partially thrombosed. The sluggish anterograde flow resulted in contrast layering appearing as a filling defect within the venous circulation (*). It is difficult to rule out the presence of thrombus given the filling defect; however, the layering of contrast posteriorly in the supine patient suggests sluggish flow.

creating a double-chambered right atrium, or isolated congenital tricuspid stenosis. The latter condition is rare and may be secondary to underdevelopment of the valve annulus, leaflets, or parachute deformity (all chordae arising from one papillary muscle).

Normally, the papillary muscles of the right ventricle are small and numerous, arising from the free wall as well as from the interventricular septum. The number of leaflets of the tricuspid valve varies from two in infancy, to three throughout most of adult life, to four in old age [33]. Tricuspid valve leaflet anatomy is difficult to ascertain on CT but annulus size can be measured and thickening/calcification of valve leaflets can be seen.

Tricuspid atresia is the result of complete absence of tricuspid valvar tissue or the presence of rudimentary valve tissue that is imperforate (Figure 16.12). Tricuspid atresia is commonly accompanied by a hypoplastic and underdeveloped right ventricle and pulmonary atresia or stenosis. Deoxygenated blood arriving at the right atrium is by necessity shunted via an atrial septal defect to the left atrium and through the mitral valve. The left ventricle functions as a single ventricular pumping chamber; a VSD is often present. Ventriculo-arterial concordance results in the pulmonary artery arising from the rudimentary right ventricle. Atresia or obstruction is often present at or below the level of the pulmonary valve. Ventriculo-arterial discordance results in the pulmonary trunk arising from the

dominant single left ventricle and the aorta arising from the hypoplastic right ventricle. Pulmonary stenosis is often present. Impedance to aortic outflow is also common because of a restrictive bulbo-ventricular foramen (embryologic term describing the connection between the left ventricle and right-sided outflow segment) or VSD. Tricuspid atresia with concomitant pulmonary atresia had been a fatal condition in infancy. A multitude of surgical techniques have been developed to treat this condition. In 1945 Blalock and Taussig initially described a palliative operation shunting systemic arterial blood from the subclavian artery to the pulmonary artery [34]. Glenn and Patino performed the first systemic venous to pulmonary arterial shunting procedure in 1954 [35] and this led to the total cavopulmonary shunting procedure described by Fontan and Baudet in 1971 [36]. This procedure has evolved through various modifications over the past three decades, most aimed at reducing postoperative arrhythmias and right atrial hypertension.

Obstruction at the right ventricular level is usually secondary to an anomalous muscle bundle extending from the crista supraventricularis beneath the infundibulum of the right ventricle to the anterior right ventricular wall at the base of the anterior papillary muscle. The muscle bundle obstructs flow into the right ventricular infundibulum and creates a double-chambered right ventricle (DCRV) (Figure 16.13). The pressure gradient across this muscle bundle varies from minimal to severe. Hypertrophy of the proximal high-pressure chamber is common. Associated defects include a perimembranous VSD (63%),

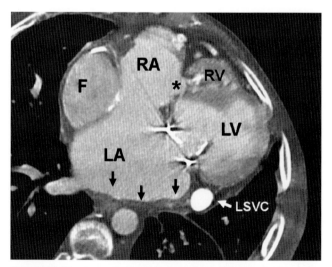

Figure 16.12. CT angiogram of a 24-year-old patient with tricuspid atresia (*) and hypoplastic right ventricle (RV). He had undergone lateral tunnel Fontan (F) conduit placement that rerouted deoxygenated systemic caval blood to the pulmonary artery. Note the large atrial septal defect between the left and right atrium (LA, RA). This patient had previously undergone bioprosthetic mitral valve replacement that resulted in mitral stenosis. He developed extensive thrombus throughout the left atrium. At this level, the dark layer of mural thrombus can be seen covering the posterior wall of the LA (black arrows). In this case, contrast was injected in the left antecubital vein. A previously undocumented left superior vena cava (LSVC) was thus revealed. A single thinly trabeculated ventricle is present, functioning as a single left ventricle (LV).

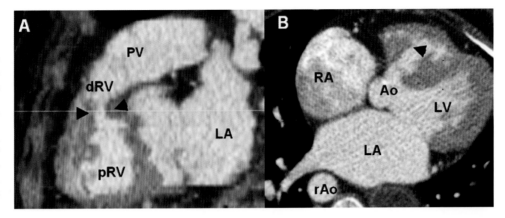

Figure 16.13. A Lateral projection of a 3-D reconstructed CTA in a patient with DCRV. The anomalous muscle bundle (black arrowhead) is clearly seen dividing the right ventricle into a proximal high-pressure chamber (pRV) and a distal low-pressure chamber (dRV). Labeled structures include left atrium (LA), and pulmonary valve (PV). **B** Axial reconstruction of EBA at the level of the anomalous muscle bundle. Additional structures: left atrium (LA), left ventricle (LV), and aorta (Ao). Note the descending aorta (rAo) is rightward.

valvar pulmonic stenosis (40%), secundum ASD (17%), and double outlet right ventricle (8%) [37]. Hypertrophy and fibrosis at the site subjected to the high-velocity left to right VSD jet has been implicated as a potential contributive mechanism. Surgical excision of the anomalous muscle bundle is recommended regardless of age if the gradient is >40 mmHg or if the patient is symptomatic. Patch repair of an associated ASD or VSD is usually done concomitantly.

In 1888, Etienne Fallot described a constellation of anatomic findings that defined a specific subset of patients with the "maladie bleue" [38], referring to the cyanosis that these patients present with. These patients all had infundibular pulmonary stenosis, VSD, overriding aorta (dextroposed), and right ventricular hypertrophy. In 1970 Van Praagh, et al. proposed that tetralogy of Fallot (TOF) is essentially a "monology," primarily the underdevelopment of the right ventricular infundibulum and its sequelae [39]. The degree of aortic override correlates with the severity of infundibular stenosis (Figure 16.14). In extreme forms of infundibulur underdevelopment, pulmonary atresia is present and the aorta arises from the right ventricle, leading to a double outlet right ventricle. The severest cases have infundibular obstruction and pulmonary atresia (Figure 16.14). Infundibular stenosis may be accompanied by sub-infundibular muscular hypertrophy as seen in double-chambered right ventricle. The pulmonary valve annulus is underdeveloped and the pulmonary valve is often deformed and stenotic. As with the degree of infundibular stenosis, the degree of pulmonary valvar stenosis is variable. Patients frequently have branch pulmonary stenoses. The ventricular septum is malaligned and a perimembranous VSD is present. These defects are generally non-restrictive and do not get smaller or close spontaneously (Figure 16.15). Surgical treatment is recommended in these patients. The surgical options are dictated by the degree of infundibular stenosis and pulmonary arterial hypoplasia. In patients with confluent and well-developed pulmonary arteries intracardiac repair is preferred. This consists of trans-annular resection and enlargement of the right ventricular infundibulum often accompanied by implantation of a tissue valve and

enlargement of any branch pulmonary artery stenoses. Patients with pulmonary atresia and non-confluent underdeveloped pulmonary arteries are cyanotic. Intracardiac repair is often not feasible. CT angiography (CTA) provides excellent visualization of the pulmonary arterial and venous systems and may be applied to evaluate pulmonary

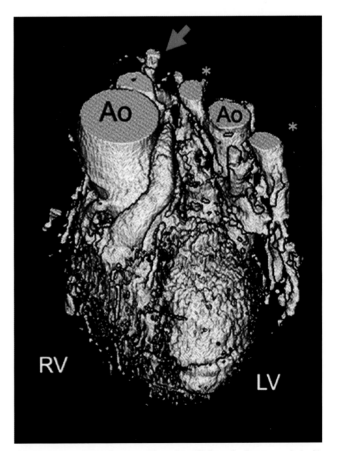

Figure 16.14. A 26-year-old woman with tetralogy of Fallot and pulmonary atresia. In this extreme form, the right ventricular infundibulum is severely underdeveloped, as is the pulmonic valve. The main pulmonary artery is hypoplastic and the left and right pulmonary arteries are completely occluded at their origin. Pulmonary blood flow is supplied by aorto-pulmonary collaterals (*), bronchial collaterals, and a right Blalock–Taussig shunt (arrow). Note the overriding (rightward shifted) and dilated ascending aorta (Ao). RV = right ventricle, LV = left ventricle.

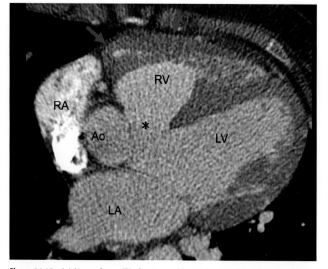

Figure 16.15. Axial image from a CTA of a 22-year-old cyanotic man with tetralogy of Fallot. Note the overriding aorta (Ao), the malaligned perimembranous ventricular septal defect (*), and the right ventricular hypertrophy (RV, arrows). RA = right atrium, LA = left atrium, LV = left ventricle.

anatomy in these patients. Aorto-pulmonary and bronchial collaterals are often present. Surgical placement of arterio-pulmonary shunts with ligation of aorto-pulmonary collaterals is a palliative option.

Isolated pulmonary valvar stenosis is characterized by fused commissures that are uncommonly dysplastic. The non-dysplastic stenotic pulmonary valves are often mobile and dome shaped. Calcium deposits may be seen at the leaflet tips. A supravalvar shelf-like narrowing may coexist. The main pulmonary artery and the proximal portions of the right and left pulmonary arteries are usually dilated and patients with significant stenosis will have varying degrees of right ventricular hypertrophy.

Congenital pulmonary vein stenosis is a rare entity with a variable clinical presentation. Patients may have single, unilateral, or complete pulmonary venous stenosis or atresia. The most severe forms are incompatible with life. The management is surgical, with pericardial patch enlargement or excision of focal stenoses [40]. More recently, percutaneous catheter-based approaches have come into use [41].

Cor triatriatum is a rare anomaly in which a restrictive fibromuscular membrane divides the left atrium into a higher pressure common pulmonary venous chamber and a lower pressure distal chamber that includes the left atrial appendage and the mitral annulus. Functionally, this lesion mimics mitral stenosis. The pulmonary veins and arteries are usually dilated. Other cardiac defects are commonly associated and include ASD, PDA, VSD, persistent left superior vena cava, partial anomalous pulmonary venous return, and coarctation of the aorta [42]. Surgical excision is the treatment of choice [43].

Isolated congenital mitral valve stenosis is an extremely rare congenital anomaly. Congenital mitral valve stenosis

is often associated with other left-sided lesions, including hypoplastic left heart syndrome [44]. Other associations are VSD, ASD, PDA, subaortic stenosis, bicuspid aortic valve, coarctation of the aorta, and supravalvar mitral membrane. In Shone's syndrome, patients may have these features along with a parachute mitral valve, in which the chordae are attached to one large papillary muscle. Congenital mitral stenosis is often diagnosed in infancy or childhood. Surgical valve repair or replacement with correction of associated abnormalities is the treatment of choice. Development of postoperative mitral stenosis or regurgitation as well as subaortic stenosis necessitates close follow-up [45]. Cardiac CT can be used to identify concomitant abnormalities prior to surgical intervention. Moreover, there may be a role for cardiac CT in identifying post-surgical changes such as subaortic stenosis.

Hypoplastic left heart syndrome refers to a small, non-functional left ventricle and underdeveloped, often atretic, mitral and aortic valves. It is an uncommon syndrome in which survival without surgery is dependent on the persistent patency of the ductus arteriosus. These patients generally have an atrial septal defect. Initial surgical treatment consists of enlargement of the atrial septal defect and primary palliation with the Norwood operation [46]. Norwood et al., in 1981, described an operation in which the distal main pulmonary artery is transected and connected to the distal aortic arch. A Gore-tex shunt is placed between the distal pulmonary artery and the new ascending aorta or subclavian artery in order to provide adequate pulmonary blood flow. The eventual goal is reparative Fontan surgery in appropriate patients (well-developed pulmonary arterial anatomy, low pulmonary vascular pressure/resistance). The traditional or modified Glenn procedures are often performed as a second stage of palliation after the Norwood operation and later converted to a total cavo-pulmonary (Fontan) conduit [47]. A growing number of these patients are surviving into adulthood, and cardiac CT may assist in the evaluation of potential long-term complications such as pulmonary venous stenosis, right ventricular enlargement and dysfunction, coarctation of the reconstructed aorta, peripheral pulmonary stenosis, or thrombus formation.

Subaortic stenosis is common in infants with congenital heart disease. It is often associated with other lesions such as VSD, coarctation of the aorta, and congenital mitral stenosis. Subaortic stenosis is visualized on CTA as a thin membrane traversing the left ventricular outflow tract. Abnormal mitral valve chordal attachments to the interventricular septum causing subaortic stenosis may be difficult to visualize. Hypertrophic cardiomyopathy is clearly evidenced by asymmetric septal hypertrophy. Valvar aortic stenosis is one of the most common congenital defects. The valve is most often bicuspid and rarely unicuspid. Even tricuspid valves may have asymmetric leaflets. The ascending aorta is generally dilated and aortic coarctation should be ruled out. Identifying the number of valve cusps is difficult with cardiac CT but valve asymmetry may

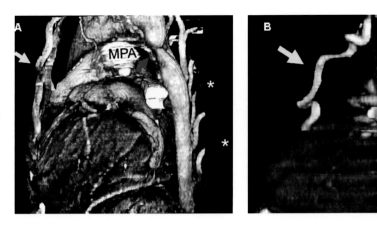

Figure 16.16. A Volume-rendered 3-D reconstruction of a CT angiogram from a 22-year-old man with severe focal coarctation of the aorta (red arrow). Note the plethora of arterial collaterals (*) and the dilated left internal mammary artery (LIMA) (yellow arrow). Main pulmonary artery (MPA). **B** A 36-year-old woman with less severe focal coarctation (red arrow). Arterioarterial collaterals (*) and LIMA (yellow arrow).

be evident. Calcium deposition within the valve leaflets may be seen in adults with bicuspid aortic valve. Supravalvar aortic stenosis is easily identified by cardiac CT. This anomaly is often associated with Williams syndrome [48]. These patients may have diffuse and progressive obstructions of the aortic arch, descending aorta, renal arteries, and pulmonary arteries. CT imaging should include evaluation of the abdominal as well as the thoracic vasculature.

Coarctation of the aorta was initially described by Morgagni in 1760. The narrowing is almost always located just distal to the origin of the left subclavian artery (Figure 16.16). There are less common, more diffuse forms of coarctation, characterized by hypoplasia of extended segments or multiple focal stenoses. The severest form is interrupted aortic arch. Possible causes include postnatal constriction of aberrant ductal tissue or aberrations of blood flow through the arch during pregnancy. It is often associated with other anomalies such as bicuspid aortic valve (85%), VSD, mitral valve abnormalities, intracranial aneurysms, and generalized arteriopathy (ectatic or hypoplastic arteries). The presence and extent of arterioarterial collaterals bridging the site of the coarctation are directly correlated with stenosis severity. The internal mammary arteries serve as collateral conduits and are often engorged and easily visible on CTA (Figure 16.16). CTA provides a plethora of essential information in this condition. The site and extent of coarctation can easily be ascertained using CTA. The dimensions of the aorta pre and post-stenosis can be accurately measured. Delineating collateral anatomy is very challenging and time-consuming during cardiac catheterization; therefore CTA is a preferred non-invasive modality for identifying collateral vessels. CTA can be an invaluable tool in patient selection and for planning of surgical and percutaneous interventions. Moreover, CTA can be used to follow the course of these patients over time and evaluate for complications such as restenosis or dissection. Patients with aortic coarctation may suffer from atherosclerotic coronary disease; therefore ECG-gated coronary CTA can be

especially useful for comprehensively evaluating cardiac anatomy in these patients.

Transpositions

D-Transposition of the great arteries (DTGA) occurs when the positions of the pulmonary artery and aorta are reversed. Normally, the aorta is posterior and medial while the pulmonary trunk is anterior and lateral. In DTGA these positions are reversed (Figure 16.17A). The ventricles retain their normal anatomic positions, with the right ventricle anterior and medial to the left ventricle. In most cases, the aorta emerges from the right ventricle and a subaortic infundibulum is usually present. The pulmonary artery emerges from the left ventricle, and there is fibrous continuity between the pulmonary valve and the anterior mitral leaflet. The position of the right pulmonary artery allows the left ventricle to empty directly into it and may account for the frequently observed dilated right pulmonary artery and increased right lung flow [49]. The atria are normally related to each other, with the right atrium anterior and medial, and the left atrium posterior and lateral.

There are a number of morphologic features easily visible on CTA that can be used to distinguish the right from the left atrium [33]:

1. The suprahepatic inferior vena cava almost always drains into the right atrium.
2. The right atrial appendage is broad and triangular whereas the left atrial appendage is narrow and finger-like.

DTGA presents as a wide spectrum of anatomic features from double outlet ventricle to single ventricle. Most commonly, patients have well-developed ventricles and the above-described great arterial relationship. VSDs are common in infancy and usually close spontaneously. Dextrocardia and subpulmonary obstruction can occur and can be investigated using CTA. The coronary anatomy is of

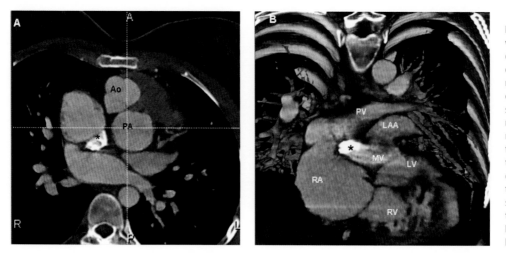

Figure 16.17. A CTA of a 21-year-old woman with DTGA who underwent a Senning procedure as an infant. Note the inverse relationship of the aorta and pulmonary artery. The iodinated contrast was injected in the right upper extremity and hence brightly opacified the superior vena cava and the systemic venous to mitral valve baffle (*). **B** 3-D volume-rendered reconstruction of the same patient viewed from an anteroposterior and cranial orientation. A large left superior pulmonary vein (PV) drains via a baffle to the right atrium (RA) then to the right ventricle (RV). The highly opacified superior vena caval blood drains via a baffle (*) to the mitral valve (MV) and thereafter to the left ventricle (LV). Left atrial appendage is also labeled (LAA).

great importance in these patients, especially if they are being considered for an arterial switch operation (Jatene procedure – see below) [50]. Occasionally, these patients may have abnormalities of the tricuspid valve such as straddling (chordae arising from both ventricles) or overriding (valve partially opens into the left ventricle without straddling). Straddling may be difficult to identify on CTA given the lack of chordal visualization. However, an overriding annulus should be evident.

Various strategies for palliation and repair are available. Atrial septostomy is often performed as a palliative measure shortly after birth. Atrial switch operations such as the Mustard (baffle made of prosthetic material or pericardium) or Senning procedure (atrial tissue sculpted to make baffle) are corrective. Caval blood is baffled from the superior vena cava and inferior vena cava to the mitral valve and pulmonary circulation. Pulmonary venous return is baffled to the tricuspid valve and the systemic circulation. The atrial switch operations maintain the right ventricle as the systemic ventricle; therefore, right ventricular enlargement, hypertrophy, and failure may occur. CTA provides excellent visualization of the baffled circulations (Figure 16.17B) and can be used to evaluate any baffle narrowing (usually near the SVC portion) or leak. CTA with cineangiography can be used to determine right ventricular ejection fraction and follow right ventricular dimensions [51].

The Rastelli operation is frequently used in patients with DTGA, VSD, and subpulmonary obstruction [52]. This operation utilizes the VSD as part of a baffled left ventricular to aortic outflow tract. The pulmonary valve is oversewn and a valved conduit is placed from the right ventricle to the pulmonary artery. Thus, the left ventricle becomes the systemic ventricle and the right ventricle becomes the pulmonary ventricle. Anatomic correction of DTGA is feasible with the arterial switch operation [50]. This is a technically challenging operation that involves transection of the aorta and pulmonary trunk above the

semilunar valves. The coronary arteries are removed with a button of surrounding aortic tissue and reimplanted in the neo-aorta (native pulmonary artery). The pulmonary artery is pulled forward and attached to the previous aortic root. Thus, anatomic correction is established, with the left ventricle supplying the systemic circulation and the right ventricle supplying the pulmonary circulation. This operation is usually performed in infancy, before regression of left ventricular muscle occurs as a result of prolonged pumping into the low-pressure pulmonary circulation. CTA with cineangiography can be used to assess bi-ventricular dimensions and function. Coronary anatomy and patency can also be accurately assessed with CTA.

"Congenitally corrected" or L-transposition of the great arteries (CCTGA or LTGA) is characterized by inverted ventricles and transposition of the great arteries. One can think of this condition as two wrongs making a right; deoxygenated blood is delivered to the lungs and oxygenated blood is delivered to the periphery. Patients are often undiagnosed until early adulthood when they present with complete heart block. The atria are normally related but the ventricles and their respective atrioventricular valves are inverted. Therefore, deoxygenated systemic venous blood returns normally to the right atrium which empties through a morphologic mitral valve into a morphologic left ventricle that is medial. This ventricle empties into an outflow tract that leads posteriorly through the pulmonary valve and into the pulmonary arteries (Figure 16.18). The morphologic left ventricle (LV) can be distinguished from the morphologic right ventricle (RV) by a number of distinct anatomic features [33], which can be visualized with CTA:

1. The LV has fine trabeculae as compared to the coarse trabeculae of the RV.

2. The LV has two large papillary muscles as compared to numerous small papillary muscles of the RV.

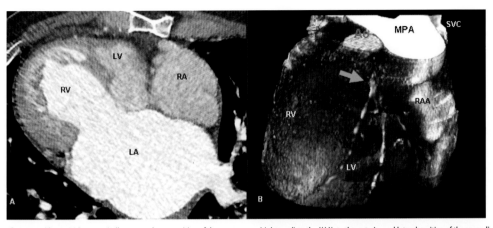

Figure 16.18. **A** Twenty-five-year-old man with congenitally corrected transposition of the great arteries and mirror image dextrocardia. The right atrium (RA) drains via a morphologic mitral valve into the pulmonic (morphologic left) ventricle (LV). The severely dilated left atrium (LA) drains into a trabeculated and hypertrophied systemic (morphologic right) ventricle (RV) via a morphologic tricuspid valve. This patient had an RV ejection fraction of 30% and severe tricuspid valve regurgitation. **B** Anteroposterior and cranial view of a volume-rendered reconstruction. The RV is lateral (rightward) to the LV. Note the anterior and lateral position of the ascending aorta (Ao) and posterior position of the main pulmonary artery (MPA). The broad right atrial appendage is labeled (RAA). The left main coronary artery (arrow) runs medially and divides into the left anterior descending and circumflex arteries. The superior vena cava (SVC) drains into the right atrium medially. This patient had abdominal situs inversus with the liver on the left side that was clearly demonstrated by the CTA.

3. Semilunar-atrioventricular fibrous continuity is present in the LV but absent in the RV.

4. The RV has one coronary as compared to two coronaries supplying the LV.

In CCTGA, the pulmonary veins drain oxygenated blood normally into a morphologic left atrium which empties via the morphologic tricuspid valve into the morphologic right ventricle located laterally. The right ventricular outflow tract is anterior and empties through an aortic valve into an anterior and lateral ascending aorta. Because mirror image dextrocardia may be present, it is important to think of the location of the anatomic structures in terms of their relationship to the vertebral column, which acts as a dividing midline. Therefore, in a patient with CCTGA and mirror image dextrocardia, the ascending aorta is anterior and rightward and the descending is to the right of the spinal column (Figure 16.18). Associated anomalies are common. Patients frequently have large perimembranous or multiple muscular VSDs, subvalvar and valvar pulmonary stenosis, and Ebstein's anomaly of the tricuspid valve. As with most forms of congenital heart disease, a thorough search for other lesions is essential. Patients less commonly have ASD, PDA, supravalvar mitral stenosis, or subaortic stenosis [53]. The tricuspid or mitral valves may be straddling the interventricular septum and associated with varying degrees of ventricular underdevelopment [54].

The coronary anatomy is reversed. The morphologic right coronary artery arises laterally from the posterior-facing sinuses of the ascending aorta and follows the atrioventricular groove to supply the morphologic right ventricular free wall via acute marginal branches. The morphologic left coronary artery arises posteriorly and travels medially, dividing into the left anterior descend-ing and circumflex branches. Adult patients commonly develop systemic ventricular or biventricular failure and severe tricuspid valve regurgitation. CTA with cineangiography may be used to assess all the pertinent anatomic features of this condition including ventricular function. Dextrocardia and abdominal situs inversus are also clearly demonstrated on CTA. These patients often develop conduction abnormalities and require permanent pacemaker placement. Those with heart failure may benefit from biventricular pacing. Coronary sinus and cardiac vein anatomy is variable, which may complicate biventricular pacing but can be clearly delineated with CTA prior to pacemaker placement. Operative repair requires atrial baffling (Senning or Mustard) and conduit placement from the right ventricle to the pulmonary artery and baffling of left ventricular outflow through a VSD to the anterior aorta. This operation is complex but carries a lower operative and overall mortality rate than conventional repair (VSD closure ± tricuspid valve repair or replacement) [55].

Anomalous pulmonary venous return can be partial or total. Total anomalous pulmonary venous return (TAPVR) occurs when all the pulmonary veins return to the pulmonic circulation. The anatomic variants can be divided into four categories [56]:

1. Supracardiac – all four pulmonary veins drain into a single common vein that may take a vertical course and drain into the innominate vein (Figure 16.19), superior vena cava, or azygos vein.

2. Cardia c – the common vein drains directly into the coronary sinus or right atrium.

3. Infradiaphragmatic – the common vein drains into the portal system.

4. Mixed

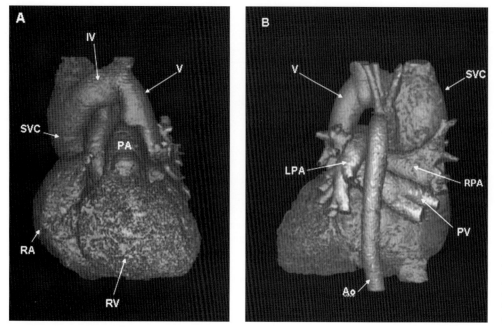

Figure 16.19. A Forty-seven-year-old woman with unrepaired total anomalous pulmonary venous return. Anteroposterior view of a surface-rendered CTA with 3-D reconstruction. Note the vertical vein (V) draining into the innominate vein (IV) and thereafter to the superior vena cava (SVC) resulting in volume overload and enlargement of the right heart. Right atrium (RA), right ventricle (RV), and pulmonary artery (PA) are labeled. **B** Posteroanterior view demonstrating a right upper lobe pulmonary vein (PV) coursing under the right pulmonary artery (RPA) to drain into a common channel that delivers all pulmonary venous drainage via a vertical vein (V) to the superior vena cava (SVC). Note the narrow circumference of the aorta (Ao) as compared to the left pulmonary artery (LPA), suggesting a large left to right shunt.

When anomalous pulmonary veins are present, their drainage may be obstructed, especially in TAPVR of the infradiaphragmatic variety. When this occurs, right ventricular hypertrophy and patent foramen ovale are usually present. CTA is ideal for determining the location, course, and patency of the pulmonary veins. Surgical repair consists of rerouting the common pulmonary vein via a large anastomosis to the left atrium. However, postoperative narrowing of this anastomosis may occur, thereby creating a functional cor triatriatum. CTA can be invaluable in directing the surgical and post-surgical management of these patients.

Partial anomalous pulmonary venous return (PAPVR) most often involves the right upper and middle lobe pulmonary veins and often occurs with a sinus venosus ASD. Isolated PAPVR is rare. The anomalous pulmonary vein/s usually drain to the superior vena caval and right atrial junction (Figure 16.4) but may also drain directly into the right atrium, inferior vena cava, coronary sinus, or innominate vein via a vertical vein [57]. Such a case is shown using 3-D reconstruction of a CTA (Figure 16.20). Surgical correction is recommended for symptomatic patients or asymptomatic patients with a pulmonary-to-systemic blood flow ratio exceeding 1.5 because of their higher likelihood of developing pulmonary vascular disease and right ventricular failure.

Persistent left superior vena cava (LSVC) is the most common thoracic venous anomaly and is often discovered accidentally. This anomaly may accompany other congenital cardiovascular anomalies such as ASD or coarctation of the aorta [58]. The persistent LSVC usually drains into the right atrium via a dilated coronary sinus. Less common

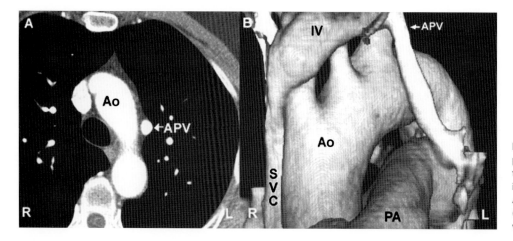

Figure 16.20. A Sixty-year-old man with partial anomalous pulmonary venous return of the left superior pulmonary vein (APV) to the innominate vein (IV). **B** The vertically oriented APV runs laterally along the arch of the aorta (Ao). PA = pulmonary artery, SVC = superior vena cava.

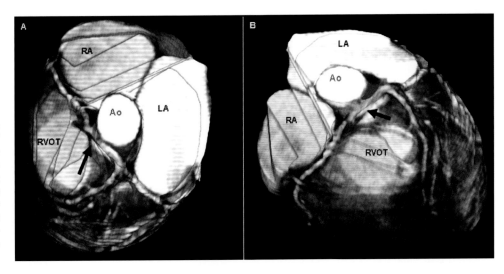

Figure 16.21. A Volume-rendered CTA of a 35-year-old man with anomalous origins of the left coronary artery (black arrow) from the right coronary cusp as viewed from a lateral steep cranial projection. Note that the long left main coronary segment courses between the aortic root (Ao) and the right ventricular outflow tract (RVOT); however, the vessel does not appear to be compressed. **B** Right anterior oblique and cranial projection. Left atrium (LA) and right atrium (RA) are labeled.

connections are directly to the left atrium, pulmonary veins, left atrial appendage, or the right atrium. A concomitant right superior vena cava (RSVC) may present with a horizontal innominate vein connecting the LSVC and RSVC. Recognition of this anomaly is of importance if a left superior venous approach to the heart is considered in patients undergoing pacemaker or defibrillator placement, and in the use of retrograde cardioplegia for surgical procedures requiring cardiopulmonary bypass. CTA clearly identifies LSVC (Figure 16.12), and all CTAs in patients with CHD should be investigated for presence/absence of LSVC.

CTA is an excellent tool for assessing coronary anomalies [59]. Anomalous origin of the left coronary artery from the right coronary cusp (Figure 16.21) and anomalous origin of the right coronary artery from the left coronary cusp are the most common variants. Rarely, the left coronary artery may emerge from the pulmonary trunk, and this often presents in childhood with congestive heart failure. Congenital arteriovenous fistula may also be imaged adequately with CTA.

Dysplasias

This category includes a miscellaneous collection of anomalies that involve malformations of various cardiac structures, most commonly arrhythmogenic right ventricular dysplasia (ARVD) in which the myocardium is replaced by fatty and fibrous infiltrates. The ventricle is enlarged and poorly functioning with increased trabeculation (Figure 16.22). These patients often develop life-threatening ventricular tachyarrhythmias requiring defibrillator placement. Fatty infiltrates may involve the left ventricular myocardium. These fatty infiltrates appear black on CT and are usually easily identified [60]. CTA can determine right ventricular ejection fraction (often reduced) and identify focal wall motion abnormalities [51].

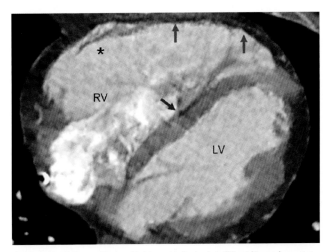

Figure 16.22. A 32-year-old man with right ventricular dysplasia. This axial image demonstrates a markedly dilated right ventricle (RV), with fat (dark areas) in the right ventricular free wall (red arrows) and interventricular septum (blue arrow). The asterisk demonstrates the increased trabeculations prevalent with this condition. LV = left ventricle.

Pulmonary Hypertension

Pulmonary hypertension (PH) related to CHD results from the effects of a long-standing increase in pulmonary blood flow which leads to pathologic changes in the pulmonary vasculature, particularly in the smaller vessels. This results in increased pulmonary vascular resistance, which in turn has deleterious effects upon the heart and larger pulmonary vascular structures.

Table 16.1 summarizes the CT findings of PH. Many of the typical CT findings of PH are not confined to a particular subset of a disease process, but rather reflect the end result of the chronic hemodynamic effect of PH upon cardiovascular anatomy [61–66]. Thus, while all PH is not due to CHD, and all CHD does not result in PH, we will attempt to demonstrate the typical findings of PH in selected cases.

Table 16.1. Summary of CT findings in pulmonary hypertension

Pulmonary arteries
Enlarged proximal vessels
Pruning of the distal vessels
Calcification
Thrombosis
Aneurysms

Heart
RV dilation
RV hypertrophy
RA dilation
decreased RV systolic function

Pulmonary hypertension is said to be more likely when the main pulmonary artery diameter is >29 mm (sensitivity 69%, specificity 100%) [61,65,67], and/or the ratio of the main pulmonary artery to ascending aorta diameter is >1 [62]. Others have demonstrated 32 mm as the upper limit of normal for main pulmonary artery diameter [66]. Rapid tapering or "pruning" of the more distal pulmonary vessels occurs as they travel toward the periphery of the lungs (Figure 16.23). Calcification of the pulmonary arteries suggests more severe disease [63]. Interestingly, one radiologic study found that pulmonary artery thromboses and aneurysms were common in patients with CHD and PH compared to patients with idiopathic pulmonary arterial

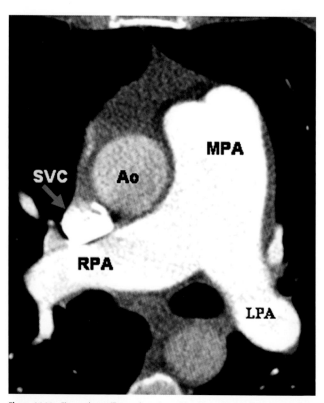

Figure 16.23. Electron beam CT scan of a patient with pulmonary hypertension reveals dilated proximal pulmonary arteries with rapid tapering distally. Ao = aorta, SVC = superior vena cava, MPA = main pulmonary artery, LPA = left pulmonary artery, RPA = right pulmonary artery.

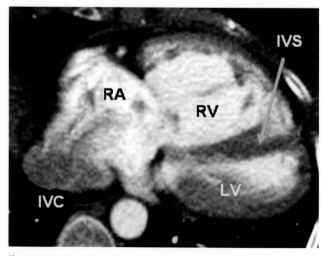

Figure 16.24. Electron beam CT scan of a patient with pulmonary hypertension demonstrating enlarged right ventricle (RV) and right atrium (RA), as well as dilated inferior vena cava (IVC). The interventricular septum (IVS) is flattened and the left ventricular cavity (LV) is small.

hypertension (IPAH), while dilation and mural calcification was seen in similar rates in both groups [64].

In patients with chronic, unrepaired systemic-to-pulmonary shunting, the CT findings can appear very similar to those found in precapillary pulmonary hypertension, including idiopathic pulmonary arterial hypertension (IPAH), and PAH associated with connective tissue disease, portal hypertension, and HIV infection. Commonly, right (or pulmonic) ventricular hypertrophy is seen, often with right ventricular enlargement, and associated right atrial enlargement (Figure 16.24). If cine-CT is performed, reduced right ventricular systolic function may also be present. The presence of retrograde opacification of the inferior vena cava or hepatic vein during contrast-enhanced CT may be a nonspecific sign of significant pulmonary hypertension and/or right ventricular dysfunction [68].

Future Directions

The future is very promising for cardiac CT. The latest generation of 64-slice CT systems, while limited in temporal resolution compared to electron beam CT, provide excellent spatial resolution. The inevitable development of faster scanners and those capable of imaging thinner slices will allow better visualization of small or thin structures such as valves, the atrial septum, the membranous ventricular septum, and small vessels.

The development of four-dimensional capability has accelerated over the last few years. The heart is a dynamic organ and is best understood when studied throughout the cardiac cycle. Hence, the development of four-dimensional CT cineangiography (time being the fourth dimension) is a milestone in the clinical application of this technology and is ideally suited for the complex dynamic dilemmas frequently encountered in congenital heart disease.

Photon emission tomography (PET) CTA allows evaluation of coronary perfusion and viability as well as anatomy and could prove specifically useful in simultaneously assessing pulmonary perfusion and arterial anatomy.

Advancements in 3-D-rendering software may soon facilitate virtual interventions and allow prediction of procedural outcomes prior to actual performance of the procedures, thus aiding in appropriate patient selection and operative planning.

It is always challenging to teach and learn congenital heart disease. Software programs capable of three-dimensional reconstruction and "virtual dissection" will promote better understanding of the variable anatomy and complex structures encountered in patients with congenital heart disease. Therefore, it is expected that the clinical and teaching applications of cardiac CT for congenital heart disease will inevitably grow.

References

1. Hoffman JI, Kaplan S. The incidence of congenital heart disease. J Am Coll Cardiol 2002;39(12):1890–1900.
2. Tworetzky W, Marshall AC. Fetal interventions for cardiac defects. Pediatr Clin North Am 2004;51(6):1503–1513.
3. Giamberti A, Mele M, DiTerlizzi M, et al. Association of Children with Heart Disease in the World. Pediatr Cardiol 2004;25:492–494.
4. Abdulla R. Congenital heart disease management in developing countries. Pediatr Cardiol 2002;23:481–482.
5. Kaemmerer H, Stern H, Fratz S, et al. Imaging in adults with congenital cardiac disease. Thorac Cardiovasc Surg 2000;48(6):328–335.
6. Wyamn RM, et al. Current complications of diagnostic and therapeutic cardiac catheterization. J Am Coll Cardiol 1988;12(6):1400–1406.
7. Fyfe DA, Parks WJ. Noninvasive diagnostics in congenital heart disease. Crit Care Nurs Q 2002;25(3):26–36.
8. Sueblinvong V. Limitations of 2-dimensional color Doppler echocardiography in the diagnosis of congenital heart disease. J Med Assoc Thai 1990;73(3):157–161.
9. Choe YH, Kang IS, Park SW, Lee JH. MR imaging of congenital heart disease in adolescents and adults. Korean J Radiol 2001;2(3):121–131.
10. Bae KT, Hong C, Whiting B. Radiation dose in multi-detector row computed tomography cardiac imaging. J Magn Reson Imaging 2004;19:859–863.
11. Grude M, Juergens KU, Wichter Y, et al. Evaluation of global left ventricular myocardial function with electrocardiogram-gated multi-detector computed tomography. Comparison with magnetic resonance imaging. Invest Radiol 2003;38(10):653–661.
12. Eliezer B, Maier S, Landzberg MJ, et al. In vivo evaluation of Fontan pathway flow dynamics by multidimensional phase-velocity magnetic resonance imaging. Circulation 1998;98:2873–2882.
13. Heidenreich PA, Steffens J, Fujita N, et al. Evaluation of mitral stenosis with velocity-encoded cine-magnetic resonance imaging. Am J Cardiol 1995;75(5):365–369.
14. Budoff MJ, et al. Clinical utility of computed tomography and magnetic resonance techniques for noninvasive coronary angiography. J Am Coll Cardiol 2003;42(11):1867–1878.
15. Criley JM. Congenital heart disease. In: Cardiology, 5th edn. Philadelphia: Lippincott Williams &Wilkins, 2004:213–220.
16. Knollmann FD, Pasic M, Zurbrugg HR, et al. Electron-beam computed tomography in heart surgery. Radiology 1998;38(12):1405–1453.
17. Campbell M. Natural History of atrial septal defect. Br Heart J 1970;32:820.
18. Du ZD, Hijazi ZM, Kleinman C, et al. Comparison between transcatheter and surgical closure of secundum atrial septal defect in children and adults. J Am Coll Cardiol 2002;39:1836–1844.
19. King TD, Mills NL. Secundum atrial septal defects: nonoperative closure during cardiac catheterization. JAMA 1976;235:2506–2509.
20. Ebeid M. Percutaneous catheter closure of secundum atrial septal defects: a review. J Invas Cardiol 2002;14:25–31.
21. Chessa M, Carminati M, Butera G, et al. Early and late complications associated with transcatheter occlusion of secundum atrial septal defect. J Am Coll Cardiol 2002;39:1061–1065.
22. Durongpisitkul K, Soongswang J, Laohaprasitipom D, et al. Comparison of atrial septal defect closure using Amplatzer septal occluder with surgery. Pediatr Cardiol 2002;23:36–40.
23. Thomson JD, Aburawi EH, Watterson KG, et al. Surgical and transcatheter closure of atrial septal defects: a prospective comparison of results and cost. Heart 2002;87:466–469.
24. Carcagni A, Presbitero P. New echocardiographic diameter for Amplatzer sizing in adult patients with secundum atrial septal defect: preliminary results. Catheter Cardiovasc Interv 2004;62(3):409–414.
25. Garrett JS, Jaschke W, Aherne T, et al. Quantitation of intracardiac shunts by cine-CT. J Comput Assist Tomogr 1988;12(1):82–87.
26. Sakakibara S, Konno S. Congenital aneurysms of the sinus of Valsalva. A clinical study. Am Heart J. 1962;63:708–719.
27. Batista RJV, Santos JLV, Takeshita N, et al. Successful reversal of pulmonary hypertension in the Eisenmenger complex. Arq Bras Cardiol 1997;68(4):279–280.
28. Osler W. The principles and practice of medicine. New York: D Appleton and Co., 1892: 667.
29. Steinberg I. Calcification of the pulmonary artery and enlargement of the right ventricle: a sign of congenital heart disease. Am J Roentgenol Radium Ther Nuc Med 1966;98(2):369–377.
30. Perloff JK, Hart EM, Greaves SM, Mines PD, Child JS. Proximal pulmonary arterial and intrapulmonary radiologic features of Eisenmenger syndrome and primary pulmonary hypertension. Am J Cardiol 2003;92:182–187.
31. Mautner SL, Mautner, GC, Froehlich J, et al. Coronary artery disease prediction with in vitro electron beam CT. Radiology 1994;192:625–630.
32. Detrano RC, Kang X, Tang W, et al. Accuracy of quantifying coronary hydroxyapatite with electron beam tomography. Invest Radiol 1994;29:733–738.
33. Van Praagh R, Van Praagh S. Morphologic anatomy. In: Nadas' Pediatric Cardiology. Philadelphia: Hanley & Belfus, 1992:17–26.
34. Blalock A, Taussig HB. The surgical treatment of malformations of the heart in which there is pulmonary stenosis or pulmonary atresia. JAMA 1945;128:189–202.
35. Glenn WW, Patino JF. Circulatory by-pass of the right heart. I. Preliminary observations on the direct delivery of vena caval blood into the pulmonary arterial circulation; azygous vein-pulmonary artery shunt. Yale J Biol Med 1954;27(3):147–151.
36. Fontan F, Baudet E. Surgical repair of tricuspid atresia. Thorax 1971;26:240–248.
37. Cil E, Saraclar M, Ozkutlus S, et al. Double-chambered right ventricle: Experience with 52 cases. Int J Cardiol 1995;50(1):19–29.
38. Fallot A. Contribution a l'anatomie pathologique de la maladie bleue (cyanose cardiaque). Marseille Med 1888;25:77, 138, 207, 270, 341, 403.
39. Van Praagh R, Van Praagh S, Nebesar R, et al. Tetralogy of Fallot: underdevelopment of the pulmonary infundibulum and its sequelae. Am J Cardiol 1970;26:25–33.
40. Spray TL, Bridges ND. Surgical management of congenital and acquired pulmonary vein stenosis. Semin Thorac Cardiovasc Surg Pediatr Card Surg Annu 1999;2:177–188.

41. Mendelsohn AM, Bove EL, Lupinetti FM, et al. Intraoperative and percutaneous stenting of congenital pulmonary artery and vein stenosis. Circulation 1993;88(5 Pt 2):II210–217.

42. Gheissari A, Malm JR, Bowman FO, Bierman FZ. Cor triatriatum sinistrum: one institution's 28-year experience. Pediatr Cardiol 1992;13(2):85–88.

43. Salomone G, Tiraboschi R, Bianchi T, et al. Cor triatriatum. Clinical presentation and operative results. J Thorac Cardiovasc Surg 1991; 101(6):1088–1092.

44. Ruckman RN, Van Praagh R. Anatomic types of congenital mitral stenosis: report of 49 autopsy cases with consideration of diagnosis and surgical implications. Am J Cardiol 1978;42:592–601.

45. Agarwal S, Airan B, Chowdhury UK, et al. Ventricular septal defect with congenital mitral valve disease: long-term results of corrective surgery. Indian Heart J 2002;54(1):67–73.

46. Norwood WI, Lang P, Casteneda AR, Campbell DN. Experience with operations for hypoplastic left heart syndrome. J Thorac Cardiovasc Surg 1981;82(4):511–519.

47. Norwood WI. Hypoplastic left heart syndrome: a review. Cardiol Clin 1989;7:377–385.

48. Beuren AJ, Apitz J, Harmjanz D. Supravalvular aortic stenosis in association with mental retardation and a certain facial appearance. Circulation 1962;26:1235.

49. Muster AJ, Paul MH, Van Grondelle A, et al. Asymmetric distribution of the pulmonary blood flow between the right and left lungs in d-transposition of the great arteries. Am J Cardiol 1976;38:352–361.

50. Jatene AD, Fontes VF, Paulista PP, et al. Anatomic correction of transposition of the great vessels. J Thorac Cardiovasc Surg 1976;72: 364–370.

51. Elegeti T, Lembecke A, Enzweiler C, et al. Comparison of electron beam CT with magnetic resonance imaging in assessment of right ventricular volumes and function. J Comput Assist Tomogr 2004; 28(5):679–685.

52. Rastelli GC, McGoon DC, Wallace RB. Anatomic correction of transposition of the great arteries with ventricular septal defect and subpulmonary stenosis. J Thorac Cardiovasc Surg 1969;58:545–552.

53. Webb CL. Congenitally corrected transposition of the great arteries: clinical features, diagnosis, and progress. Prog Pediatr Cardiol 1999; 10:17–30.

54. Fyler DC. "Corrected" transposition of the great arteries. In: Nadas' Pediatric Cardiology. Philadelphia: Hanley & Belfus, 1992: 701–706.

55. Yeh T, Connelley MS, Coles JG, et al. Atrioventricular discordance: results of repair in 127 patients. J Thorac Cardiovasc Surg 1999;117: 1190–1203.

56. Fyler DC. Total anomalous pulmonary venous return. In: Nadas' Pediatric Cardiology. Philadelphia: Hanley & Belfus, 1992: 683–691.

57. AboulHosn JA, Criley JM, Stringer WW. Partial anomalous pulmonary venous return: case report and review of the literature. Catheter Cardiovasc Interv 2003;58(4):548–552.

58. Gonzalez-Juanatey C, Testa A, Vidan J, et al. Persistent left superior vena cava draining into the coronary sinus: Report of 10 cases and literature review. Clin Cardiol 2004;27:515–518.

59. Hong C, Woodard PK, Bae KT. Congenital coronary artery anomaly demonstrated by three dimensional 16 slice spiral CT angiography. Heart 2004;90(5):478.

60. Kimura F, Sakai F, Sakomura Y, et al. Helical CT features of arrhythmogenic right ventricular cardiomyopathy. Radiographics 2002;22: 1111–1124.

61. Tan RT, Kuzo R, Goodman LR, et al. Utility of CT scan evaluation for predicting pulmonary hypertension in patients with parenchymal lung disease. Chest 1998;113:1250–1256.

62. Ng CS, Wells AU, Padley SP. A CT sign of chronic pulmonary arterial hypertension: the ratio of main pulmonary artery to aortic diameter. J Thorac Imaging 1999;14:270–278.

63. Chatterjee K, De Marco T, Alpert JS. Pulmonary hypertension: hemodynamic diagnosis and management. Arch Intern Med 2002;162: 1925–1933.

64. Perloff JK, Hart EM, Greaves SM, Miner PD, Child JS. Proximal pulmonary arterial and intrapulmonary radiologic features of Eisenmenger syndrome and primary pulmonary hypertension. Am J Cardiol 2003;92:182–187.

65. Kuo PC, Plotkin JS, Johnson LB, et al. Distinctive clinical features of portopulmonary hypertension. Chest 1997;112:980–986.

66. Edwards PD, Bull RK, Coulden R. CT measurement of main pulmonary artery diameter. Br J Radiol 1998;71:1018–1020.

67. Kuriyama K, Gamsu G, Stern RG, Cann CE, Herfkens RJ, Brundage BH. CT-determined pulmonary artery diameters in predicting pulmonary hypertension. Invest Radiol 1984;19:16–22.

68. Yeh BM, Kurzman P, Foster E, Qayyum A, Joe B, Coakley F. Clinical relevance of retrograde inferior vena cava or hepatic vein opacification during contrast-enhanced CT. Am J Roentgenol 2004;183: 1227–1232.

17

Nuclear Cardiology and Cardiac Computed Tomography in Assessment of Patients with Known or Suspected Chronic Coronary Artery Disease

Daniel S. Berman, Rory Hachamovitch, Leslee J. Shaw, Guido Germano, Nathan D. Wong, and Alan Rozanski

Introduction

Non-invasive cardiac imaging is now central to the diagnosis and management of patients with known or suspected chronic coronary artery disease (CAD). Among these methods, nuclear cardiology plays a central role in risk stratification. Cardiac computed tomography (CT) measurement of coronary calcification has been shown to be highly valuable in the early detection and assessment of coronary atherosclerosis and more recently CT coronary angiography is becoming accepted for the assessment of coronary stenosis and potentially coronary plaque characterization. This chapter examines the current applications and interactions of these non-invasive cardiac imaging approaches.

Which of these methods is most appropriate as the initial test depends on the clinical question being asked. Among patients with a relatively low likelihood of CAD, the clinical question frequently revolves around the presence of subclinical coronary atherosclerosis for delineation of *long-term* risk for developing clinical CAD. The answer to this question will help determine who needs aggressive medical management. But as a priori risk for cardiac disease increases, a second question becomes increasingly important: "What is the *shorter-term* risk of myocardial infarction (MI) or cardiac death?"; this question appears to be best answered by the amount of inducible ischemia or potentially by the assessment of the extent and severity of coronary stenoses. In all stages of atherosclerosis, it would be desirable to be able to evaluate the effects of therapy non-invasively.

Assessment of Subclinical Atherosclerosis by Coronary Calcium Scanning

Blankenhorn and Stern first described the importance of coronary artery calcium as a marker of coronary atherosclerosis in 1959 [1]. For many years, the assessment of coronary artery calcium (CAC) using fluoroscopy was recognized as providing clinically useful information. In fact, Diamond et al. incorporated a subjective fluoroscopic assessment of CAC into their original algorithm for assessing the likelihood of angiographically significant coronary artery disease [2] by Bayesian analysis. The advent of CT scanning provided a technique that was potentially quantifiable, avoiding the subjectivity of fluoroscopy. While CAC measurements were first described using electron beam CT (EBT), increasingly investigators are considering that recent generation multidetector (MDCT) and EBT provide comparable measurements for practical clinical purposes [3,4]. In standard practice, the presence and extent of coronary calcium is expressed by the Agatston coronary calcium score (CCS), related to the extent and the density of calcification in the coronary tree. Examples of coronary calcium scans obtained with EBT are shown in Figure 17.1.

Measuring Coronary Calcium by CT

The scoring of these scans typically involves a reproducible semi-automatic computer method as exemplified in Figure 17.2. The CCS is defined for each focus of calcium in the

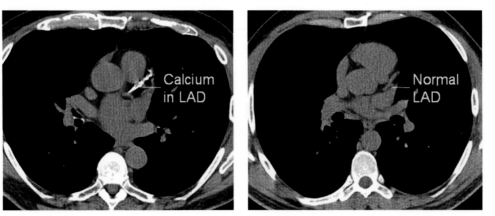

Figure 17.1. Examples of normal and abnormal coronary calcium scans obtained by electron beam tomography. LAD = left anterior descending artery.

coronary tree, with areas containing calcium being defined by having Hounsfield units (HU) >130. The software calculates lesion-specific scores as the product of the area of each calcified focus and peak CT number (scored as 1 if 131 to 199 HU, 2 if 200 to 299 HU, 3 if 300 to 399 HU, and 4 if 400 HU or greater) according to the Agatston method [5]. These are summed across all lesions identified in the coronary arteries to provide the total CCS.

In common practice, this score is often also expressed as a coronary calcium percentile score based on age and gender using one of many available databases [6–8]. While initially developed for EBT, methods for approximating the density-weighted Agatston score using MDCT have been developed. As noted above, the scores derived from recent generation MDCT and EBT are now widely considered the same for practical purposes. Most of the available software programs also often provide a *calcified volume score* developed by Callister [9], which has been described as more

useful for following the progression (or regression) of the calcification over time [10]. With the use of calcium phantoms as standards, the mass of calcium in the coronary tree can also be accurately measured by EBT or MDCT; whether calcified coronary mass will become the standard assessment of the future is not yet clear.

Early Detection and Quantification of Coronary Atherosclerosis: The Role of Coronary Calcium Scanning

Assessment of the presence of subclinical coronary atherosclerosis provides an opportunity to identify asymptomatic patients who are at risk for developing clinical coronary heart disease over the long term. While consideration of conventional risk factors for atherosclerosis –

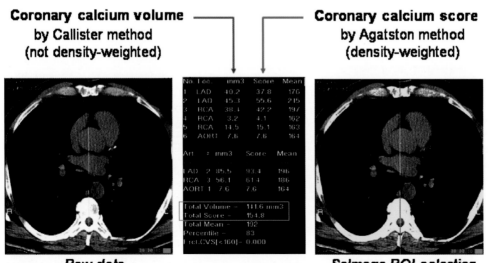

Figure 17.2. Illustration of measurement of the coronary calcium volume (Callister method) and the coronary calcium score (Agatston method).

increased serum cholesterol levels, hypertension, smoking, etc. – are important in overall assessment, this approach does not provide an actual marker of the pathologic disease state. Conventionally, these risk factors are aggregated into a global score of risk such as the Framingham Risk Score (FRS), which is expressed as a number reflecting the likelihood of developing cardiac death or non-fatal myocardial infarction (MI) over a 10-year period [11]. The FRS has been proposed as a guide to risk assessment and the need for aggressive anti-atherosclerotic treatment among asymptomatic patients, but this algorithm, developed in healthy epidemiological cohorts, has not been widely tested as a screening algorithm among patients typically eligible for cardiac stress testing. Moreover, the FRS does not take into account family history of early heart disease, of known importance but not accurately recorded in the initial FRS database, as well as other factors (such as visceral obesity) which might be of importance for certain patients. It also may underestimate long-term risk in women – and even if a wide range of FRS (e.g. 6–20% 10-year risk of CHD) is used to define intermediate risk, still <5% of adult women would be eligible for screening. As an alternative, coronary calcium scanning or carotid intima-to-media thickness measurements (IMT) using ultrasound [12,13] have become increasingly used to screen for atherosclerosis among patients with relatively low likelihood of hemodynamically significant CAD.

From the currently available information, in a Bethesda conference on imaging of coronary atherosclerosis [14], it was concluded that CT CAC provides the most accurate method currently available for the early detection of coronary atherosclerosis. The amount of coronary calcium correlates strongly with the overall amount of coronary plaque (calcified and non-calcified) as determined at postmortem examination [15] (Figure 17.3). The slope of this correlation was 0.2, implying that approximately 80% of plaque is non-calcified and 20% is calcified in the untreated patient. While microscopic calcification of coronary plaque appears very early in the atherosclerotic process, macroscopic calcification (the amount required for detection by the EBT/MDCT) occurs somewhat after cholesterol and inflammatory cell accumulation, apparently triggered by the inflammatory process [16]. Nonetheless, it is very uncommon for extensive atherosclerosis to be presented with no evidence of calcification on the coronary calcium scan. Of note, in a manuscript currently under review, only 1 of 276 patients scanned prior to admission with a suspected acute coronary syndrome was then found to have an acute syndrome in the absence of coronary calcium by EBT [17].

It became clear from early coronary calcium scanning experience that whereas CAC was almost always present in the presence of angiographically significant CAD (≥50% stenosis), CAC had low specificity; that is, calcification implies atherosclerosis but not necessarily the presence of a stenosis. This phenomenon is explained by a process referred to as the Glagov phenomenon [18] (Figure 17.4).

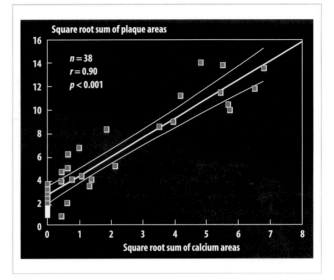

Figure 17.3. Relationship between coronary calcium areas (mm) by electron beam tomography and atherosclerotic plaque areas (mm) by postmortem examination for each of the individual coronary arteries in patients who died of non-cardiac cause. (Adapted with permission from Rumberger et al. [15]).

Characteristically, in the early stages of coronary atherosclerosis, and often in the more advanced stages, plaque accumulation produces an outward remodeling (expansion) of the external elastic membrane. During this phase of disease, there is little or no encroachment of the plaque on the vascular lumen. In simplistic terms, in most circumstances, only after maximal outward remodeling does a narrowing of the lumen develop. Due to this process, there is only a weak relationship between plaque burden and the proportion of the coronary artery tree supplied by vessels with greater than 50% stenosis. However, if more mild luminal narrowing is considered, as demonstrated by Schmermund et al. [19], the total coronary calcium score as determined from EBT correlates strongly ($r = 0.77$) with the number of segments by coronary angiography demonstrating ≥20% stenosis (Figure 17.5). From the extensive available data it can be concluded that assessment of coronary calcium allows detection of atherosclerotic lesions often long before they become hemodynamically significant.

In contrast, stress nuclear cardiology techniques (as with all stress imaging methods) require the presence of a hemodynamically significant lesion, either fixed or dynamic, before abnormality becomes evident. Thus, it is not surprising that once the CCS was known, Schmermund et al. [19] found that nuclear testing provided no additional information regarding the presence of atherosclerosis, although this has yet to be validated in a sufficiently powered patient sample. The results of a multivariate analysis for predicting the number of segments with mild coronary narrowing are illustrated in Table 17.1. In the absence of the coronary calcium data, stress myocardial perfusion SPECT (MPS) provided significant information for the prediction of the number of segments with 20% or

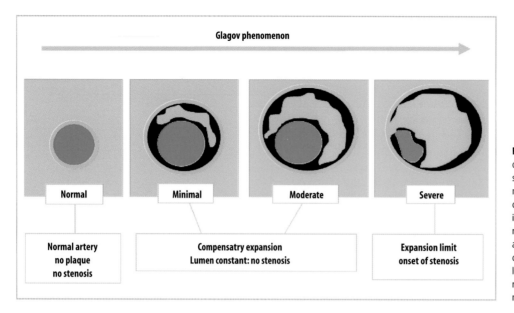

Figure 17.4. Diagrammatic representation of a possible sequence of changes in atherosclerotic arteries leading eventually to lumen narrowing. The artery enlarges initially in association with plaque accumulation, maintaining an adequate, if not normal, lumen area. At more than 40% stenosis, however, the plaque area continues to increase to involve the entire circumference of the vessel, and the artery no longer enlarges at a rate sufficient to prevent narrowing of the lumen. (Adapted with permission from Glagov et al. [18]).

greater maximal coronary stenosis at angiography, along with age, male gender, and cholesterol measurements in a multivariate model. However, once the CCS was known, the radionuclide perfusion score and conventional risk factors were no longer a significant predictor. While this study represents only one of a number of studies that have demonstrated that the CCS provides independent and incremental information over risk factors for predicting the extent of angiographic CAD, it gives insight into the perceived discordance between angiographic and CAC results, and is illustrative of the concept that the presence of CAC is expected to be more sensitive than MPS or even the angiographic "gold standard" in the detection of early coronary atherosclerosis.

Table 17.2 summarizes the use of coronary calcium measurements by EBT/MDCT for early detection and quantification of coronary atherosclerosis.

Table 17.1. Multiple linear regression analysis to determine independent predictors of the number of angiographic segments with 20% or greater maximum stenosis (CAGE ≥20 score)

Predictors of segments with CAGE ≥20 scores	p value	R^2
Model 1		
Age	0	0.32
Male sex	0	
Total/HDL cholesterol	0.03	
LDL cholesterol (calculated)	0.03	
Model 2		
Age	0	0.37
Male sex	0.01	
Total/HDL cholesterol	0.01	
Radionuclide perfusion score	0	
Model 3		
Age	0.01	0.60
Male sex	0.22	
Total/HDL cholesterol	0.08	
Radionuclide perfusion score	0.14	
Total calcium score (log$_e$-transformed)	0	

Source: Adapted with permission from Schmermund et al. [19].
CAGE = coronary artery greater even; HDL = high-density lipoprotein; LDL = low-density lipoprotein.

Table 17.2. Early detection and quantification of atherosclerosis

Most accurate non-invasive test for early detection: abnormal study implies coronary atherosclerosis
Strong quantitative relationship between coronary calcium score and plaque burden
High sensitivity for ≥50% angiographic stenosis (but low specificity)
Independent and incremental information over risk factors for predicting extent of angiographic CAD

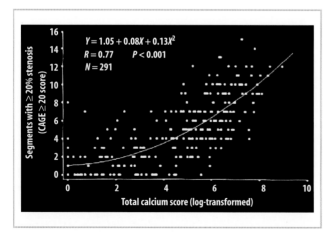

Figure 17.5. Relation between number of segments with coronary artery narrowing greater or equal to 20% (CAGE) scores (y-axis) and log$_e$-transformed total calcium scores (x-axis). (Adapted with permission from Schmermund et al. [19]).

Detection of Angiographically Significant CAD

The Role of MPS

The diagnostic applications of non-invasive stress testing to detect the presence of CAD are based on a hemodynamically significant anatomic endpoint: the detection of flow-limiting coronary stenoses. Generally, this is considered to be ≥50% diameter stenosis (translating to a 75% cross-sectional area reduction). This criterion is operationally important to invasive cardiologists as it is considered to represent the level required to cause a reduction in maximal hyperemia and thus a minimal criterion for the consideration of revascularization with either percutaneous coronary intervention (PCI) or coronary artery bypass grafting (CABG).

By current guidelines [20], the consideration of using a stress imaging study is preceded by assessment of the pretest likelihood of CAD. Specifically, prior to stress testing, the likelihood of CAD can be assessed by Bayesian analyses of patient age, sex, risk factors, and symptoms, as initially developed by Diamond and colleagues [2,21]. Patients with an intermediate likelihood of CAD following the analyses of the above factors are considered the best candidates for stress testing with or without imaging. Patients reclassified as "low likelihood" patients following stress testing will still require modifications of coronary risk factors, which may follow along either primary or secondary prevention guidelines. Patients who are reclassified as having a high likelihood of CAD following stress testing may become appropriate referrals for cardiac catheterization depending on the magnitude of inducible ischemia on stress testing. There is no consensus as to the exact range for this intermediate likelihood, with various recommendations ranging from 10–90% to 30–70%. This diagnostic application has resulted in class I indications in the recent ACC/AHA/ASNC guidelines [22]. Patients with an initially high likelihood of CAD prior to stress testing are unique in that the issue with them is more a prognostic one – are they of sufficient risk to merit aggressive intervention? As a consequence, such high-likelihood patients also commonly benefit from MPS as the next step in their clinical evaluation, because a normal MPS study identifies them as low-risk patients relative to cardiac events [23,24]. Conversely, the more abnormal the MPS study is, the greater the likelihood that a patient would benefit from revascularization (e.g. PCI, CABG) [25].

This approach is embodied in multiple ACC/AHA guidelines in which stress testing, with or without stress imaging, is considered a class I indication in many patients with an intermediate likelihood of CAD but a class IIb indication (usefulness/efficacy is less well established by evidence/opinion) for diagnostic testing in patients with either high or low pretest probability of CAD [20,22,26,27].

The Role of CCS

The coronary calcium scan can also be thought of in terms of its ability to detect angiographically significant CAD. In this regard, the presence of any coronary calcification is considered to have a sensitivity of 95% after correction for verification bias, based on a CAC score >0 [28]. In the largest single study to date, the sensitivity has been reported to be 99%, with equally high sensitivity in both genders in a large study of consecutive patients being sent to coronary angiography for clinical reasons [29]. This implies that many patients with CAC score of 0 might be spared from unnecessary coronary angiography if there are not compelling clinical reasons to suspect the presence of disease. An approach that incorporates age, gender, and CCS in prediction of likelihood of angiographically significant CAD has been described [28], and the approach could be further refined by incorporation of the presence or absence of chest discomfort and its type as well as the results of stress testing. In general, if the pretest likelihood of CAD is less than 50%, a CAC score of 0 provides very strong evidence against the presence of CAD and can be used confidently for clinical decision-making.

Unlike abnormal MPS, however, the presence of coronary calcium alone is not an accurate prediction of angiographically significant stenosis. This is because the specificity of CCS for defining obstructive CAD (i.e. 50% stenosis) is low. Extensive atherosclerosis is known to occur before there is any luminal encroachment by the plaque, as explained by the Glagov phenomenon [18]. While the higher the CCS, the greater the likelihood of angiographically significant CAD [29], and while the incorporation of age and gender can improve the angiographic predictions, asymptomatic patients even with very high CCS (>1000) are generally sent for stress imaging rather than for catheterization in the absence of other evidence of ischemia.

The Role of CT Coronary Angiography

Beyond its use in assessment of coronary calcium, cardiac CT scanning has now become increasingly used for non-invasive CT coronary angiography (CTA) and has demonstrated high sensitivity and specificity for detecting coronary stenosis [30–32]. While virtually all EBT scanners and most recent generation MDCT scanners are capable of the CCS measurements, only the latest generation scanners have been successful in providing clinically useful CTA. EBT scanners are limited in their z-axis resolution (1.5 mm), diminishing their value. In 2004, 64-slice MDCT with rotation time of 330 milliseconds was introduced for routine clinical use. Since tomography with CT requires approximately 210° acquisition (slightly more than SPECT), this speed implies single beat acquisition times of approximately 180 milliseconds. With heart rates of <65 beats/minute (usually through the use of beta blockers) and regular rhythm, high-resolution coronary angiograms with as low as 0.4 mm isotropic resolution can be routinely obtained with these scanners. Newest data with 64-slice scanners have been recently reported [33]. Results showing approximately 90% sensitivity and 90% specificity for coronary stenosis visualized by invasive angiography have been consistently reported with 16-slice scanners. With the 64-slice scanners, covering between 20 and 40 mm with each rotation, fewer heartbeats are required for acquisition, and contrast volumes of less than 100 mL are routine. The low contrast dose minimizes problems associated with higher contrast loads in terms of potential nephrotoxicity, particularly if the CT findings result in diagnosis of a condition that needs urgent contrast coronary angiography. The entire procedure can be performed in approximately 10 minutes, and the rapid reconstruction possible with new computer systems makes the study immediately available for final interpretation. The amount of radiation associated with these procedures is comparable to that received with the standard nuclear cardiology procedures. Of note, the assessments possible from a single first pass acquisition of the chest CT data can be expanded to include assessment of ventricular function. Potentially, this approach can also become of value in the emergency department setting, possibly providing assessments of pulmonary embolism, acute coronary syndrome, and aortic dissection in a single study.

The principal limitation of the CTA method, given the most recent generation scanners, is the presence of dense calcification of the coronary arteries. While mild amounts of calcification do not pose a problem for these scanners, with dense calcification it is not possible to assess the degree of luminal obstruction within the calcified zone. Despite multiple different evaluation methods (Chapter 4), to date, these approaches are not able to evaluate the presence of stenosis in densely calcified plaques.

Whereas the relationship between CCS and MPS is fairly well understood, the relative roles of MPS and CTA have not yet been defined. As CTA becomes more widely available, it is likely that this technology will compete with stress imaging methods (MPS or stress echo) in patients with an intermediate likelihood of CAD. For purposes of risk assessment, for patients with known disease, or for those known or likely to have extensive coronary calcium, MPS is likely to remain the dominant approach.

Patients who might benefit from the further assessment by CTA include those with a strong clinical suspicion of CAD, but an apparent low-risk MPS and CCS, even if there is no evidence of coronary calcium. Isolated cases of patients with critical stenoses associated with soft plaque only have been reported. Examples of patients in this category may include symptomatic patients with diabetes or the metabolic syndrome [34] or patients with marked test discordance (e.g. a high-risk treadmill test with a normal MPS). Other patients might be those in whom multiple risk factors are found to be associated with left main coronary calcium by EBT but a CCS <400. Since MPS has the rare but important limitation of at times missing balanced reduction of coronary flow such as might be observed in patients with left main coronary artery disease (Figures 17.6 and 17.7), assessment by MDCT/EBT coronary angiography may be useful in identifying these patients. In this regard, there have recently been several publications documenting high sensitivity and specificity of non-invasive EBT/MDCT coronary angiography [35,36]. EBT can also be of use in patients with suspected non-ischemic cardiomyopathy (Figure 17.8), patients with coronary anomalies, and patients with prior CABG.

With the rapid development of faster and higher resolution CT scanners, non-invasive MDCT coronary angiography is becoming more commonly employed for clinical purposes. The availability of this powerful new modality will add further complexity to the concepts regarding appropriate selection of tests. It may be that the utilization of PET/CT in the cardiac patient will help solve much of this dilemma. With the development of cardiac dedicated CT/PET and CT/SPECT systems, it may be that a large body of data will be available in the future in which patients will

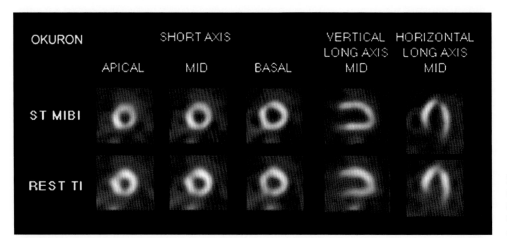

Figure 17.6. Exercise MPS in an asymptomatic 70-year-old diabetic man shows mild decreased uptake in the anterior and lateral walls. The overall study was considered equivocal.

Nuclear Cardiology and Cardiac Computed Tomography in Assessment of Patients with Known or Suspected Chronic Coronary Artery Disease

245

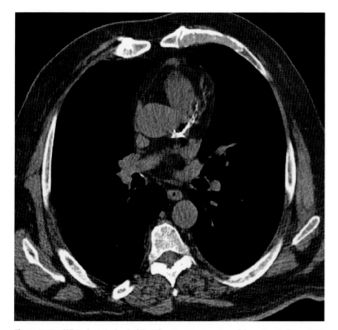

Figure 17.7. EBT study at the level of the left main coronary artery of the patient in Figure 17.6. There is severe calcification in the left main and left anterior descending (LAD) coronary arteries. The CCS was 1295 (87th percentile). Coronary angiogram revealed 75% stenosis in the left main artery and 60% stenosis in mid LAD. The patient underwent successful CABG.

have information regarding coronary calcium, coronary stenoses, and stress-induced ischemia, potentially providing large databases that can be a source of evidence regarding which test or combination of tests is most appropriate in a given setting. The PET/CT is likely to provide the highest sensitivity and specificity for myocardial perfusion testing, with its higher resolution than SPECT and routine attenuation correction, and potentially to offer absolute quantitative measures, eliminating the problem of occasionally missing balanced reduction in flow. At the same

time, since rest/stress PET studies could be performed as a routine in conjunction with CT coronary angiography, the possibility of taking "all comers" regardless of the amount of coronary calcium that they have would enhance the usefulness of non-invasive coronary angiography.

The Role of Cardiac Magnetic Resonance in Detection of CAD

On a research basis, great strides have been made in cardiac magnetic resonance (CMR) for purposes of non-invasive investigation of coronary stenosis. A variety of approaches are available for this purpose, and initial reports have suggested that the sensitivity and specificity of the approach comes close to that of CTA. However, there are several obstacles impeding the routine use of CMR for non-invasive coronary angiography. CMR is intrinsically far more complex from the technical and interpretive standpoint than cardiac CT. Since unlike cardiac CT, CMR is not yet truly three-dimensional, there is the need for separate prescription of the planes for imaging, a step that extends the study time and takes considerable expertise. The acquisitions are obtained over several heartbeats, increasing the possibility of misregistration. Intrinsically, CMR does not achieve as high spatial resolution as CT. While over time CMR coronary angiography could become more common, at present it is widely accepted that CT scanning has at the minimum a multiple year lead in this application.

Non-invasive Risk Stratification in Chronic CAD

Classification of Patients into Risk Categories

Non-invasive testing can provide information that can be useful for risk stratification in the chronic CAD patient. For CAD patients who have limiting anginal symptoms, consideration of revascularization is routine, and non-invasive imaging methods are generally not needed. However, for the asymptomatic or mildly symptomatic patient, non-invasive assessment of patient risk is increasingly being used to select patients for catheterization with consideration of revascularization. This application applies to patients deemed clinically to be at intermediate risk. Patients at the extremes of risk – high or low risk of adverse cardiovascular events – are not generally considered appropriate candidates for risk stratification, because they are already stratified sufficiently for clinical decision-making [37–39].

Prognostic Applications of MPS

Stress-gated MPS is the most commonly used and best-documented non-invasive method for risk stratification. It

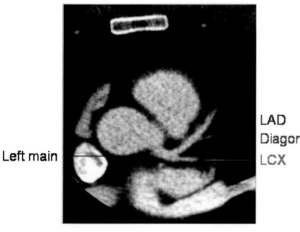

Left main | LAD
Diagonal
LCX

Figure 17.8. Single frame from an EBT non-invasive coronary angiogram in a 45-year-old man with suspected non-ischemic cardiomyopathy. There was no coronary artery calcium and the non-invasive angiogram was normal. The normal study obviated the need for contrast-enhanced electron beam tomography. LAD = left anterior descending artery; LCX = left circumflex artery.

is most cost-effective in patients with a clinically intermediate risk of a subsequent cardiac event. This directly parallels the diagnostic application of MPS in patients with an intermediate likelihood of suspected CAD [22]. In general, low prognostic risk has been defined as a less than 1% cardiac mortality rate per year and high risk as a more than 3% cardiac mortality rate per year [26]. Intermediate risk generally refers to the 1% to 3% cardiac mortality rate per year range [26]. In chronic CAD, it has been suggested that a more than 3% per year mortality rate can be used to identify patients with minimal symptoms whose mortality rate can be improved by myocardial revascularization [22,40]. Since the mortality risk associated with revascularization procedures is at least 1% [22,41], patients whose symptoms can be controlled medically and are at low (<1%) risk of cardiac death are not generally considered candidates for revascularization procedures. This 1–3% range would be scaled up for patients who are very elderly or have serious co-morbidities, due to increased mortality in all subgroups of these patients. Also, patients whose known or suspected CAD is seriously affecting quality of life or functional status should be considered catheterization candidates irrespective of risk status.

Post-MPS Patient Outcomes

Two basic tenets, confirmed by extensive literature evidence, are behind the acceptance of MPS for risk stratification: a normal MPS study defines patients at low risk for subsequent cardiac events [38,39] and risk increases exponentially with worsening perfusion abnormality [42]. Because of this evidence, physicians today can comfortably manage most patients with normal MPS without resorting to myocardial revascularization, confident that angiographic assessment is unlikely to yield further benefit. At the other end of the spectrum, extensive and/or severe perfusion defects define high risk independent of age, sex, prior revascularization or MI, type of stress performed and underlying cardiac risk factors, and usually leads to coronary angiography.

In recent years, it has become apparent that MPS can be used to define separate risks for MI and cardiac death in patients referred for clinical study [43]. These findings can be used to refine important decisions relative to optimal patient management. For example, Hachamovitch et al. [43] demonstrated in a large population that cardiac mortality rate progressively increased with increasing scan abnormality (Figure 17.9). When the MPS scan was mildly abnormal (summed stress score (SSS) 4–8: 5–10% of the myocardium with stress perfusion defect), the rate of MI was generally intermediate although the risk of cardiac death, in general, is low. Thus, once the patient has an MPS study with any degree of abnormality, they are at risk for subsequent MI, and need intensive preventive therapy toward that end (e.g. aspirin, statins, ACE inhibitors, etc.), since these therapies have been demonstrated to reduce the

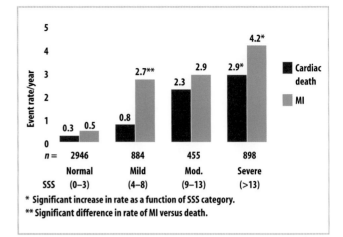

Figure 17.9. Relationship between the annualized cardiac death rate (red) and MI rate (green) of a large group of patients undergoing stress myocardial perfusion SPECT (two thirds exercise stress, one third adenosine stress). *$p < 0.001$ for each endpoint across scan categories; **$p < 0.01$ for cardiac death versus myocardial infarction in mildly abnormal scans. (Adapted with permission from Lippincoff Williams & Wilkins. [43]).

risk of MI. However, the risk of cardiac death, which would imply the need to consider revascularization to prolong survival, did not begin to rise until there was at least a moderately elevated SSS (>8: >10% myocardium abnormal at stress).

Since the time of this initial large prognostic study, we have found that there are subgroups of patients with mild perfusion abnormalities who might need to be considered for revascularization based on other high-risk scan information (e.g. patients with a low ejection fraction [44], transient ischemic dilation of the left ventricle [45], increased lung uptake) or other clinical information suggesting high risk (e.g. diabetes [46], atrial fibrillation [47], those undergoing adenosine stress [43], high pretest likelihood of CAD [24,48], very abnormal stress ECG [49]). As an example, Figure 17.10 illustrates how for any stress MPS result, the

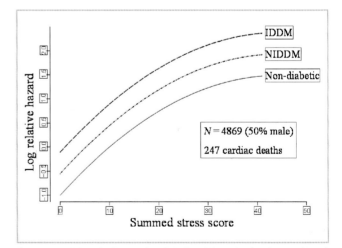

Figure 17.10. Relationship between log relative hazard for predicted cardiac mortality and summed stress score in insulin-dependent diabetes mellitus (IDDM), non-insulin-dependent diabetes mellitus (NIDDM), and non-diabetics ($p < 0.001$). (Adapted with permission from Berman et al. [46]).

risk of cardiac death is higher in diabetic than in non-diabetic patients, and highest when there is insulin dependence [46].

Many different subgroups have been analyzed with respect to risk-assessment by MPS; most of these subgroups are well summarized in the 2003 Revised Guidelines for the Use of Radionuclide Imaging of the ACC/AHA/ASNC [22]. MPS has been shown to be effective for risk stratification in several subsets including women, the elderly, diabetics, left bundle branch block, left ventricular hypertrophy, intermediate risk Duke treadmill scores, patients with a high pretest likelihood of CAD, patients with borderline coronary angiographic findings, prior MI, those who have undergone PCI or CABG, and patients undergoing non-cardiac surgery. In virtually all of these subsets, a relationship has been shown between the extent and severity of stress perfusion defects and prognosis. In overall patient groups, similar findings to those observed with Tc-99m sestamibi stress MPS have been shown with Tl-201 [50] and more recently Tc-99m tetrofosmin [51]. These findings have resulted in a large number of class I indications for myocardial perfusion SPECT in risk assessment of patients with an intermediate or high likelihood of CAD [22].

Potential Underestimation of Prognostic Power of MPS

We have suggested that most of the current MPS data regarding risk stratification underestimates the strength of the modality [38]. First, most studies have excluded patients undergoing early revascularization from prognostic assessment, thus eliminating many of the sickest patients with the most abnormal MPS scans who without revascularization are likely to have had the worst outcomes. The impact of this referral bias has been recently assessed [23]. Further, if patients with very high-risk MPS do not undergo early revascularization, at a minimum they are much more likely than the average patient to receive very aggressive medical therapy which would decrease their observed event rates and thus reduce the apparent extra prognostic information provided by MPS in these observational studies. Finally, recent technical advances and measures from MPS other than perfusion defects have generally not been included in these prognostic studies. These other factors include lung uptake, transient dilation of left ventricle [45], and ventricular function results, the latter now routinely measured with gated SPECT.

Gated LVEF and Volume Assessments and the Prognostic Efficacy of MPS

It is generally assumed that physicians appropriately weigh the various patient characteristics available after a stress MPS study in formulating their final management decision.

This assumption has been shown to be the case with respect to referral for catheterization and revascularization, as a function of patient sex, age, prior CAD, and other factors [25,46,52,53]. However, questions have arisen as to how decision-making is influenced by knowledge of left ventricular ejection fraction (LVEF). Specifically, we have recently observed that an unusual referral bias *against* revascularization exists in patients with reduced ejection fraction, even in the presence of extensive ischemia, despite the observation that this group benefits most from successful revascularization [48] (Figure 17.11). This referral bias may help explain the findings of Miller and colleagues from the Mayo Clinic [54], who found that in a cohort of 77 patients with congestive heart failure, LEVF <45%, and large reversible perfusion defects by SPECT, the 5-year revascularization rate was only 13% despite a 57.6% mortality rate over this same period of time.

Several reports have now addressed the added value of gated SPECT for risk stratification. For example, Sharir et al. [44] demonstrated incremental prognostic value of post-stress gated SPECT LVEF when added to MPS perfusion defect analysis in a cohort of over 2600 patients (mean follow up 21 ± 5 months). The strongest predictor of cardiac death was LVEF (Figure 17.12). The cardiac death rate was low until the LVEF was reduced, and rose exponentially when the LVEF fell below 35%. Patients with normal left ventricular function had a less than 1% risk of death unless there was extensive ischemia. Patients with mild to moderate reduction of ejection fraction (30–50%) had less than 1% risk of death only when small amounts of ischemia were present. When LVEF was less than 30%, from a standpoint of risk assessment (as opposed to assessment of therapeutic benefit discussed below) all groups had high risk of cardiac death regardless of the amount of ischemia

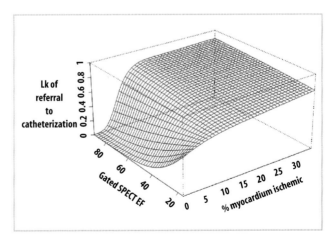

Figure 17.11. Multivariable, risk-adjusted relationship between gated ejection fraction and percent myocardium ischemic with respect to prediction of likelihood of referral to catheterization based on a logistic regression model. Increase in likelihood $p < 0.0001$. Lk = likelihood; EF = ejection fraction. (Adapted with permission from Hachamovitch et al. [48]). Note that when EF was normal, the amount of ischemia strongly influenced the decision for angiography; however, when EF was reduced, the amount of ischemia did not influence the rate of catheterization, despite evidence that the patients with low EF and extensive ischemia benefit the most from revascularization in terms of survival.

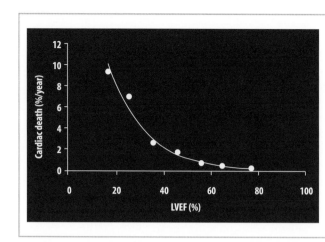

Figure 17.12. Relationship between post-stress EF by MPS and rate of cardiac death in 2686 consecutive patients with known or suspected CAD. (Reprinted by permission of the Society of Nuclear Medicine. From Sharir T, Germano G, Kang X, et al. Prediction of myocardial infarction versus cardiac death by gated myocardial perfusion SPECT. J Nucl Med 2001;42:831–837, Figure 2.)

[44]. Regarding LV volumes, Sharir et al. [55], analyzing the Cedars-Sinai gated MPS database, reported that when post-stress end-systolic volume is taken into account, the larger the end-systolic volume, the higher the cardiac death rate, for any given ejection fraction (Figure 17.13), as had been shown previously with contrast ventriculography [56]. Thus, risk assessment with MPS is improved if functional assessments of ejection fraction and end-systolic volume are taken into account. Similarly it has also been shown that risk assessment by MPS is improved by considering transient ischemic dilation of the left ventricle [45] as well as non-nuclear parameters such as the hemodynamic responses to adenosine [57] or exercise [58].

Using MPS for Deciding Between Medical and Revascularization Therapy

As noted above, until recently, all reports of MPS for risk stratification removed (censored) patients undergoing revascularization early after MPS, thus excluding the highest risk group from prognostic analysis. In a recent study, we examined the relationship between the extent and severity of ischemia and the survival benefit associated with subsequent revascularization [25] in a manner that avoided this problem. In order to express the extent and severity of MPS perfusion defects in a more intuitive manner, and in order to employ a system that could be applied with either 17- or 20-segment systems, we introduced in this study a new approach which derives the percent myocardium abnormal from the summed stress, summed rest, and summed difference scores. To this end, the summed perfusion scores are expressed as a percentage of maximal, defined by multiplying the number of segments scored by the maximal score (e.g. in a 0–4 score/20-segment model, the maximum score would be 80), resulting in a percentage that is intuitively understood and independent of the number of segments scored [42]. In 10,627 patients without prior MI or revascularization

who underwent stress MPS and were followed up for a mean of 1.9 years (4% lost to follow-up) [25], cardiac death occurred in 146 patients (1.4% mortality). Patient treatment was defined on the basis of that received within 60 days post-MPS (revascularization (671 patients, 2.8% mortality) versus medical therapy (9956 patients, 1.3% mortality; $p = 0.0004$)) and a risk-adjusted approach was used including a propensity score to adjust for non-randomization of treatment assignment.

Based on a Cox proportional hazards model most predictive of cardiac death ($\chi^2 = 539, p < 0.0001$), in the setting of no or mild ischemia, patients undergoing medical therapy as their initial treatment had superior survival to those patients referred for revascularization. On the other hand, when moderate to severe ischemia (>10% of the total myocardium ischemic) was detected by MPS, patients undergoing revascularization had an increasing survival benefit over patients undergoing medical therapy (Figure

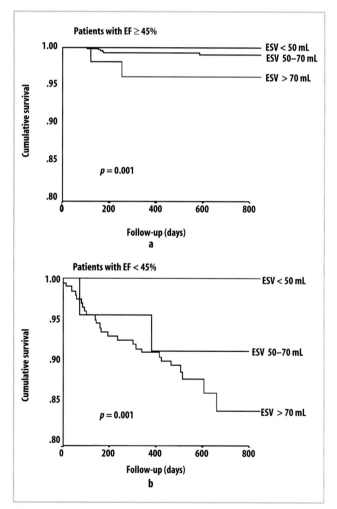

Figure 17.13. In the first paper on the prognostic value of gated SPECT, Sharir et al., studying 1680 patients, demonstrated that end-systolic volume (ESV), as measured by gated SPECT, provided significant information about the extent and severity of perfusion defect as measured by the summed stress score in prediction of cardiac death [55]. **a** Patients with normal LVEF by gated SPECT; **b** patients with abnormal LVEF by gated SPECT. Within each EF group, patients are then subdivided by the gated SPECT end-systolic volume. In both EF groups, ESV further stratified patients with respect to survival. (Adapted with permission from Lippincoff Williams & Wilkins [55]).

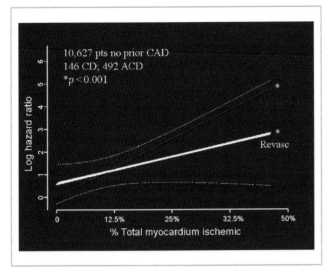

Figure 17.14. Log hazard ratio for revascularization versus medical therapy as a function of percent myocardium ischemic based on final Cox proportional hazards model. Revasc = revascularization. Model $p < 0.0001$, interaction $p = 0.0305$ (Adapted with permission from Lippincoff Williams & Wilkins [25]).

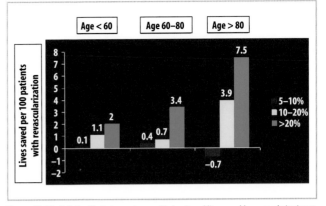

Figure 17.16. Relationship between degree of ischemia and lives saved by revascularization as a function of age.

17.14). The survival advantage for revascularization over medical therapy as the amount of ischemia increased was accentuated in the presence of greater clinical risk (elderly patients, women, diabetic patients, and patients undergoing pharmacologic stress) (Figures 17.15 and 17.16).

Preliminary data presented at the American Heart Association in 2002 extended these findings to include information regarding gated MPS ejection fraction [59] showing that LVEF, % ischemic and % infarcted myocardium were all predictors of cardiac death. However, only inducible ischemia by MPS identified patients who would benefit from revascularization. With increasing amounts of inducible ischemia, an increasing survival benefit for revascularization over medical therapy was found across the range of LVEF. The findings of these two studies suggest a new paradigm: rather than identify patient *risk*, the goal of MPS in terms of testing strategy is to identify which patients may or may not *benefit* from revascularization.

This approach promises to yield an enhanced role for non-invasive testing in patient management strategies.

Using MPS for risk stratification or risk/benefit assessment markedly broadens the patient population in whom MPS might be applicable, beyond the intermediate likelihood of CAD group appropriate for diagnostic purposes. For example, two studies from separate institutions have shown that patients without known CAD but with a high pretest likelihood of CAD (defined by two different approaches – one based on clinical risk and the other conventional pretest likelihood of CAD) are excellent candidates for initial testing with stress MPS [23,24]. Further, this approach was shown to be more cost-effective in these patients than initial referral for either exercise treadmill test (ETT) or catheterization [23,24].

Prognostic Applications of CCS

As with MPS, measuring CCS has potentially wide prognostic applications, but in contrast to MPS, which provides useful information across the spectrum of patients with *known* as well as suspected CAD, it is not likely that assessment of CCS will provide incremental prognostic discrimination in patients with known CAD, because prognosis in such patients is governed more by functional parameters, such as ischemia and LV function, rather than measurements of atherosclerotic disease burden. Rather, the principal prognostic value of CCS is likely to reside in patients with a low-intermediate likelihood of CAD (e.g. 15% to 50% range). Studies in this regard demonstrate that CCS provides incremental information over conventional risk factors in assessing the risk of hard cardiac events. For example, a recent publication of results in over 10,000 asymptomatic patients followed over 5 years for all-cause mortality demonstrated that in both men and women the previously described categories for degrees of CCS abnormality were strongly predictive of all-cause mortality and that CCS provided significant incremental information over that provided by conventional risk factor analysis alone (Figures 17.17 and 17.18) [60]. Similarly, Kondos et

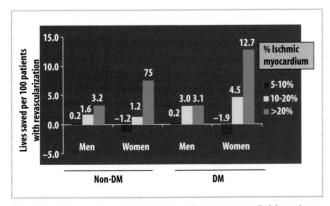

Figure 17.15. Lives saved per 100 treated with revascularization versus medical therapy in men and women with versus without diabetes mellitus as a function of percent myocardium ischemic. Revasc = revascularization. Results based on Cox proportional hazards model. Statistical significance as per model.

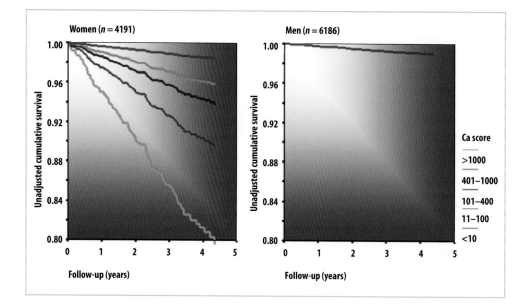

Figure 17.17. Unadjusted all-cause survival according to calcium score subsets in women and men. Survival rate is proportionally worse as calcium score increases. Ca = coronary calcium score by Agatston method. (Adapted with permission from RSNA [60]).

al. [61] demonstrated in 37-month follow-up of 5635 initially asymptomatic low- to intermediate-risk adults (1484 women) that cardiac events (death, MI, or revascularization) were predicted by the CCS in both genders using multivariable analysis. In men, cardiac events were also predicted by diabetes and smoking, whereas in women, risk factors were not significant predictors in their study. O'Malley et al. have performed a meta-analysis of several studies dealing with the prognostic value of EBT in asymptomatic populations [62]. While there is variability in these reports, in general it has been documented that the risk ratio for patients with an abnormal EBT is higher than 1 in all of the publications cited [63]. Of note, in a recent publication, Park et al. [64] found CCS levels to provide incremental information over that of high sensitivity C-reactive protein (CRP) levels in subjects primarily at intermediate risk. Of interest is a report by Park that the CCS and CRP were additive, suggesting that a marker of inflammation

(likely related to plaque stability) may provide additional value in risk assessment.

In others works, Greenland et al. [65] recently demonstrated that the CCS adds to the Framingham Risk Score (FRS) in prediction of non-fatal MI or cardiac death in asymptomatic individuals. In a population of 1029 asymptomatic subjects with at least one coronary risk factor but no diabetes, the CCS was predictive of risk among subjects with a FRS of ≥10% (implying ≥1%/year risk of hard cardiac event). Their data suggested that the CCS did not provide useful added risk assessment for subjects with FRS of <10% (n = 89 low risk). Their conclusion from their data is consistent with the recommendations from the Bethesda conference supporting the concept that the CCS is useful for risk assessment in patients with an intermediate risk category.

Regarding the definition of the intermediate risk category, while the consensus document of the Bethesda conference suggested this category should be expanded to 6–20% rate of hard cardiac event over 10 years (which would detect more women than the more commonly used 10–20% range), others still consider that this range should be 10–20%, since even with the relatively narrow range, there is a large proportion of the adult population of the United States (11.9%) that would be in need of testing [66,67]. It appears to be emerging that CCS is justified for the risk assessment of asymptomatic patients with intermediate risk on clinical grounds, and there is now general support that third party carriers should pay for testing in this patient group, rather than having it be a test only for patients who can afford to pay for it on their own.

Several reports have shown that approximately 95% of patients suffering a first MI have an abnormal CCS within days of the MI, too early for the CCS to have developed in response to the new event [6,68–70]. These data imply that it is highly unusual for coronary atherosclerosis to result in acute MI before the development of coronary calcification.

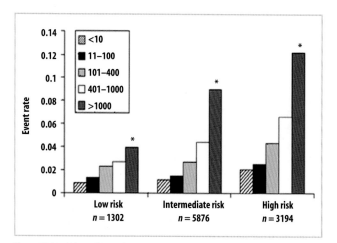

Figure 17.18. Risk stratification for each category of Framingham risk (from low to high) according to calcium score. Event rate is predicted mortality at 5 years. (Adapted with permission from RSNA [60]). (* = p < 0.0001)

They suggest that CCS can be a useful test for ruling out (or markedly reducing the likelihood of) an acute ischemic syndrome in patients presenting with chest pain in the emergency room [17,68].

Guiding Patient Management Decisions by CCS in Diagnostic Patients

One of the important applications of non-invasive testing is in determining the appropriate therapy in an individual patient. In patients with suspected but without known CAD, the CCS may be of particular use in this regard. On the basis of available data, the extent of CAC by MDCT/EBT may be used to determine the appropriateness and aggressiveness of medical therapies, such as statin use, or need for stress testing, among patients presenting with an intermediate 10-year risk of MI or cardiac death by the FRS. One example of this involves assessment of patients with the metabolic syndrome, many of whom are at intermediate risk. Approximately one-fifth of such patients actually have an FRS indicating >20% 10-year risk of CHD and one-fourth have CAC ≥75th percentile, which has been designated by the National Cholesterol Educational Program as a criterion to stratify the patient into more intensive risk factor management. Nearly half of such patients have either or both criteria that could justify them for intensive secondary prevention medical therapy (e.g. treatment of LDL-cholesterol to <100 mg/dL) as a high-risk (e.g. CHD risk equivalent) patient [34]. In our experience, this application of CCS is one of the most common reasons that the test is currently ordered by physicians.

Part of guiding management decisions is the manner in which a test result affects the choice of subsequent testing. From the above discussion, it would seem clear that asymptomatic patients with extensive coronary atherosclerosis by CCS would benefit from additional testing for ischemia. This concept fits with recommendations made years ago by Rumberger et al. [71]. For purposes of cost-effectiveness, it would not be appropriate for all patients with atherosclerosis by EBT to be referred for further testing.

To date, there are now three published reports that have been helpful in this regard. He et al. [72] evaluated the frequency of stress-induced ischemia by MPS in patients who had undergone EBT scanning. These investigators evaluated 292 males and 78 females undergoing both MPS and EBT for coronary calcification. They divided their patients into the traditional categories of no (CCS 0), minimal (CCS 1–10), mild (CCS 11–100), moderate (CCS 101–399), and extensive coronary calcium (CCS >400) [71]. Only one patient in more than 100 with CCS of 100 or less had abnormal MPS; 12% of patients with moderate CCS had abnormal MPS and 47% of patients with extensive CCS had abnormal MPS (Figure 17.19). Moser et al. [73] recently reported results of combined SPECT and CCS testing in 102 patients, with these investigators employing MDCT for CCS. In this smaller group, none of 19 patients

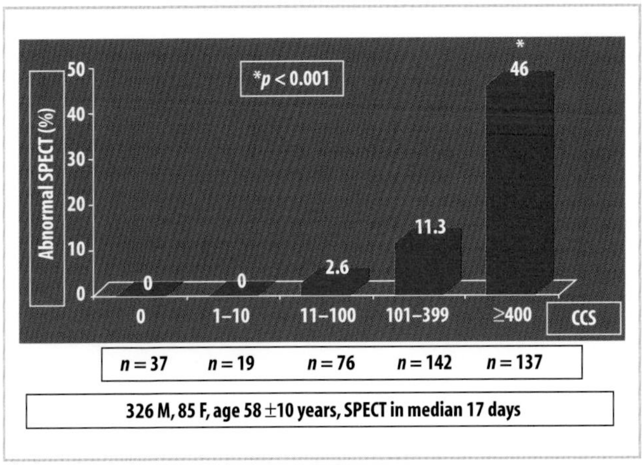

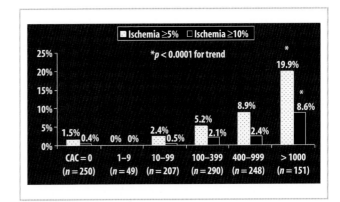

Figure 17.19. SPECT results based on total CCS. Few subjects with CCS <400 had abnormal SPECT (6.6%), and most (99.3%) had only small (<15%) perfusion defect size (PDS). CCS = coronary calcium score. (Adapted with permission from He et al. [72]).

with a CCS <100, 6 of 51 (12%) of patients with CCS 100–400, and 13 of 32 (41%) of patients with CCS ≥400 had an abnormal SPECT study. They concluded that a CCS threshold of >400 was useful in determining the need for subsequent MPS.

Recent data from our institution have confirmed the findings of previous studies with respect to the patients with CCS ≥400 [74]. In 1195 consecutive patients with no history of CAD who had EBT and MPS, among the patients with a CCS <100, MPS ischemia was rare, occurring in less than 2% of such patients [74]. This low frequency of ischemia with a CCS <100 was present in patients with and without clinical symptoms, although a trend toward more ischemia in symptomatic patients with scores 10–99 was observed. As the CCS increased in magnitude above 100, the frequency of myocardial ischemia on MPS increased progressively (Figure 17.20). Among patients with CCS exceeding 1000, 20% manifested an ischemia by MPS. Our results further indicate that the likelihood of myocardial ischemia by MPS is more tightly related to the absolute CCS rather than age-gender-stratified CCS percentile. For

Figure 17.20. The frequency of an ischemic MPS (≥5% ischemic) and of a moderate to severe ischemia (>10% ischemic) for patients divided into six coronary artery calcium (CAC) score groupings. (Adapted with permission from Berman et al. [74]).

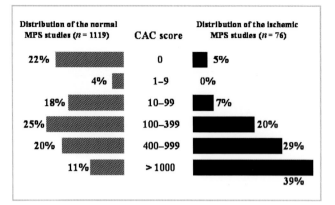

Figure 17.21. Distribution of CAC scores for the 1119 patients manifesting a normal MPS (left) and the 76 patients with an ischemic MPS (right). (Adapted with permission from Berman et al. [74]).

example, among patients with CCS exceeding 400, the frequency of myocardial ischemia was comparably high over a wide range of percentile rankings. A large proportion had high enough CCS that there would be consensus that aggressive medical management is warranted: 56% had CCS >100 and 31% had CCS >400 (Figure 17.21). These findings suggest that if testing begins with MPS in a given patient, further assessment of atherosclerotic burden by CAC testing may be useful in assessment of the need for aggressive attempts to prevent coronary events.

The data from these studies provide information which indicates an important distinction. Whereas a low CCS with a high percentile ranking in young patients may be indicative of *long-term* risk for developing cardiac events [14,75,76], this same score is probably not predictive of *short-term* risk, given the finding that such patients rarely have evidence of ischemia on MPS. Thus, further testing by MPS of patients found to have high CCS percentile but a CCS <100 would not appear to be needed in most patients.

Based on the available data, the following three summary statements might be made regarding combined MPS and CAC testing:

1. It appears that the referral of patients for MPS is generally not needed when the CCS is <100 due to the very low likelihood of observing inducible myocardial ischemia in such patients. Conversely, when the CCS exceeds 400, stress imaging would appear to be generally beneficial, because the frequency of inducible ischemia is substantial within this CCS range, even in asymptomatic patients.

2. CCS in the range of 100 to 400 constitutes a "gray zone" relative to the issue of who may require stress test referral following CAC imaging. For CCS in this range, clinical factors, such as gender, concomitant chest pain, or specific combinations of coronary risk factors, are likely to determine whether ischemia testing is needed, but prospective study is needed in this regard.

3. The wide range of CCS in patients with normal MPS studies exposes an important limitation relevant to all forms of stress testing: they do not effectively screen for subclinical atherosclerosis [74]. Along these lines, there are no available data to yet compare the relative short- and long-term risk for cardiac events among patients with various combinations of MPS results and CCS, such as those presenting with the combination of very high CCS but normal MPS results. It is reasonable to hypothesize that such patients might be at low *short-term* risk but high *long-term* risk for cardiac events, as supported by a preliminary analysis [77]. If borne out by further study, CAC could then be unmasking a subgroup of patients who would receive more aggressive anti-atherosclerotic intervention than would have been indicated based on the results of MPS testing alone. Accordingly, future study that incorporates the prognostic follow-up data from patients undergoing both studies would now be of interest, to determine which patients with normal stress imaging tests are best suited for undergoing *subsequent* CAC scanning.

Given the results described above, we have developed a conceptual approach to the use of EBT and nuclear testing in CAD diagnosis and risk stratification (Figure 17.22). First, the pretest likelihood of angiographically significant CAD is assessed, at low (less than 10%), low-intermediate (10–50%), high-intermediate (50–85%) and high (greater than 85%), employing age, gender, risk factors, and symptoms, as initially suggested by Diamond et al. [2,21]. The low likelihood group generally corresponds to the less than 10%, 10-year risk by Framingham, the low-intermediate with the 10–20% risk, and the high-intermediate and high groups to the greater than 20%, 10-year risk of MI or cardiac death by Framingham. Then, patients are assigned to groups – corresponding to the <10%, 10–20%, and >20% 10-year risk of MI or cardiac death categories recently advocated as low, intermediate, and high risk [78]. Patients with a low likelihood of CAD (in our experience <15%) or low 10-year risk (<10%) require only primary prevention guidelines regarding coronary risk factors (Adult Treatment Panel III) [37]. Patients with a low-intermediate likelihood of CAD (15–50%), a group which by ACC/AHA guidelines might be selected for exercise testing, in this approach become excellent candidates for CCS measurement. This group tends to include the patients who would be classified as having an intermediate risk of developing a clinical cardiovascular event over 10 years (10–20%) [78]. Since CCS provides a far more sensitive, quantitative measurement of subclinical CAD in this population, we consider it more useful than the exercise ECG in selecting patients for aggressive medical management. Patients would then have the intensiveness of their medical therapy guided by the degree of CCS abnormality. As shown in Figure 17.22, scores <100 are generally considered low enough that aggressive medical therapy may not be needed. Scores >100 are generally accepted as the cutoff for recommending

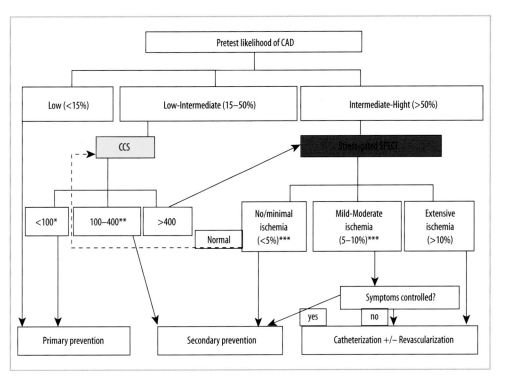

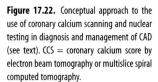

Figure 17.22. Conceptual approach to the use of coronary calcium scanning and nuclear testing in diagnosis and management of CAD (see text). CCS = coronary calcium score by electron beam tomography or multislice spiral computed tomography.

aggressive medical therapy with target LDL <70 mg/dL and the target blood pressure would be 120/80 [78]. Patients with scores ≥10 but <100 might be considered as appropriate for aggressive medical therapy when CCS is ≥90th percentile for age and gender [74], although the exact thresholds remain controversial.

Regarding further testing, patients with CCS >400 would be candidates for further testing with MPS for purposes of risk/benefit assessment with respect to the possible need to consider revascularization. The exact cutoff above which patients should be referred for stress imaging is unclear. In the presence of symptoms referral for nuclear testing might be appropriate with any abnormal score. In asymptomatic patients, the threshold for referral of 400 may be appropriate. In the CCS category 100–400 it would not be cost-effective to refer all patients for myocardial perfusion scanning; however, if tailoring this referral to the individual patient, based on age, sex, and risk factors, selective referral for stress imaging might be appropriate. In this regard, a recent report has shown that the category of 100–400 would warrant testing in diabetic patients [79], and preliminary data have suggested that this would also be appropriate in patients with the metabolic syndrome [80].

As shown in Figure 17.22, patients deemed to have a high-intermediate (50–85%) or a high (greater than 85%) likelihood of CAD benefit from MPS for purposes of determining the need for consideration of revascularization. These patients in general have a >20% 10-year risk of CAD. We have demonstrated that directly testing with MPS,

rather than either CCS or direct catheterization, may be cost-effective and appropriate, unless the patient has limiting symptoms [23]. These findings have also been shown recently by the Mayo Clinic group [81], who reported that even in patients with a normal resting ECG, if the clinical risk of CAD is high, a low-risk treadmill test alone is insufficient to result in a low risk of cardiac events. If the resting ECG is abnormal or otherwise uninterpretable (e.g. digoxin or left bundle branch block) or the patient cannot exercise adequately, there is concordance of opinion that direct referral to a stress imaging procedure is appropriate [22,27].

As shown in Figure 17.22, we also consider that patients with a high-intermediate likelihood of ischemia are also excellent candidates to go directly to MPS, but we acknowledge that this has yet to be shown to be cost-effective. These patients are generally identified clinically by the presence of atypical angina or lesser symptoms with multiple CAD risk factors. It may be that patients in this group can be effectively screened with the CCS.

After stress imaging, patients with extensive ischemia by nuclear testing, or those who are for other reasons considered to be at high risk by clinical assessment after stress imaging, would be candidates for coronary angiography. Patients with ischemia of lesser magnitude might be candidates for angiography depending on the clinical presentation. In this regard, we have described that there are a number of clinical and non-perfusion MPS indicators of risk that should be considered in making the decision regarding the need for coronary angiography (Table 17.3).

Table 17.3. Non-nuclear and nuclear variables shown to be of importance in guiding management decisions in chronic CAD, illustrating the importance of integrating clinical and test results

Non-nuclear	Nuclear
Symptoms/clinical presentation	Extent and severity of perfusion stress, rest, late defects
Exercise duration	Lung uptake
Exercise hypotension	Transient ischemic dilation of the left ventricle
Heart Rate Recovery	LV function:
Duke Treadmill Score	LVEF
Type of stress	LV volume
Hemodynamic response to pharmacologic stress	
ECG evidence of ischemia	

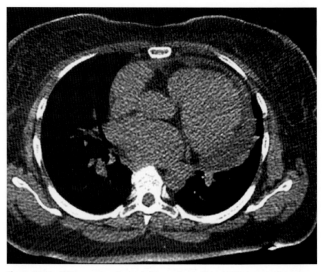

Figure 17.24. EBT image at cardiac level of the patient in Figure 17.19 shows cardiac enlargement and a moderate to large pericardial effusion. There is no evidence of coronary atherosclerosis. The coronary calcium score is 0.

Patients considered to be at high risk despite having only 5–10% ischemia include those with low LVEF [44], transient ischemic dilation of the left ventricle [45], lung uptake [82], diabetes [46,83], and atrial fibrillation [84].

In selected patients with normal or nearly normal nuclear scans, CCS might be appropriate in order to evaluate the extent of atherosclerosis and help guide medical management decisions [85], and to avoid missing extensive atherosclerosis simply because there is no stress-induced ischemia. While this would not be needed in patients who are already following an aggressive medical management approach using secondary prevention guidelines, a CCS in this setting may help motivate patients to follow medical approaches to the control of CAD as well as to guide the intensity of medical management in settings in which the need for secondary prevention is not clear. Examples of the application of EBT are shown in Figures 17.6–17.8, 17.23, and 17.24. We have found that CCS after MPS is very effective in defining further management in patients with equivocal MPS results.

Evaluating Response to Treatment

Another application for which non-invasive testing is frequently used is assessing the response to therapy. Work by Callister et al. [10] and others [75,86] suggest that serial assessment of the calcified coronary volume score (CVS) as determined by EBT can be effective in documenting that therapy has slowed the accumulation of CAC in individual patients.

CCS to Track Progression of Atherosclerotic Disease

Serial CCS measurement may be of use to track the progression of disease, although the data in this regard are less

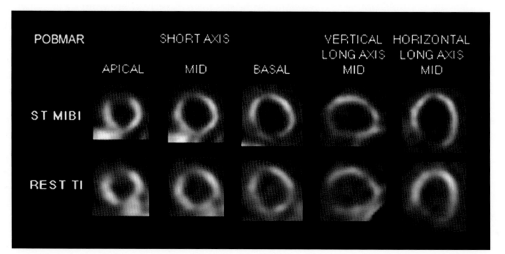

Figure 17.23. Adenosine stress MPS in an asymptomatic 54-year-old diabetic woman shows dilated non-ischemic cardiomyopathy. The mild anterior wall defect is considered likely to be a normal variant or artifact from left bundle branch block.

well documented than in guiding the intensity of medical management. Using this technique, a second scan is performed approximately 2 years after initial testing, and changes between the first and second scan are assessed. Callister et al. [10] examined the value of statin therapy in slowing the progression of CCS. Untreated individuals had an average yearly increase in CCS of 52% ± 36%, whereas in those receiving statin therapy the increase was only 5% ± 28% ($p < 0.001$). Of patients who achieved an LDL <120 mg/dL, regression was actually achieved with a change in the CCS of –7% ± 23% ($p = 0.01$). In other work [76], 817 patients were serially tested. The yearly absolute and percent change in the CVS were significantly higher in 45 patients who developed an MI after the second coronary calcium scan than in the 772 patients who did not. More data are needed assessing the clinical usefulness of such findings. In a further report, Budoff et al. evaluated 299 intermediate-high FRS patients and noted a yearly CCS increase ranging from 35% to 40%, with treated individuals exhibiting a significantly slower rate of atherosclerotic progression (~15%/year, $p < 0.0001$) [87]. In a crossover design, randomized controlled trial, Achenbach et al. [86] evaluated the use of cerivastatin at 0.3 mg/day using serial CCS measurements taken 1 year apart in patients with a baseline LDL >130 mg/dL. Concurrent with a marked reduction in LDL-cholesterol averaging 35%, treatment with this statin resulted in a median CCS progression of 8.9% per year versus 25% per year noted during the untreated phase of this trial ($p < 0.0001$). Although there have been several reports noting no treatment benefit [88,89], the majority of the evidence supports a therapeutic dampening in CCS progression with statin therapy. Wong ND et al. [90] recently showed in a large observational study of subjects scanned twice over a 7-year period, that good HDL-cholesterol control, but not LDL-cholesterol control, was associated with less progression of CAC over 7 years. Additional clinical trials such as the St Francis Heart Study and the Beyond Endorsed Lipid Lowering with EBT Scanning (BELLES) trial, soon to be published, should further add to this evidence on the use of CCS for serial monitoring of disease progression [91].

Recent studies have evaluated the prognostic significance of CCS changes. In a series of 817 asymptomatic intermediate-risk patients undergoing serial CCS measurement, those having an acute MI after the second scan had an average rate of progression of 47% ± 50%, a rate of increase that was nearly double that of event-free survivors (26% ± 32%/year, $p < 0.001$) [76]. In a follow-up report from these investigators, a total of 495 asymptomatic individuals underwent serial EBT scanning and were followed for 3 years for the occurrence of first acute MI [92]. LDL control (mean = 119 mg/dL) was similar for those patients having an event as for those non-event individuals. However, CCS progression was 42% ± 23% per year for those patients hospitalized for an acute MI as compared with 17% ± 25% for those event-free survivors ($p < 0.001$). Thus, early data suggests that a change in CCS

over time may be an important determiner of outcome and perhaps of greater prognostic value than the degree of LDL control.

MPS to Evaluate Therapy

In patients with documented ischemic abnormalities, nuclear cardiology techniques have been demonstrated to be effective in monitoring the effects of medical or invasive therapies over time (Figure 17.25) [93,94]. It is possible that reassessment of a patient after institution of therapy could provide early evidence regarding alteration of patient risk, although this application has only achieved class IIb in the current guidelines [22]. There are also some data with MPS and a greater amount with pharmacologic myocardial perfusion PET suggesting that these methods may reveal abnormalities at a stage when atherosclerosis is non-obstructive depending on the activity of the disease [94–96]. In patients undergoing revascularization after MPS, a post-revascularization study can objectively document the effectiveness of the revascularization procedure. While this is often of research interest, it is not considered generally necessary for clinical care. In selected high-risk patients where improvement in risk needs to be documented (e.g. diabetic patients with silent ischemia subjected to PCI) such testing may be warranted. However, if improvement is noted early after PCI, such patients may also merit assessment at 4–6 months after PCI.

Conclusion

This review has indicated that there is an interaction between the assessment of coronary anatomic abnormality – through the CCS or possibly even the non-invasive coronary angiogram – and the assessment of the functional consequences of atherosclerosis using gated MPS. Additional information of clinical importance may come from assessment of biomarkers of inflammation such as high-sensitivity CRP. It is considered likely that with an increased emphasis on prevention and a concomitant aging of the population, many forms of non-invasive cardiac imaging will continue to grow. The CCS and non-invasive CT coronary angiography approaches are likely to grow greatly in the preventive arena for the early detection of coronary atherosclerosis, in guiding the aggressiveness of medical therapy in these patients, and in detection of significant CAD. Gated MPS is likely to have its greatest growth in the increasing numbers of patients with known CAD, as the most effective method to identify which of these patients are most likely to benefit from medical therapy versus coronary revascularization or myocardial reshaping procedures.

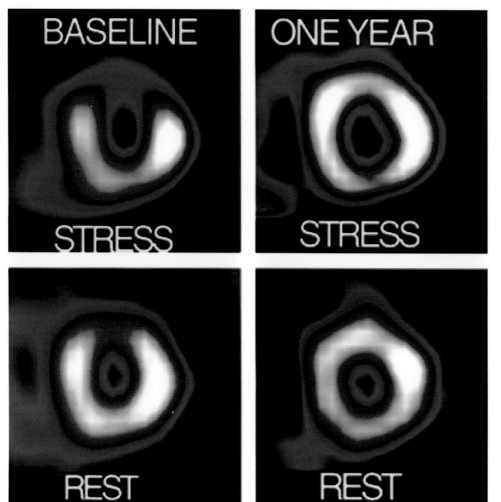

Figure 17.25. Baseline pharmacologic stress (dipyridamole; top) and rest (thallium; bottom) single photon emission computed tomography images before medical therapy alone (left) and dual-isotope (thallium and technetium sestamibi) images with adenosine stress 1 year later (right). Complete resolution of the baseline stress-induced anterior wall defect is obvious. (Adapted with permission from Lippincoff Williams & Wilkins [93]).

References

1. Blankenhorn DH, Stern D. Calcification of the coronary arteries. Am J Roentgenol, Radium Ther Nuc Med 1959;81:772–777.

2. Diamond GA, Staniloff HM, Forrester JS, Pollock BH, Swan HJ. Computer-assisted diagnosis in the noninvasive evaluation of patients with suspected coronary artery disease. J Am Coll Cardiol 1983;1:444–455.

3. Becker CR, Kleffel T, Crispin A, et al. Coronary artery calcium measurement: agreement of multirow detector and electron beam CT. Am J Roentgenol 2001;176:1295–1298.

4. Daniell AL, Friedman JD, Ben-Yosef N, et al. Concordance of coronary calcium estimation between multi-detector and electron beam CT (abstr). Circulation 2002;106:II-479.

5. Agatston AS, Janowitz WR, Hildner FJ, Zusmer NR, Viamonte M Jr, Detrano R. Quantification of coronary artery calcium using ultrafast computed tomography. J Am Coll Cardiol. 1990;15:827–832.

6. Raggi P, Callister TQ, Cooil B, et al. Identification of patients at increased risk of first unheralded acute myocardial infarction by electron-beam computed tomography. Circulation 2000;101:850–855.

7. Cheng YJ, Church TS, Kimball TE, et al. Comparison of coronary artery calcium detected by electron beam tomography in patients with to those without symptomatic coronary heart disease. Am J Cardiol 2003;92:498–503.

8. Hoff JA, Chomka EV, Krainik AJ, Daviglus M, Rich S, Kondos GT. Age and gender distributions of coronary artery calcium detected by electron beam tomography in 35,246 adults. Am J Cardiol 2001; 87:1335–1339.

9. Callister TQ, Cooil B, Raya SP, Lippolis NJ, Russo DJ, Raggi P. Coronary artery disease: improved reproducibility of calcium scoring with an electron-beam CT volumetric method. Radiology 1998;208: 807–814.

10. Callister TQ, Raggi P, Cooil B, Lippolis NJ, Russo DJ. Effect of HMG-CoA reductase inhibitors on coronary artery disease as assessed by electron-beam computed tomography. N Engl J Med 1998;339: 1972–1978.

11. Grundy SM, Bazzarre T, Cleeman J, et al. Beyond secondary prevention: identifying the high-risk patient for primary prevention: medical office assessment: Writing Group I. Circulation 2000;101: E3–E11.

12. O'Leary DH, Polak JF, Kronmal RA, Manolio TA, Burke GL, Wolfson SK Jr. Carotid-artery intima and media thickness as a risk factor for myocardial infarction and stroke in older adults. Cardiovascular Health Study Collaborative Research Group. N Engl J Med 1999;340: 14–22.

13. Hodis HN, Mack WJ, LaBree L, et al. The role of carotid arterial intima-media thickness in predicting clinical coronary events. Ann Intern Med 1998;128:262–269.

14. Taylor AJ, Merz CN, Udelson JE. 34th Bethesda Conference: Executive summary – can atherosclerosis imaging techniques improve the

detection of patients at risk for ischemic heart disease? J Am Coll Cardiol 2003;41:1860–1862.

15. Rumberger JA, Simons DB, Fitzpatrick LA, Sheedy PF, Schwartz RS. Coronary artery calcium area by electron-beam computed tomography and coronary atherosclerotic plaque area. A histopathologic correlative study. Circulation 1995;92:2157–2162.

16. Stary HC. The sequence of cell and matrix changes in atherosclerotic lesions of coronary arteries in the first forty years of life. Eur Heart J 1990;11(Suppl E):3–19.

17. Laudon DA, Behrenbeck TR, Vukov LF, Sheedy PF, Rumberger JA, Breen JF. Coronary artery calcification scanning for chest pain in the emergency department: a prospective blinded study (abstr). J Am Coll Cardiol 2001;37:428A.

18. Glagov S, Weisenberg E, Zarins CK, Stankunavicius R, Kolettis GJ. Compensatory enlargement of human atherosclerotic coronary arteries. N Engl J Med 1987;316:1371–1375.

19. Schmermund A, Denktas AE, Rumberger JA, et al. Independent and incremental value of coronary artery calcium for predicting the extent of angiographic coronary artery disease: comparison with cardiac risk factors and radionuclide perfusion imaging. J Am Coll Cardiol 1999;34:777–786.

20. Gibbons RJ, Abrams J, Chatterjee K, et al. ACC/AHA 2002 guideline update for the management of patients with chronic stable angina – summary article: a report of the American College of Cardiology/American Heart Association Task Force on Practice Guidelines (Committee on the Management of Patients With Chronic Stable Angina). Circulation 2003;107:149–158.

21. Diamond GA, Forrester JS. Analysis of probability as an aid in the clinical diagnosis of coronary-artery disease. N Engl J Med 1979; 300:1350–1358.

22. Klocke FJ, Baird MG, Lorell BH, et al. ACC/AHA/ASNC Guidelines for the Clinical Use of Cardiac Radionuclide Imaging – Executive Summary. A Report of the American College of Cardiology/American Heart Association Task Force on Practice Guidelines (ACC/AHA/ASNC Committee to Revise the 1995 Guidelines for the Clinical Use of Cardiac Radionuclide Imaging). Circulation 2003;108: 1404–1418.

23. Hachamovitch R, Hayes SW, Friedman JD, Cohen I, DS. B. Stress myocardial perfusion SPECT is clinically effective and cost-effective in risk-stratification of patients with a high likelihood of CAD but no known CAD. J Am Coll Cardiol 2004;43:200–208.

24. Poornima IG, Miller TD, Christian TF, Hodge DO, Bailey KR, Gibbons RJ. Utility of myocardial perfusion imaging in patients with low-risk treadmill scores. J Am Coll Cardiol 2004;43:194–199.

25. Hachamovitch R, Hayes SW, Friedman JD, Cohen I, Berman DS. Comparison of the short-term survival benefit associated with revascularization compared with medical therapy in patients with no prior coronary artery disease undergoing stress myocardial perfusion single photon emission computed tomography. Circulation. 2003;107:2900–2907.

26. Gibbons RJ, Chatterjee K, Daley J, et al. ACC/AHA/ACP-ASIM guidelines for the management of patients with chronic stable angina: a report of the American College of Cardiology/American Heart Association Task Force on Practice Guidelines (Committee on Management of Patients With Chronic Stable Angina). J Am Coll Cardiol 1999;33:2092–2197.

27. Gibbons RJ, Balady GJ, Bricker JT, et al. ACC/AHA 2002 guideline update for exercise testing: summary article: a report of the American College of Cardiology/American Heart Association Task Force on Practice Guidelines (Committee to Update the 1997 Exercise Testing Guidelines). Circulation. 2002;106:1883–1892.

28. Budoff MJ, Diamond GA, Raggi P, et al. Continuous probabilistic prediction of angiographically significant coronary artery disease using electron beam tomography. Circulation. 2002;105:1791–1796.

29. Haberl R, Becker A, Leber A, et al. Correlation of coronary calcification and angiographically documented stenoses in patients with suspected coronary artery disease: results of 1,764 patients. J Am Coll Cardiol. 2001;37:451–457.

30. Budoff MJ, Achenbach S, Duerinckx A. Clinical utility of computed tomography and magnetic resonance techniques for noninvasive coronary angiography. J Am Coll Cardiol 2003;42:1867–1878.

31. Ropers D, Baum U, Pohle K, et al. Detection of coronary artery stenoses with thin-slice multi-detector row spiral computed tomography and multiplanar reconstruction. Circulation. 2003;107:664–666.

32. Nieman K, Cademartiri F, Lemos PA, Raaijmakers R, Pattynama PM, de Feyter PJ. Reliable noninvasive coronary angiography with fast submillimeter multislice spiral computed tomography. Circulation 2002;106:2051–2054.

33. Ropers D, Anders K, Lell M, et al. Noninvasive coronary artery imaging using 64-slice spiral computed tomography: initial experiences. (abstr). Circulation 2004;110:III-522.

34. Wong ND, Sciammarella MG, Polk D, et al. The metabolic syndrome, diabetes, and subclinical atherosclerosis assessed by coronary calcium. J Am Coll Cardiol 2003;41:1547–1553.

35. Achenbach S, Giesler T, Ropers D, et al. Detection of coronary artery stenoses by contrast-enhanced, retrospectively electrocardiographically-gated, multislice spiral computed tomography. Circulation 2001;103:2535–2538.

36. Rensing BJ, Bongaerts A, van Geuns RJ, van Ooijen P, Oudkerk M, de Feyter PJ. Intravenous coronary angiography by electron beam computed tomography: a clinical evaluation. Circulation 1998;98: 2509–2512.

37. Berman DS, Hachamovitch R, Kiat H, et al. Incremental value of prognostic testing in patients with known or suspected ischemic heart disease: a basis for optimal utilization of exercise technetium-99m sestamibi myocardial perfusion single-photon emission computed tomography [published erratum appears in J Am Coll Cardiol 1996 Mar 1;27(3):756]. J Am Coll Cardiol. 1995;26:639–647.

38. Berman DS, Hachamovitch R, Shaw LJ, Hayes SW, Germano G. Nuclear cardiology. In: Fuster V AR, O'Rourke RA, Roberts R, King SB, Wellens HJJ (eds) Hurst's The heart, 11th edn. New York: McGraw-Hill, 2004.

39. Hachamovitch R, Shaw L, Berman DS. Methodological considerations in the assessment of noninvasive testing using outcomes research: pitfalls and limitations. Prog Cardiovasc Dis 2000;43:215–230.

40. Yusuf S, Zucker D, Peduzzi P, et al. Effect of coronary artery bypass graft surgery on survival: overview of 10-year results from randomised trials by the Coronary Artery Bypass Graft Surgery Trialists Collaboration. Lancet 1994;344:563–570.

41. Comparison of coronary bypass surgery with angioplasty in patients with multivessel disease. The Bypass Angioplasty Revascularization Investigation (BARI) Investigators. N Engl J Med 1996;335:217–225.

42. Berman DS, Abidov A, Kang X, et al. Prognostic validation of a 17-segment score derived from a 20-segment score for myocardial perfusion SPECT interpretation. J Nucl Cardiol 2004;11:414–423.

43. Hachamovitch R, Berman DS, Shaw LJ, et al. Incremental prognostic value of myocardial perfusion single photon emission computed tomography for the prediction of cardiac death: differential stratification for risk of cardiac death and myocardial infarction. Circulation 1998;97:535–543.

44. Sharir T, Germano G, Kang X, et al. Prediction of myocardial infarction versus cardiac death by gated myocardial perfusion SPECT: risk stratification by the amount of stress-induced ischemia and the post-stress ejection fraction. J Nucl Med 2001;42:831–837.

45. Abidov A, Bax JJ, Hayes SW, et al. Transient ischemic dilation ratio of the left ventricle is a significant predictor of future cardiac events in patients with otherwise normal myocardial perfusion SPECT. J Am Coll Cardiol 2003;42:1818–1825.

46. Berman DS, Kang X, Hayes SW, et al. Adenosine myocardial perfusion single-photon emission computed tomography in women compared with men. Impact of diabetes mellitus on incremental prognostic value and effect on patient management. J Am Coll Cardiol 2003;41:1125–1133.

47. Santos MM, Abidov A, Hayes SW, et al. Prognostic implications of myocardial perfusion SPECT in patients with atrial fibrillation (abstr). J Nucl Med 2002;43:98P.

48. Hachamovitch R, Hayes SW, Friedman JD, et al. Is there a referral bias against revascularization of patients with reduced LV ejection fraction? influence of ejection fraction and inducible ischemia on post-SPECT management of patients without history of CAD. J Am Coll Cardiol 2003;42:1286–1294.

49. Hachamovitch R, Berman DS, Kiat H, Cohen I, Friedman JD, Shaw LJ. Value of stress myocardial perfusion single photon emission computed tomography in patients with normal resting electrocardiograms: an evaluation of incremental prognostic value and cost-effectiveness. Circulation 2002;105:823–829.

50. Vanzetto G, Ormezzano O, Fagret D, Comet M, Denis B, Machecourt J. Long-term additive prognostic value of thallium-201 myocardial perfusion imaging over clinical and exercise stress test in low to intermediate risk patients : study in 1137 patients with 6-year follow-up. Circulation 1999;100:1521–1527.

51. Galassi AR, Azzarelli S, Tomaselli A, et al. Incremental prognostic value of technetium-99m-tetrofosmin exercise myocardial perfusion imaging for predicting outcomes in patients with suspected or known coronary artery disease. Am J Cardiol 2001;88:101–106.

52. Hachamovitch R, Berman DS, Kiat H, et al. Gender-related differences in clinical management after exercise nuclear testing. J Am Coll Cardiol 1995;26:1457–1464.

53. Hachamovitch R, Berman DS, Morise AP, Diamond GA. Statistical, epidemiological and fiscal issues in the evaluation of patients with coronary artery disease. Q J Nucl Med. 1996;40:35–46.

54. Miller WL, Tointon SK, Hodge DO, Nelson SM, Rodeheffer RJ, Gibbons RJ. Long-term outcome and the use of revascularization in patients with heart failure, suspected ischemic heart disease, and large reversible myocardial perfusion defects. Am Heart J 2002;143:904–909.

55. Sharir T, Germano G, Kavanagh PB, et al. Incremental prognostic value of post-stress left ventricular ejection fraction and volume by gated myocardial perfusion single photon emission computed tomography. Circulation 1999;100:1035–1042.

56. White HD, Norris RM, Brown MA, Brandt PW, Whitlock RM, Wild CJ. Left ventricular end-systolic volume as the major determinant of survival after recovery from myocardial infarction. Circulation 1987;76:44–51.

57. Abidov A, Hachamovitch R, Hayes SW, et al. Prognostic impact of hemodynamic response to adenosine in patients older than age 55 years undergoing vasodilator stress myocardial perfusion study. Circulation 2003;107:2894–2899.

58. Azarbal B, Hayes SW, Lewin HC, Hachamovitch R, Cohen I, Berman DS. The incremental prognostic value of percentage of heart rate reserve achieved over myocardial perfusion single-photon emission computed tomography in the prediction of cardiac death and all-cause mortality: superiority over 85% of maximal age-predicted heart rate. J Am Coll Cardiol 2004;44:423–430.

59. Hachamovitch R, Hayes SW, Cohen I, Germano G, Berman DS. Inducible ischemia is superior to EF for identification of short-term survival benefit with revascularization vs. medical therapy (abstr). Circulation 2002;106:II-523.

60. Shaw LJ, Raggi P, Schisterman E, Berman DS, Callister TQ. Prognostic value of cardiac risk factors and coronary artery calcium screening for all-cause mortality. Radiology 2003;228:826–833.

61. Kondos GT, Hoff JA, Sevrukov A, et al. Electron-beam tomography coronary artery calcium and cardiac events: a 37-month follow-up of 5635 initially asymptomatic low- to intermediate-risk adults. Circulation 2003;107:2571–2576.

62. O'Malley PG, Taylor AJ, Jackson JL, Doherty TM, Detrano RC. Prognostic value of coronary electron-beam computed tomography for coronary heart disease events in asymptomatic populations. Am J Cardiol 2000;85:945–948.

63. Pletcher MJ, Tice JA, Pignone M, Browner WS. Using the coronary artery calcium score to predict coronary heart disease events: a systematic review and meta-analysis. Arch Intern Med 2004;164:1285–1292.

64. Park R, Detrano R, Xiang M, et al. Combined use of computed tomography coronary calcium scores and C-reactive protein levels in predicting cardiovascular events in nondiabetic individuals. Circulation 2002;106:2073–2077.

65. Greenland P, LaBree L, Azen SP, Doherty TM, Detrano RC. Coronary artery calcium score combined with Framingham score for risk prediction in asymptomatic individuals. JAMA 2004;291:210–215.

66. Wilson PW, Smith SC Jr, Blumenthal RS, Burke GL, Wong ND. 34th Bethesda Conference: Task force #4 – How do we select patients for atherosclerosis imaging? J Am Coll Cardiol 2003;41:1898–1906.

67. Berman DS, Wong ND. Implications of estimating coronary heart disease risk in the United States population. J Am Coll Cardiol 2004;43:1797–1798.

68. Schmermund A, Baumgart D, Gorge G, et al. Coronary artery calcium in acute coronary syndromes: a comparative study of electron-beam computed tomography, coronary angiography, and intracoronary ultrasound in survivors of acute myocardial infarction and unstable angina. Circulation 1997;96:1461–1469.

69. Schmermund A, Schwartz RS, Adamzik M, et al. Coronary atherosclerosis in unheralded sudden coronary death under age 50: histopathologic comparison with "healthy" subjects dying out of hospital. Atherosclerosis 2001;155:499–508.

70. Pohle K, Ropers D, Maffert R, et al. Coronary calcifications in young patients with first, unheralded myocardial infarction: a risk factor matched analysis by electron beam tomography. Heart 2003;89:625–628.

71. Rumberger JA, Brundage BH, Rader DJ, Kondos G. Electron beam computed tomographic coronary calcium scanning: a review and guidelines for use in asymptomatic persons. Mayo Clin Proc 1999;74:243–252.

72. He ZX, Hedrick TD, Pratt CM, et al. Severity of coronary artery calcification by electron beam computed tomography predicts silent myocardial ischemia. Circulation 2000;101:244–251.

73. Moser KW, O'Keefe JH, Bateman TM, McGhie IA. Coronary calcium screening in asymptomatic patients as a guide to risk factor modification and stress myocardial perfusion imaging. J Nucl Cardiol 2003;10:590–598.

74. Berman DS, Wong ND, Gransar H, et al. Relationship between stress-induced myocardial ischemia and atherosclerosis measured by coronary calcium tomography. J Am Coll Cardiol 2004;44:923–930.

75. Budoff MJ, Raggi P. Coronary artery disease progression assessed by electron-beam computed tomography. Am J Cardiol 2001;88:46E–50E.

76. Raggi P, Cooil B, Shaw LJ, et al. Progression of coronary calcium on serial electron beam tomographic scanning is greater in patients with future myocardial infarction. Am J Cardiol 2003;92:827–829.

77. Berman DS, Gransar H, Rozanski A, et al. Does coronary calcium add incremental value for predicting cardiac events when myocardial perfusion SPECT is normal? (abstr). Circulation. 2004;110:111–561.

78. Grundy SM, Cleeman JI, Merz CN, et al. Implications of recent clinical trials for the National Cholesterol Education Program Adult Treatment Panel III guidelines. Circulation 2004;110:227–239.

79. Anand DV, Lim E, Raval U, Lipkin D, Lahiri A. Prevalence of silent myocardial ischemia in asymptomatic individuals with subclinical atherosclerosis detected by electron beam tomography. J Nucl Cardiol 2004;11:450–457.

80. Wong ND, Gransar H, Hayes S, et al. Higher coronary calcium scores identify greater likelihood of myocardial ischemia in patients with metabolic syndrome (abstr). Circulation. 2004;110:111–168.

81. Gibbons RJ, Hodge DO, Berman DS, et al. Long-term outcome of patients with intermediate-risk exercise electrocardiograms who do not have myocardial perfusion defects on radionuclide imaging. Circulation 1999;100:2140–2145.

82. Kaminek M, Myslivecek M, Skvarilova M, et al. Increased prognostic value of combined myocardial perfusion SPECT imaging and the

quantification of lung Tl-201 uptake. Clin Nucl Med 2002;27:255–260.

83. Kang X, Berman DS, Lewin HC, et al. Incremental prognostic value of myocardial perfusion single photon emission computed tomography in patients with diabetes mellitus. Am Heart J 1999;138:1025–1032.

84. Abidov A, Hachamovitch R, Rozanski A, et al. Prognostic implications of atrial fibrillation in patients undergoing myocardial perfusion single-photon emission computed tomography. J Am Coll Cardiol 2004;44:1062–1070.

85. Berman DS, Hayes S, Friedman J, et al. Normal myocardial perfusion SPECT does not imply the absence of significant atherosclerosis (abstr). Circulation 2003;108:IV-562.

86. Achenbach S, Ropers D, Pohle K, et al. Influence of lipid-lowering therapy on the progression of coronary artery calcification: a prospective evaluation. Circulation 2002;106:1077–1082.

87. Budoff MJ, Lane KL, Bakhsheshi H, et al. Rates of progression of coronary calcium by electron beam tomography. Am J Cardiol 2000;86:8–11.

88. Hecht HS, Harman SM. Comparison of the effects of atorvastatin versus simvastatin on subclinical atherosclerosis in primary prevention as determined by electronbeam tomography. Am J Cardiol 2003;91:42–45.

89. Hecht HS, Harman SM. Evaluation by electron beam tomography of changes in calcified coronary plaque in treated and untreated asymptomatic patients and relation to serum lipid levels. Am J Cardiol 2003;91:1131–1134.

90. Wong ND, Kawakubo M, LaBree L, Azen SP, Xiang M, Detrano R. Relation of coronary calcium progression and control of lipids according to National Cholesterol Education Program guidelines. Am J Cardiol 2004;94:431–436.

91. Raggi P, Callister TQ, Davidson M, et al. Aggressive versus moderate lipid-lowering therapy in postmenopausal women with hypercholesterolemia: Rationale and design of the Beyond Endorsed Lipid Lowering with EBT Scanning (BELLES) trial. Am Heart J 2001;141:722–726.

92. Raggi P, Callister TQ, Shaw LJ. Progression of coronary artery calcium and risk of first myocardial infarction in patients receiving cholesterol-lowering therapy. Arterioscler Thromb Vasc Biol 2004;24:1272–1277.

93. O'Rourke RA, Chaudhuri T, Shaw L, Berman DS. Resolution of stress-induced myocardial ischemia during aggressive medical therapy as demonstrated by single photon emission computed tomography imaging. Circulation 2001;103:2315.

94. Schwartz RG, Pearson TA, Kalaria VG, et al. Prospective serial evaluation of myocardial perfusion and lipids during the first six months of pravastatin therapy: coronary artery disease regression single photon emission computed tomography monitoring trial. J Am Coll Cardiol 2003;42:600–610.

95. Hernandez-Pampaloni M, Keng FY, Kudo T, Sayre JS, Schelbert HR. Abnormal longitudinal, base-to-apex myocardial perfusion gradient by quantitative blood flow measurements in patients with coronary risk factors. Circulation 2001;104:527–532.

96. Sdringola S, Nakagawa K, Nakagawa Y, et al. Combined intense lifestyle and pharmacologic lipid treatment further reduce coronary events and myocardial perfusion abnormalities compared with usual-care cholesterol-lowering drugs in coronary artery disease. J Am Coll Cardiol 2003;41:263–272.

18

CT Imaging: Cardiac Electrophysiology Applications

Jerold S. Shinbane and Matthew J. Budoff

Diagnosis and treatment of electrophysiologically related cardiovascular disease requires detailed understanding and characterization of an individual patient's cardiovascular substrate. Cardiac computed tomographic (CT) angiography allows for comprehensive assessment of cardiovascular structure and function through non-invasive simultaneous three-dimensional (3-D) visualization of cardiac chambers, coronary vessels, and thoracic vasculature. This technique enables assessment of structures particularly germane to electrophysiology including: the coronary veins, pulmonary veins, and left atrium (Figure 18.1). Studies can provide identification of ventricular and vascular substrates associated with sudden death and can provide detailed definition of atrial anatomy. In addition to providing substrate identification and characterization, CT angiography can provide relevant roadmaps for catheter ablation, implantable pacemaker and defibrillator placement, intra-procedure correlation with electrophysiologic findings, and follow-up for complications.

In regard to imaging patients with electrophysiologically relevant issues, heart rate and ectopy are important factors. Multidetector CT requires slower ventricular rates (<60–70 beats/minute) during imaging, while electron beam CT can image patients with a greater spectrum of ventricular rates. Ectopy can be problematic with both modalities. In contradistinction to cardiovascular magnetic resonance imaging (CMR), patients with pacemakers and implantable cardiac defibrillators can be studied.

Identification and Characterization of Anatomic Substrates Associated with Sudden Cardiac Death

Sudden cardiac death is associated with a variety of cardiovascular structural and/or electrophysiologic abnormalities, often with the first manifestation of disease being sudden death due to ventricular arrhythmias or non-arrhythmic hemodynamic compromise. Etiologies associated with grossly identifiable anatomic substrates are multiple and include: acute coronary syndromes [1–3], anomalous coronary arteries [4], dilated and ischemic cardiomyopathy [5], hypertrophic cardiomyopathy [6,7], right ventricular dysplasia [8,9], critical aortic stenosis [10], aortic aneurysms [11,12], and complex congenital heart disease [13]. Additional substrates not always associated with gross anatomic abnormalities are primarily diagnosed through electrocardiographic or electrophysiologic evaluation including Wolff–Parkinson–White syndrome [14], long QT syndromes [15], Brugada syndrome [16–18], and significant bradycardia or high-grade atrioventricular block. CT angiographic evaluation can identify anatomic substrates associated with sudden cardiac death and potentially facilitate approaches to therapeutic interventions associated with these diagnoses.

Coronary Artery Disease and Anomalies

Due to the ability to assess the proximal coronary arteries and their relation to the aorta and other thoracic vasculature, anomalous coronary arteries can be diagnosed with CT (Figure 18.2) [19,20]. Anomalous origin of the coronary arteries is a rare cause of sudden cardiac death, with the initial presentation often occurring as sudden death during exertion in a young patient [21,22]. Some anatomies, although anomalous, are not associated with an increased risk of sudden cardiac death. Specific anatomies associated with sudden death risk include takeoff of the left coronary artery from the pulmonary trunk, left coronary artery from the right aortic sinus, and right coronary artery from the left aortic sinus [23].

Significant proximal vessel and left main disease can lead to significant ischemia, ventricular arrhythmias, and hemodynamic collapse with exertion. CT angiography is

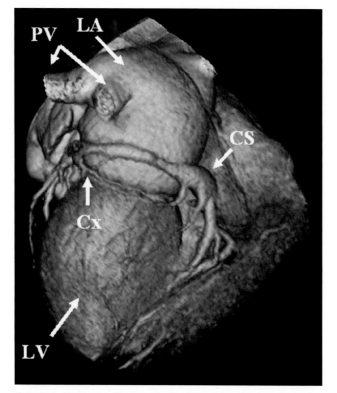

Figure 18.1. CT angiogram with 3-D posterior view demonstrating coronary vasculature including simultaneous imaging of coronary arteries, coronary veins, and their relationships to the left atrium (LA) and left ventricle (LV). CS = coronary sinus, Cx = circumflex, PV = pulmonary vein.

useful for the diagnosis of proximal to mid vessel coronary artery disease [24–34]. Additionally, this technique can assess for patency and stenoses of coronary artery bypass grafts. In regard to electrophysiologic procedures involving induction of ventricular arrhythmias, where left main or

left main equivalent disease would be contraindicated, information on proximal coronary artery disease and graft patency may have great relevance.

Sudden death due to plaque rupture and thrombosis often occurs in coronary arterial segments without obstructive disease [1,2]. The focus of cardiac CT has been assessment of plaque burden through calcium scoring. With CT angiography, calcium scoring provides a measure of overall plaque burden, with high Agatston calcium scores (>500) associated with high event rates for myocardial infarction and cardiovascular death, while scores of 0 are associated with extremely low rates of myocardial infarction and cardiovascular death [35]. CT angiography can assess soft plaque, with correlation of findings to intravascular ultrasound, but requires further investigation [36].

Dilated Ischemic and Non-ischemic Cardiomyopathy

Sudden death prevention and treatment in recent years has focused on dilated ischemic and non-ischemic cardiomyopathy with multicenter prospective studies demonstrating benefit to implantable cardiac defibrillator (ICD) therapy when placed solely on anatomic/functional substrate of ischemic cardiomyopathy. The MADIT II study demonstrated a significant decrease in overall mortality with prophylactic ICD placement with criteria for implantation being a substrate of ischemic cardiomyopathy with an ejection fraction of less than or equal to 30% [5]. Recently, data from the Sudden Cardiac Death in Heart Failure Trial have broadened the indications for prophylactic ICD therapy as a primary prevention modality to non-ischemic dilated cardiomyopathy [37]. The results of these studies place particular emphasis on the need for precise quantitative functional assessment of cardiomyopathic substrates, as algorithms for device placement based on these studies allow for implant decisions based on anatomic substrate and ventricular function.

CT angiography can provide detailed assessment of cardiomyopathic cardiac substrates with reproducible quantitative measurement of slice-by-slice volumetric biventricular volumes and ejection fraction, wall thickness, and regional wall motion (Figure 18.3) [38–40]. CT technology helps to differentiate ischemic from non-ischemic dilated cardiomyopathy based on coronary calcium scores [41]. CT angiography can directly visualize coronary arteries, which may potentially facilitate differentiation between ischemic and non-ischemic cardiomyopathy.

In addition to characterization of cardiomyopathy, CT angiography may potentially be useful in facilitation of resynchronization therapy for heart failure in ischemic and non-ischemic dilated cardiomyopathy. In patients with dilated ischemic and non-ischemic cardiomyopathy,

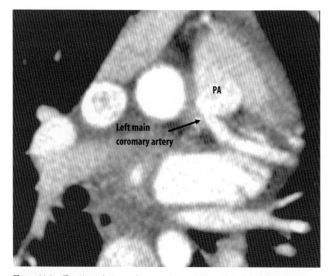

Figure 18.2. CT angiography image demonstrating anomalous origin of the left coronary artery off of the pulmonary artery (arrow), which is a substrate associated with sudden cardiac death. PA = pulmonary artery.

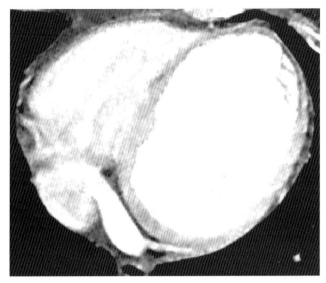

Figure 18.3. Axial slice demonstrating biventricular enlargement in a patient with ischemic cardiomyopathy secondary to previous anterior myocardial infarct. The left ventricular end-diastolic volume was quantified at 179 mL, left ventricular mass at 76 grams, and left ventricular ejection fraction at 35% with anteroapical severe hypokinesis. Thinning of the left ventricular apex is seen.

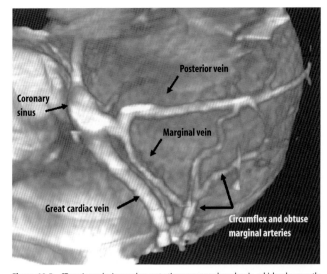

Figure 18.5. CT angiography image demonstrating a coronary branch vein, which subsequently bifurcates into a posterior and marginal branch. The circumflex and obtuse marginal branch arteries are also visualized.

ventricular conduction abnormalities, and moderate to severe heart failure, resynchronization therapy has been shown to decrease heart failure symptoms, improve quality of life, improve ventricular function, and decrease hospitalizations [42–44].

In biventricular pacing, left ventricular pacing is usually achieved via an endocardial approach by placing a chronic pacing lead in a coronary sinus branch vessel (Figure 18.4). Placement of the coronary venous lead can be challenging, as the coronary sinus needs to be cannulated and lead posi-tion is limited to the individual location and variation of the existing coronary venous anatomy. CT angiography, due to its ability to visualize coronary veins, can provide detailed assessment of the coronary venous anatomy, with coronary sinus dimensions, branch vessel locations, branch vessel diameters, and branch vessel angulations off of the coronary sinus/great cardiac vein (Figure 18.5) [45–48]. Additionally, 3-D reconstructions can identify specific myocardial segments associated with a particular coronary venous site (Figure 18.6).

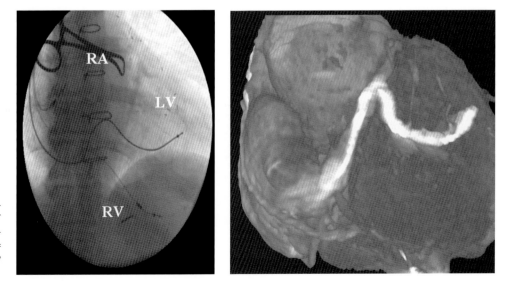

Figure 18.4. Fluoroscopy image demonstrating biventricular pacing leads and CT image demonstrating the position of the coronary sinus lead. RA = right atrial lead, RV = right ventricular lead, and LV = coronary venous lead.

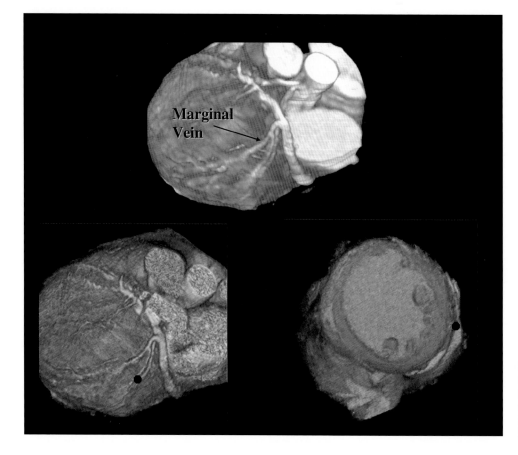

Figure 18.6. CT coronary angiogram demonstrating the coronary venous system (top panel). Three-dimensional localization of the myocardial segment associated with a particular segment of the marginal vein is displayed (black circle, lower panels).

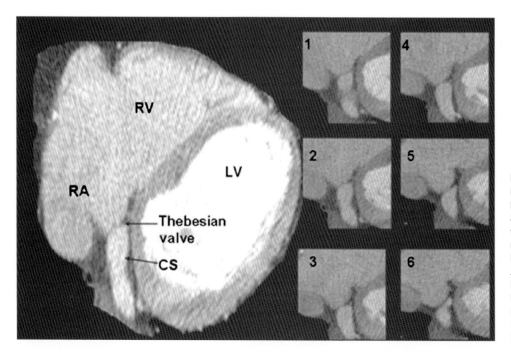

Figure 18.7. Serial CT angiography axial images at the coronary sinus os level, numbered from superior to inferior, demonstrating a prominent Thebesian valve (coronary sinus os valve) on all slices. CS = coronary sinus, RA = right atrium, RV = right ventricle, and LV = left ventricle. (Reprinted from: Shinbane JS, Girsky MJ, Mao S, Budoff MJ. Thebesian valve imaging with electron beam CT angiography: implications for resynchronization therapy. Pacing Clin Electrophysiol 2004;27: 1566–1567, with permission from Blackwell Publishing, USA.)

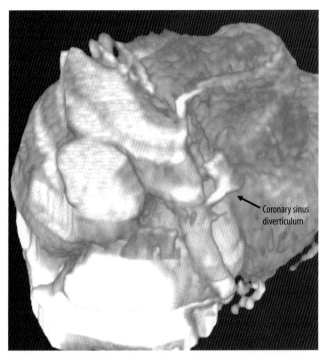

Figure 18.8. CT angiogram demonstrating a coronary sinus diverticulum (arrow).

CT angiography can also visualize details of coronary veins, such as Thebesian valves (prominent coronary vein os valves), which can obstruct access to the coronary sinus (Figure 18.7) [49]. Other abnormalities such as coronary sinus diverticula (Figure 18.8), and anomalous connection such as left superior vena cava to coronary sinus connections (Figure 18.9) can be visualized. The ability to provide venous roadmaps, as well as to assess the spatial relationships between the coronary veins and adjacent cardiac structures, requires further investigation in order to assess its utility in facilitation of coronary venous interventions.

Hypertrophic Cardiomyopathy

Hypertrophic cardiomyopathy can lead to sudden cardiac death due to a variety of mechanisms including atrial and ventricular arrhythmias, bradyarrhythmias, and ischemia [6,50,51]. Echocardiography is the main diagnostic modality for the diagnosis of hypertrophic cardiomyopathy and in addition to anatomy can assess resting and exercise gradients and associated valve function [52,53]. The diagnosis can be also be made by CT angiography with similar left ventricular measures to magnetic resonance imaging, although without hemodynamic gradient data (Figure 18.10) [54].

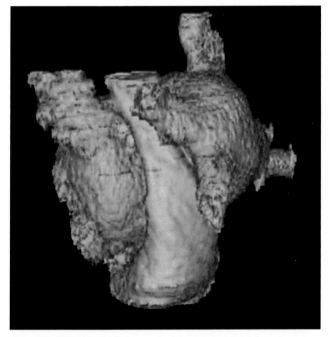

Figure 18.9. Three-dimensional volume-rendered view demonstrating a left superior vena cava with connection to an aneurysmal coronary sinus. A right-sided superior vena cava was not present.

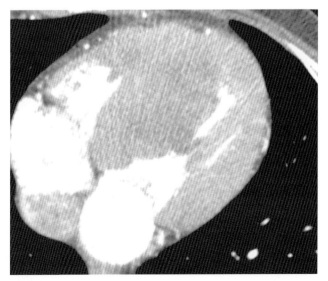

Figure 18.10. CT angiogram demonstrating hypertrophic cardiomyopathy with a profoundly hypertrophied septum.

Right Ventricular Pathology

The diagnosis of right ventricular dysplasia can be challenging, and often the initial presentation is sudden death [8,55]. Imaging is only one component of the diagnosis, which also involves: clinical history of palpitations, syncope or right heart failure symptoms, family history of right ventricular dysplasia or sudden cardiac death from suspected right ventricular dysplasia, ECG criteria, and electrophysiologic testing results [56]. Even with these techniques, the diagnosis can be elusive. Additionally, some right ventricular arrhythmias, such as right ventricular outflow tract tachycardia, are not associated with significant right ventricular pathology and do not confer risk of sudden death. Since similar right ventricular arrhythmias can be associated with either right ventricular dysplasia or right ventricular outflow tract tachycardia, it extremely important to differentiate normal from pathologic right ventricular structure and function.

Cardiovascular magnetic resonance (CMR) is the diagnostic imaging modality of choice for the diagnosis of arrhythmogenic right ventricular dysplasia, due to the ability to differentiate fat and myocardium, as well as the ability to define right ventricular morphology and size, regional wall motion, and ejection fraction. Initial efforts to diagnose right ventricular dysplasia focused on characterization of CMR intramyocardial fat patterns, but there is great variation in these patterns in normal subjects [57,58]. Additionally, CMR findings of myocarditis can mimic arrhythmogenic right ventricular dysplasia [59]. Therefore, diagnosis has focused on right ventricular wall motion abnormalities, right ventricular ejection fraction, and ventricular wall morphologic changes.

CT angiography has been assessed for the ability to diagnose anatomic features associated with right ventricular dysplasia, such as epicardial and myocardial fat, low-attenuation trabeculations, and right ventricular free wall scalloping, but has not been evaluated as a screening tool (Figure 18.11) [60–62]. When right ventricular dysplasia is clinically considered as a mechanism of ventricular arrhythmias, comprehensive evaluation with CMR needs to be considered prior to ICD placement, as this modality cannot be used subsequent to device placement. Cardiac CT, although not currently the diagnostic procedure of choice, can be performed when the diagnosis is considered in patients with devices already implanted.

Congenital Heart Disease

A variety of arrhythmic processes are associated with specific congenital anatomies and sudden cardiac death is often associated with worsening of ventricular function late after surgical repair [13]. CT imaging can assess 3-D anatomy and provide comprehensive characterization of native and operated congenital heart disease including ventricular function, myocardial scar, anomalous vascular connections, and shunts [63–65]. Ventricular arrhythmias can be associated with worsening hemodynamic and ventricular function and can also be associated with reentrant circuits involving surgical scars [13]. A spectrum of atrial arrhythmias including atrial tachycardia, a variety of atrial flutter types including incisional reentry in previously operated patients, and atrial fibrillation can occur [66–68]. CT can provide 3-D roadmaps of complex congenital heart disease for pre-procedure planning of surgical or endovascular interventions [63,69].

Aorta and Aortic Valve Pathology

Aortic aneurysm is associated with risk for sudden death due to aortic dissection or rupture associated with connective tissue disorders or acquired cardiovascular disease [70]. CT angiography can diagnose aortic aneurysm, dissection, and wall abnormalities such as penetrating ulcers, calcification or thrombus with ability to assess all aortic segments (Figure 18.12) [71]. From the procedural standpoint, these studies can provide comprehensive assessment for aortic pathology which may affect decisions as to whether a retrograde aortic approach is contraindicated for ablations of left ventricular tachycardias or left-sided accessory pathways.

Severe to critical aortic stenosis can lead to sudden cardiac death and is typically diagnosed by echocardiography. CT can only indirectly assess aortic valve stenosis as aortic valve calcium is a marker for significant aortic valve stenosis. Patients with elevated aortic valve calcium

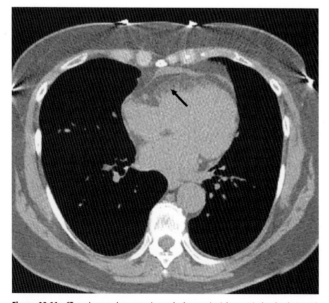

Figure 18.11. CT angiogram demonstrating arrhythmogenic right ventricular dysplasia with fatty replacement of the right ventricular myocardium (arrow).

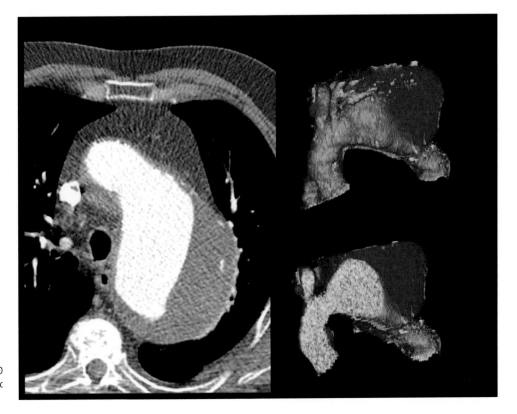

Figure 18.12. Axial 2-D image and 3-D reconstructions demonstrating a large aortic aneurysm with intramural thrombus.

scores should be further assessed for aortic valve disease [72].

Assessment of Atrial Anatomy Associated with Supraventricular Arrhythmias

Cardiac CT angiography can assess atrial anatomy, pulmonary venous anatomy, and coronary venous anatomy, all with great relevance to left atrial arrhythmias including atrial fibrillation, atypical atrial flutter circuits, and focal atrial tachycardias. Catheter-based techniques for ablation of atrial fibrillation have focused on ablation of the pulmonary veins with either segmental ablation or complete circumferential electrical isolation of the pulmonary veins [73–75]. CT imaging can characterize these features through 3-D volume-rendered and endocardial images, including number of veins, location in the atrium, vein size, vein morphology, and vein os complexity (Figures 18.13–18.15) [76]. Preoperative CT angiography can provide a roadmap of atrial and pulmonary vein structure to guide electrophysiologic study and ablation of atrial fibrillation [76,77]. Additionally, integration of 3-D images obtained pre-procedure with real-time catheter position, and electrophysiologic recordings may potentially facilitate ablation procedures [78].

Assessment for atrial thrombi is important to the evaluation, management, and pre-procedure assessment of patients with atrial fibrillation and atrial flutter. CT angiography can visualize the left atrial appendage in detail and has been reported to be able to visualize atrial thrombi [79,80]. Contrast electron beam CT has also been preliminarily compared to transesophageal echocardiography in a series of 96 patients, with detection of all 9 thrombi seen on transesophageal echocardiography studies, although 4 additional false-positive studies were obtained with CT [79]. Further study will be required to assess the utility of CT to rule out atrial thrombus. The ability to assess for atrial thrombus would greatly enhance the comprehensive nature of pre-procedure CT angiography prior to atrial fibrillation ablation.

Pulmonary vein stenosis is a potential complication of atrial fibrillation ablation. The incidence of stenosis has not been completely defined and is dependent on technique and degree of surveillance. CT and MRI have been used to diagnose pulmonary vein stenosis [81–85]. The time course of pulmonary vein stenosis has not been fully defined and long-term studies need to be performed. In addition to significant stenoses, mild to moderate degrees of stenosis can be documented. The long-term possible progression of these stenoses requires further study [86]. Preoperative studies, in addition to providing a roadmap for intervention, can provide templates for follow-up studies assessing for pulmonary vein stenosis.

The 3-D relationship between the left atrium and esophagus may have relevance to atrial fibrillation ablation

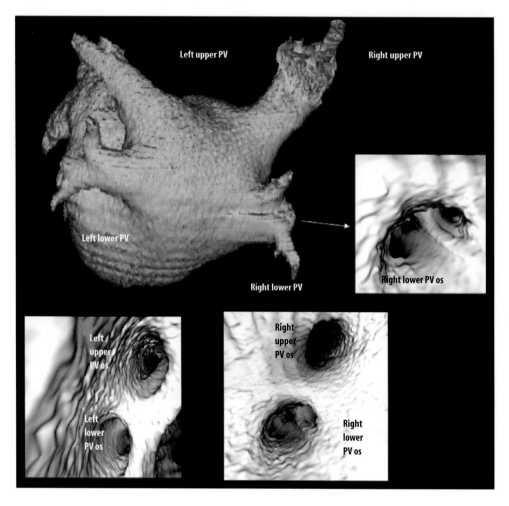

Figure 18.13. Three-D CT angiography volume-rendered view of the posterior left atrium demonstrating the pulmonary veins. Endocardial views demonstrate venous anatomy, relationships between veins, and pulmonary vein os details. PV = pulmonary vein.

approaches, as left atrial-esophageal fistula has been reported as a fatal complication of left atrial ablation for atrial fibrillation [87]. There is variability in the course of the esophagus and degree of contact between the posterior left atrium/pulmonary veins and the esophagus, which can be visualized prior to ablation [88].

As mentioned previously, CT angiography is effective for visualization of the coronary sinus and its tributaries [89]. Coronary sinus anatomy and its relationship to other cardiac structures is important in a variety of supraventricular electrophysiologic procedures, including mapping and ablation of accessory pathways and focal left atrial arrhythmias [90–92]. Coronary sinus anatomy is important in ablation of posteroseptal accessory pathways, as these pathways are often associated with coronary sinus

diverticula with successful ablation often performed in the coronary sinus diverticulum. CT angiography can visualize coronary sinus diverticula (Figure 18.8). Additionally, understanding the relationship of coronary veins, coronary arteries, and myocardium may be important if ablation in a coronary vein is considered in order to avoid coronary artery complications, especially if a coronary artery courses between the coronary vein and epicardium. CT angiography can define these relationships including the relationship between the circumflex coronary artery and coronary sinus/great cardiac vein (Figures 18.16–18.18) [47,48].

Congenital anomalies affecting the atria such as atrial septal defect, [93,94] and Ebstein anomaly [95], which can be associated with accessory pathways, can be

Figure 18.14. **a** CT angiography 3-D volume-rendered image of the left atrium demonstrating the spatial relationships between the pulmonary veins, atrial appendage, and atrium on a posterior view. There is a small additional pulmonary vein near the os of the right lower pulmonary vein. PV = pulmonary vein. **b** Endocardial image demonstrating left atrial endocardial anatomy with spatial relationship between the right upper and right lower pulmonary vein. The small additional os near the right lower pulmonary vein is also visualized. **c** Endocardial image demonstrating left atrial endocardial anatomy with spatial relationship between the left upper and left lower pulmonary vein, as well as the relationship between the left upper pulmonary vein and the left atrial

appendage. A closer view better defines the muscular ridge between the left upper and left lower pulmonary veins. **d** Axial 2-D images of the left upper, left lower, right upper, and right lower pulmonary veins, and an additional vein near the right lower pulmonary vein. These images are helpful for quantitation of pulmonary vein size, and understanding of these images is enhanced through reference to the 3-D images. (**a** and **b** reprinted from: Shinbane JS, Girsky MJ, Chau A, Mao S, Budoff MJ. Three-dimensional computed tomography imaging of left atrial anatomy for atrial fibrillation ablation. Clin Cardiol 2005;28:100, with permission from Clinical Cardiology Publishing Company, Inc., Mahwah, NJ, USA.)

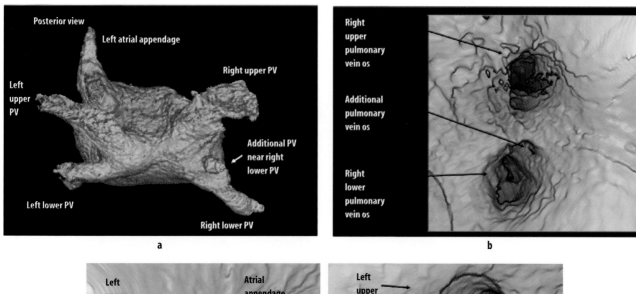

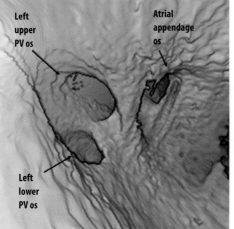

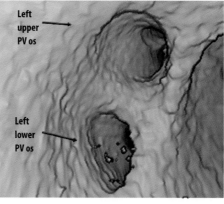

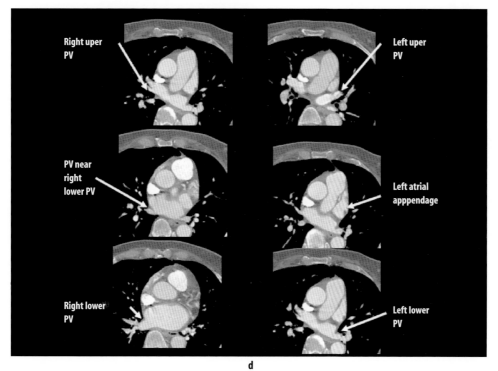

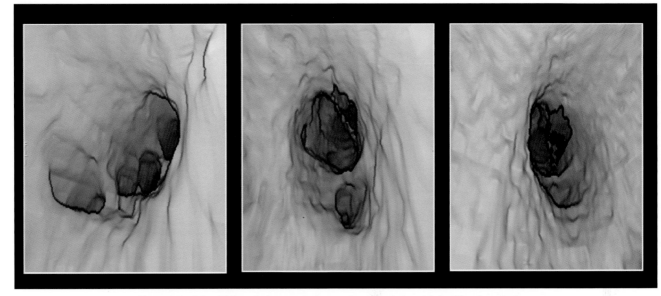

Figure 18.15. Endocardial views of pulmonary veins demonstrating variation in the complexity of the pulmonary vein os.

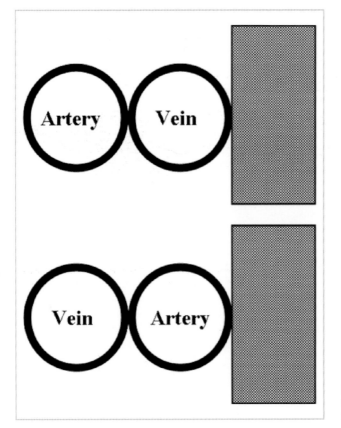

Figure 18.16. Schematic diagram of 3-D spatial arrangements between the coronary arteries and coronary veins in overlapping segments in reference to the epicardium. The medial vessel is the vessel closer to epicardium in overlapping segments.

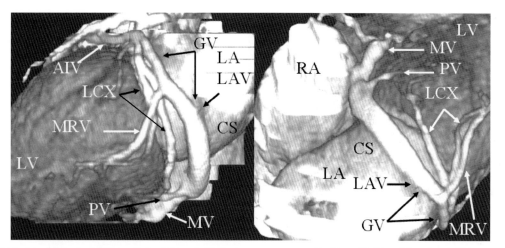

Figure 18.17. The left-lateral view (left panel) and diaphragmatic view (right panel) of the heart. The left circumflex coronary artery and coronary veins are clearly displayed. The great cardiac vein is seen overlying the left circumflex coronary artery for a short (<30 mm) segment. The marginal vein is dominant and the posterior vein is small in size. AIV = anterior interventricular vein, CS = coronary sinus, GV = great cardiac vein, LA = left atrium, LAV = left atrial vein, LCX = left circumflex coronary artery, LV = left ventricle, MV = middle cardiac vein, MRV = marginal vein, PV = posterior vein. (Reprinted from: Mao S, Shinbane JS, Girsky MJ, Child J, Carson S, Flores F, Oudiz RJ, Budoff MJ. Three-dimensional coronary venous imaging with computed tomographic angiography. Am Heart J 2005;150:315–322, with permission of Elsevier, Philadelphia, PA, USA.)

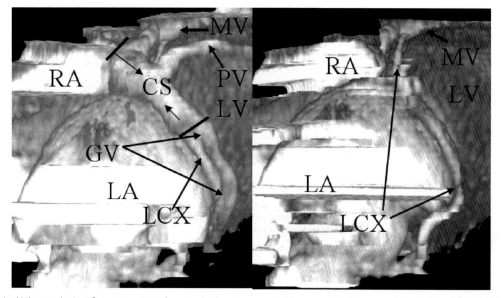

Figure 18.18. The relationship between the circumflex coronary artery and coronary sinus/great cardiac vein is displayed. The great cardiac vein is lateral and covering the circumflex for almost the entire circumflex course. After editing the 3-D images to remove the coronary sinus/great cardiac vein, the circumflex is displayed. The coronary sinus boundary is clear and the coronary sinus distance is marked between arrows (→ ←). The posterior vein is dominant and marginal vein is not present. CS = coronary sinus, GV = great cardiac vein, MV = middle vein, MRV = marginal vein, PV = posterior vein, LA = left atrium, LAV = left atrial vein, LCx = left circumflex coronary artery, LV = left ventricle, and RA = right atrium. (Reprinted from: Mao S, Shinbane JS, Girsky MJ, Child J, Carson S, Flores F, Oudiz RJ, Budoff MJ. Three-dimensional coronary venous imaging with computed tomographic angiography. Am Heart J 2005; In press, with permission of Elsevier, Philadelphia, PA, USA.)

characterized by CT angiography. Anomalous venous return to the atria such as persistent left superior vena cava often with connection to the coronary sinus can be imaged and has great relevance to the approach to placement of pacemakers and ICDs (Figure 18.9) [96].

Summary

The ability of CT angiography to comprehensively assess cardiovascular structure and function makes it a robust technology for the assessment, treatment, and follow-up of patients with electrophysiologically related disease processes. Cardiovascular CT angiographic imaging holds the promise to continue to advance the field of cardiac electrophysiology through understanding of electrophysiologically relevant pathologic substrates and facilitation of novel interventional approaches. This effort will be enhanced by a multidisciplinary approach to diagnosis and therapeutic intervention in patients with electrophysiologically relevant issues.

References

1. Naghavi M, Libby P, Falk E, et al. From vulnerable plaque to vulnerable patient: a call for new definitions and risk assessment strategies: Part I. Circulation 2003;108:1664–1672.

2. Naghavi M, Libby P, Falk E, et al. From vulnerable plaque to vulnerable patient: a call for new definitions and risk assessment strategies: Part II. Circulation 2003;108:1772–1778.

3. Burke AP, Farb A, Malcom GT, Liang Y, Smialek JE, Virmani R. Plaque rupture and sudden death related to exertion in men with coronary artery disease. JAMA 1999;281:921–926.

4. Basso C, Corrado D, Thiene G. Congenital coronary artery anomalies as an important cause of sudden death in the young. Cardiol Rev 2001;9:312–317.

5. Moss AJ, Zareba W, Hall WJ, et al. Prophylactic implantation of a defibrillator in patients with myocardial infarction and reduced ejection fraction. N Engl J Med 2002;346:877–883.

6. Elliott PM, Poloniecki J, Dickie S, et al. Sudden death in hypertrophic cardiomyopathy: identification of high risk patients. J Am Coll Cardiol 2000;36:2212–2218.

7. Maron BJ. Hypertrophic cardiomyopathy: a systematic review. JAMA 2002;287:1308–1320.

8. Corrado D, Thiene G, Nava A, Rossi L, Pennelli N. Sudden death in young competitive athletes: clinicopathologic correlations in 22 cases. Am J Med 1990;89:588–596.

9. Corrado D, Basso C, Thiene G, et al. Spectrum of clinicopathologic manifestations of arrhythmogenic right ventricular cardiomyopathy/dysplasia: a multicenter study. J Am Coll Cardiol 1997;30:1512–1520.

10. Wolfe RR, Driscoll DJ, Gersony WM, et al. Arrhythmias in patients with valvar aortic stenosis, valvar pulmonary stenosis, and ventricular septal defect. Results of 24-hour ECG monitoring. Circulation 1993;87:I89–101.

11. Fikar CR, Koch S. Etiologic factors of acute aortic dissection in children and young adults. Clin Pediatr (Phila) 2000;39:71–80.

12. Glorioso J Jr, Reeves M. Marfan syndrome: screening for sudden death in athletes. Curr Sports Med Rep 2002;1:67–74.

13. Ghai A, Silversides C, Harris L, Webb GD, Siu SC, Therrien J. Left ventricular dysfunction is a risk factor for sudden cardiac death in adults late after repair of tetralogy of Fallot. J Am Coll Cardiol 2002;40:1675–1680.

14. Sharma AD, Yee R, Guiraudon G, Klein GJ. Sensitivity and specificity of invasive and noninvasive testing for risk of sudden death in Wolff–Parkinson–White syndrome. J Am Coll Cardiol 1987;10:373–381.

15. Towbin JA. Molecular genetic basis of sudden cardiac death. Cardiovasc Pathol 2001;10:283–295.

16. Brugada P, Brugada J. Right bundle branch block, persistent ST segment elevation and sudden cardiac death: a distinct clinical and electrocardiographic syndrome. A multicenter report. J Am Coll Cardiol 1992;20:1391–1396.

17. Brugada J, Brugada P, Brugada R. The syndrome of right bundle branch block ST segment elevation in V1 to V3 and sudden death – the Brugada syndrome. Europace 1999;1:156–166.

18. Antzelevitch C, Brugada P, Brugada J, Brugada R, Towbin JA, Nademanee K. Brugada syndrome: 1992–2002: a historical perspective. J Am Coll Cardiol 2003;41:1665–1671.

19. Ropers D, Moshage W, Daniel WG, Jessl J, Gottwik M, Achenbach S. Visualization of coronary artery anomalies and their anatomic course by contrast-enhanced electron beam tomography and three-dimensional reconstruction. Am J Cardiol 2001;87:193–197.

20. Van Ooijen PM, Dorgelo J, Zijlstra F, Oudkerk M. Detection, visualization and evaluation of anomalous coronary anatomy on 16-slice multidetector-row CT. Eur Radiol 2004;14(12):2163–2171.

21. Basso C, Maron BJ, Corrado D, Thiene G. Clinical profile of congenital coronary artery anomalies with origin from the wrong aortic sinus leading to sudden death in young competitive athletes. J Am Coll Cardiol 2000;35:1493–1501.

22. Maron BJ, Shirani J, Poliac LC, Mathenge R, Roberts WC, Mueller FO. Sudden death in young competitive athletes. Clinical, demographic, and pathological profiles. JAMA 1996;276:199–204.

23. Frescura C, Basso C, Thiene G, et al. Anomalous origin of coronary arteries and risk of sudden death: a study based on an autopsy population of congenital heart disease. Hum Pathol 1998;29:689–695.

24. Moshage WE, Achenbach S, Seese B, Bachmann K, Kirchgeorg M. Coronary artery stenoses: three-dimensional imaging with electrocardiographically triggered, contrast agent-enhanced, electron-beam CT. Radiology 1995;196:707–714.

25. Schmermund A, Rensing BJ, Sheedy PF, Bell MR, Rumberger JA. Intravenous electron-beam computed tomographic coronary angiography for segmental analysis of coronary artery stenoses. J Am Coll Cardiol 1998;31:1547–1554.

26. Reddy GP, Chernoff DM, Adams JR, Higgins CB. Coronary artery stenoses: assessment with contrast-enhanced electron-beam CT and axial reconstructions. Radiology 1998;208:167–172.

27. Achenbach S, Moshage W, Ropers D, Nossen J, Daniel WG. Value of electron-beam computed tomography for the noninvasive detection of high-grade coronary-artery stenoses and occlusions. N Engl J Med 1998;339:1964–1971.

28. Budoff MJ, Oudiz RJ, Zalace CP, et al. Intravenous three-dimensional coronary angiography using contrast enhanced electron beam computed tomography. Am J Cardiol 1999;83:840–845.

29. Achenbach S, Ropers D, Regenfus M, Muschiol G, Daniel WG, Moshage W. Contrast enhanced electron beam computed tomography to analyse the coronary arteries in patients after acute myocardial infarction. Heart 2000;84:489–493.

30. Lu B, Shavelle DM, Mao S, et al. Improved accuracy of noninvasive electron beam coronary angiography. Invest Radiol 2004;39:73–79.

31. Budoff MJ, Lu B, Shinbane JS, et al. Methodology for improved detection of coronary stenoses with computed tomographic angiography. Am Heart J 2004;148:1085–1090.

32. Nieman K, Cademartiri F, Lemos PA, Raaijmakers R, Pattynama PM, de Feyter PJ. Reliable noninvasive coronary angiography with fast submillimeter multislice spiral computed tomography. Circulation 2002;106:2051–2054.

33. Ropers D, Baum U, Pohle K, et al. Detection of coronary artery stenoses with thin-slice multi-detector row spiral computed tomography and multiplanar reconstruction. Circulation 2003;107:664–666.

34. Budoff MJ, Achenbach S, Duerinckx A. Clinical utility of computed tomography and magnetic resonance techniques for noninvasive coronary angiography. J Am Coll Cardiol 2003;42:1867–1878.

35. Georgiou D, Budoff MJ, Kaufer E, Kennedy JM, Lu B, Brundage BH. Screening patients with chest pain in the emergency department using electron beam tomography: a follow-up study. J Am Coll Cardiol 2001;38:105–110.

36. Achenbach S, Moselewski F, Ropers D, et al. Detection of calcified and noncalcified coronary atherosclerotic plaque by contrast-enhanced, submillimeter multidetector spiral computed tomography: a segment-based comparison with intravascular ultrasound. Circulation 2004;109:14–17.

37. Bardy GH, Lee KL, Mark DB, et al. Amiodarone or an implantable cardioverter-defibrillator for congestive heart failure. N Engl J Med 2005;352:225–237.

38. Rich S, Chomka EV, Stagl R, Shanes JG, Kondos GT, Brundage BH. Determination of left ventricular ejection fraction using ultrafast computed tomography. Am Heart J 1986;112:392–396.

39. Rumberger JA, Behrenbeck T, Bell MR, et al. Determination of ventricular ejection fraction: a comparison of available imaging methods. The Cardiovascular Imaging Working Group. Mayo Clin Proc 1997;72:860–870.

40. Schmermund A, Rensing BJ, Sheedy PF, Rumberger JA. Reproducibility of right and left ventricular volume measurements by electron-beam CT in patients with congestive heart failure. Int J Card Imaging 1998;14:201–209.

41. Budoff MJ, Shavelle DM, Lamont DH, et al. Usefulness of electron beam computed tomography scanning for distinguishing ischemic from nonischemic cardiomyopathy. J Am Coll Cardiol 1998;32:1173–1178.

42. Abraham WT, Fisher WG, Smith AL, et al. Cardiac resynchronization in chronic heart failure. N Engl J Med 2002;346:1845–1853.

43. Saxon LA, De Marco T, Schafer J, Chatterjee K, Kumar UN, Foster E. Effects of long-term biventricular stimulation for resynchronization on echocardiographic measures of remodeling. Circulation 2002; 105:1304–1310.

44. St John Sutton MG, Plappert T, Abraham WT, et al. Effect of cardiac resynchronization therapy on left ventricular size and function in chronic heart failure. Circulation 2003;107:1985–1990.

45. Gerber TC, Sheedy PF, Bell MR, et al. Evaluation of the coronary venous system using electron beam computed tomography. Int J Cardiovasc Imaging 2001;17:65–75.

46. Girsky MJ, Mao S, Shinbane JS, et al. Electron beam computed tomographic angiography: Three-dimensional characterization of anatomy for coronary vein intervention. Heart Rhythm 2004;1:S26 Abstract.

47. Shinbane JS, Mao S, Girsky MJ, et al. Computed tomographic angiography can define three-dimensional relationships between coronary veins and coronary arteries relevant to coronary venous procedures. Circulation 2004;110:702.

48. Mao S, Shinbane JS, Girsky MJ, et al. Three-dimensional coronary venous imaging with computed tomographic angiography. Am Heart J 2005;150:315–322.

49. Shinbane JS, Girsky MJ, Mao S, Budoff MJ. Thebesian valve imaging with electron beam CT angiography: implications for resynchronization therapy. Pacing Clin Electrophysiol 2004;27:1566–1567.

50. Maron BJ, Shen WK, Link MS, et al. Efficacy of implantable cardioverter-defibrillators for the prevention of sudden death in patients with hypertrophic cardiomyopathy. N Engl J Med 2000; 342:365–373.

51. Maron MS, Olivotto I, Betocchi S, et al. Effect of left ventricular outflow tract obstruction on clinical outcome in hypertrophic cardiomyopathy. N Engl J Med 2003;348:295–303.

52. Klues HG, Schiffers A, Maron BJ. Phenotypic spectrum and patterns of left ventricular hypertrophy in hypertrophic cardiomyopathy: morphologic observations and significance as assessed by two-dimensional echocardiography in 600 patients. J Am Coll Cardiol 1995;26:1699–1708.

53. Charron P, Dubourg O, Desnos M, et al. Diagnostic value of electrocardiography and echocardiography for familial hypertrophic cardiomyopathy in a genotyped adult population. Circulation 1997;96: 214–219.

54. Stone DL, Petch MC, Verney GI, Dixon AK. Computed tomography in patients with hypertrophic cardiomyopathy. Br Heart J 1984;52: 136–139.

55. Tabib A, Loire R, Chalabreysse L, et al. Circumstances of death and gross and microscopic observations in a series of 200 cases of sudden death associated with arrhythmogenic right ventricular cardiomyopathy and/or dysplasia. Circulation 2003;108:3000–3005.

56. Wilde AA, Antzelevitch C, Borggrefe M, et al. Proposed diagnostic criteria for the Brugada syndrome: consensus report. Circulation 2002;106:2514–2519.

57. Tandri H, Calkins H, Nasir K, et al. Magnetic resonance imaging findings in patients meeting task force criteria for arrhythmogenic right ventricular dysplasia. J Cardiovasc Electrophysiol 2003;14:476–482.

58. di Cesare E. MRI assessment of right ventricular dysplasia. Eur Radiol 2003;13:1387–1393.

59. Chimenti C, Pieroni M, Maseri A, Frustaci A. Histologic findings in patients with clinical and instrumental diagnosis of sporadic arrhythmogenic right ventricular dysplasia. J Am Coll Cardiol 2004;43:2305–2313.

60. Dery R, Lipton MJ, Garrett JS, Abbott J, Higgins CB, Schienman MM. Cine-computed tomography of arrhythmogenic right ventricular dysplasia. J Comput Assist Tomogr 1986;10:120–123.

61. Hamada S, Takamiya M, Ohe T, Ueda H. Arrhythmogenic right ventricular dysplasia: evaluation with electron-beam CT. Radiology 1993;187:723–727.

62. Tada H, Shimizu W, Ohe T, et al. Usefulness of electron-beam computed tomography in arrhythmogenic right ventricular dysplasia. Relationship to electrophysiological abnormalities and left ventricular involvement. Circulation 1996;94:437–444.

63. Chen SJ, Li YW, Wang JK, et al. Three-dimensional reconstruction of abnormal ventriculoarterial relationship by electron beam CT. J Comput Assist Tomogr 1998;22:560–568.

64. Chen SJ, Wang JK, Li YW, Chiu IS, Su CT, Lue HC. Validation of pulmonary venous obstruction by electron beam computed tomography in children with congenital heart disease. Am J Cardiol 2001; 87:589–593.

65. Choe KO, Hong YK, Kim HJ, et al. The use of high-resolution computed tomography in the evaluation of pulmonary hemodynamics in patients with congenital heart disease: in pulmonary vessels larger than 1 mm in diameter. Pediatr Cardiol 2000;21:202–210.

66. Cosio FG, Martin-Penato A, Pastor A, Nunez A, Goicolea A. Atypical flutter: a review. Pacing Clin Electrophysiol 2003;26:2157–2169.

67. Balaji S, Harris L. Atrial arrhythmias in congenital heart disease. Cardiol Clin 2002;20:459–468, vii.

68. Kirsh JA, Walsh EP, Triedman JK. Prevalence of and risk factors for atrial fibrillation and intra-atrial reentrant tachycardia among patients with congenital heart disease. Am J Cardiol 2002;90:338–340.

69. Haramati LB, Glickstein JS, Issenberg HJ, Haramati N, Crooke GA. MR imaging and CT of vascular anomalies and connections in patients with congenital heart disease: significance in surgical planning. Radiographics 2002;22:337–347; discussion 348–349.

70. Lu B, Dai RP, Jing BL, et al. Electron beam tomography with three-dimensional reconstruction in the diagnosis of aortic diseases. J Cardiovasc Surg (Torino) 2000;41:659–668.

71. Hartnell GG. Imaging of aortic aneurysms and dissection: CT and MRI. J Thorac Imaging 2001;16:35–46.

72. Shavelle DM, Budoff MJ, Buljubasic N, et al. Usefulness of aortic valve calcium scores by electron beam computed tomography as a marker for aortic stenosis. Am J Cardiol 2003;92:349–353.

73. Nakagawa H, Aoyama H, Beckman KJ, et al. Relation between pulmonary vein firing and extent of left atrial-pulmonary vein connection in patients with atrial fibrillation. Circulation 2004;109:1523–1529.

74. Pappone C, Rosanio S, Oreto G, et al. Circumferential radiofrequency ablation of pulmonary vein ostia: A new anatomic approach for curing atrial fibrillation. Circulation 2000;102:2619–2628.

75. Oral H, Knight BP, Ozaydin M, et al. Segmental ostial ablation to isolate the pulmonary veins during atrial fibrillation: feasibility and mechanistic insights. Circulation 2002;106:1256–1262.

76. Scharf C, Sneider M, Case I, et al. Anatomy of the pulmonary veins in patients with atrial fibrillation and effects of segmental ostial ablation analyzed by computed tomography. J Cardiovasc Electrophysiol 2003;14:150–155.

77. Kato R, Lickfett L, Meininger G, et al. Pulmonary vein anatomy in patients undergoing catheter ablation of atrial fibrillation: lessons learned by use of magnetic resonance imaging. Circulation 2003; 107:2004–2010.

78. Solomon SB, Dickfeld T, Calkins H. Real-time cardiac catheter navigation on three-dimensional CT images. J Interv Card Electrophysiol 2003;8:27–36.

79. Tani T, Yamakami S, Matsushita T, et al. Usefulness of electron beam tomography in the prone position for detecting atrial thrombi in chronic atrial fibrillation. J Comput Assist Tomogr 2003;27:78–84.

80. Alam G, Addo F, Malik M, Levinsky R, Lieb D. Detection of left atrial appendage thrombus by spiral CT scan. Echocardiography 2003;20:99–100.

81. Robbins IM, Colvin EV, Doyle TP, et al. Pulmonary vein stenosis after catheter ablation of atrial fibrillation. Circulation 1998;98:1769–1775.

82. Taylor GW, Kay GN, Zheng X, Bishop S, Ideker RE. Pathological effects of extensive radiofrequency energy applications in the pulmonary veins in dogs. Circulation 2000;101:1736–1742.

83. Yang M, Akbari H, Reddy GP, Higgins CB. Identification of pulmonary vein stenosis after radiofrequency ablation for atrial fibrillation using MRI. J Comput Assist Tomogr 2001;25:34–35.

84. Qureshi AM, Prieto LR, Latson LA, et al. Transcatheter angioplasty for acquired pulmonary vein stenosis after radiofrequency ablation. Circulation 2003;108:1336–1342.

85. Dill T, Neumann T, Ekinci O, et al. Pulmonary vein diameter reduction after radiofrequency catheter ablation for paroxysmal atrial fibrillation evaluated by contrast-enhanced three-dimensional magnetic resonance imaging. Circulation 2003;107:845–850.

86. Saad EB, Rossillo A, Saad CP, et al. Pulmonary vein stenosis after radiofrequency ablation of atrial fibrillation: functional characterization, evolution, and influence of the ablation strategy. Circulation 2003;108:3102–3107.

87. Scanavacca MI, D'Avila A, Parga J, Sosa E. Left atrial-esophageal fistula following radiofrequency catheter ablation of atrial fibrillation. J Cardiovasc Electrophysiol 2004;15:960–962.

88. Lemola K, Sneider M, Desjardins B, et al. Computed tomographic analysis of the anatomy of the left atrium and the esophagus: implications for left atrial catheter ablation. Circulation 2004;110:3655–3660.

89. Schaffler GJ, Groell R, Peichel KH, Rienmuller R. Imaging the coronary venous drainage system using electron-beam CT. Surg Radiol Anat 2000;22:35–39.

90. Lesh MD, Van Hare G, Kao AK, Scheinman MM. Radiofrequency catheter ablation for Wolff–Parkinson–White syndrome associated with a coronary sinus diverticulum. Pacing Clin Electrophysiol 1991;14:1479–1484.

91. Shinbane JS, Lesh MD, Stevenson WG, et al. Anatomic and electrophysiologic relation between the coronary sinus and mitral annulus: implications for ablation of left-sided accessory pathways. Am Heart J 1998;135:93–98.

92. Hwang C, Wu TJ, Doshi RN, Peter CT, Chen PS. Vein of marshall cannulation for the analysis of electrical activity in patients with focal atrial fibrillation. Circulation 2000;101:1503–1505.

93. Mochizuki T, Ohtani T, Higashino H, et al. Tricuspid atresia with atrial septal defect, ventricular septal defect, and right ventricular hypoplasia demonstrated by multidetector computed tomography. Circulation 2000;102:E164–165.

94. Skotnicki R, MacMillan RM, Rees MR, et al. Detection of atrial septal defect by contrast-enhanced ultrafast computed tomography. Cathet Cardiovasc Diagn 1986;12:103–106.

95. Garrett JS, Schiller NB, Botvinick EH, Higgins CB, Lipton MJ. Cine-computed tomography of Ebstein anomaly. J Comput Assist Tomogr 1986;10:664–666.

96. Gerber TC, Kuzo RS. Images in cardiovascular medicine. Persistent left superior vena cava demonstrated with multislice spiral computed tomography. Circulation 2002;105:e79.

Index